An Atlas of the Human Brain for Computerized Tomography

Takayoshi Matsui, M. D.

Assistant Professor, Department of Neurosurgery,
Teikyo University School of Medicine, Tokyo

Division of Neuropathology, Montefiore Hospital
and Medical Center, New York

Consultant, Department of Neurosurgery,
University of Tokyo Faculty of Medicine, Tokyo

Asao Hirano, M. D.

Head, Devision of Neuropathology, Montefiore Hospital
and Medical Center, New York

Professor, Department of Pathology and Neuroscience
Albert Einstein College of Medicine, New York

In Cooperation with

Terukuni Imai, M.D.   Tamotsu Osugi, M.D.

Josefina F. Llena, M.D.   Makoto Iwata, M.D.

Keiji Kawamoto, M.D.   Shuntaro Hojo, M.D.

With a foreword by

H. M. Zimmerman, M. D.

IGAKU-SHOIN   Tokyo · New York

Published and distributed by

IGAKU-SHOIN Ltd.
  5-24-3 Hongo, Bunkyo-ku, Tokyo
IGAKU-SHOIN Medical Publishers, Inc.
  50 Rockefeller Plaza, New York, N.Y. 10020

ISBN: 0-89640-027-1
Library of Congress Catalog Card Number: 77-95453

Printed and bound in Japan

To our wives
MIHOKO and KEIKO

Foreword

A giant step forward was taken but a few years ago in neuroradiologic diagnosis of intracranial lesions with the development of the computerized scanner. This has already had a great impact on the field of neurosurgery, let alone radiology, and but to only a slightly less degree the field of neurology. Almost daily new applications are found for the scanner, so that its invention for the primary purpose of locating the extent and exact position of an intracranial space-occupying lesion has been extended to define cerebral hemorrhage, cerebral edema, infarction and now, most recently, the demyelinating processes as in multiple sclerosis. And this is probably just the beginning of the discoveries of its many applications in the neurosciences. With refinements in technique, even more applications will undoubtedly be discovered so that the future of this approach to diagnosis is most challenging.

There are other aspects to computerized tomography that account for its rapidly spreading employment as a tool in diagnosis. One is its non-invasive character that makes it practically free of morbidity. Another is its safety as regards exposure to x-radiation, which permits repeated scans possible. The non-invasive and radiation safety features of this procedure place it at a decided advantage over cerebral angiography. Indeed, experience shows that there is a diminished need for angiography in diagnosis when computerized scanning is available. And an even lesser need exists for pneumoencephalography in this circumstance.

Another advantage of cerebral scanning is that it is a relatively comfortable procedure for the patient and can be employed on an ambulatory basis. This, of course, is important in these days of high costs of everything, including hospitalization. Unfortunately, however, the procedure is so costly that it would be out of the reach of many patients were it not that third party payments come to their aid. The high expense involved is due to the initial cost of the rather complicated apparatus, the need for highly skilled technicians to operate the equipment, and the attempt to amortize the equipment in a brief period before the next, improved model appears on the market. And in some cases, undoubtedly, the cost per test is high because it provides income for the institution that helps meet other less financially rewarding operations.

As refinements are developed in the technique of computerized cerebral scanning, it becomes imperative for the interpreter to be thoroughly familiar with the anatomical minutiae of the brain and its coverings. A specialized knowledge of cerebral anatomy is requisite which goes beyond merely that of gross anatomy. It requires complete familiarity with the brain in section in many planes and at different angles. This volume by Doctors Takayoshi Matsui and Asao Hirano provides the familiarity that is requisite to the neuroradiologist, the neurosurgeon, the neurologist and the neuropathologist. We owe the authors of this book a debt of gratitude beyond measure for the many illustrations that help illumine each brain scan. The excellence and variety of the explanatory figures are matched by the perfection of the printer's achievement in this volume. These features make this book well high indispensable.

H.M. Zimmerman, M.D.

Preface

The use of the CT scanner for the purpose of localizing intracranial lesions is becoming more widespread. However, the elucidation of the anatomy of the brain from the point of view of the scanner is essential for exploiting this remarkable new instrument to its fullest extent.

For that purpose we have sectioned approximately 500 brains in the preparation of this Atlas. Sectioning was performed at various angles including those most commonly used in the CT scanner.

The internal structures as well as the gyri and sulci revealed at each level are described. In addition, we have devised a "Level Index" which is designed to enable the CT user to predict the structure to be seen at any level for a given angle regardless of the absolute size of the cranium.

We hope that this Atlas will be of help in the evaluation of the images produced by CT scanner.

T. Matsui, M.D.
A. Hirano, M.D.

Acknowledgment

The authors and collaborators are indebted to a large number of individuals both within and outside our department who made this work possible. It is not possible to list them all, but we wish to thank them now. Among these men and women there are some who deserve our special gratitude. These include, Dr. L.G. Koss, Chairman and Professor of the Department of Pathology, Albert Einstein College of Medicine at Montefiore Hospital for his support and encouragement and Dr. Norman E. Leeds, Head of the Neuroradiology Division, Department of Radiology, at Montefiore Hospital, and his associate Dr. Thomas P. Naidich were especially helpful by providing the CT scanning photographs and helpful advice. Dr. H.M. Zimmerman has graciously agreed to write the foreward and has encouraged us throughout this undertaking. We are also grateful to Dr. Robert S. Ledley, President, National Biomedical Research Faundation, and Dr. Alfred J. Luessenhop, Chairman of Neurosurgery Department, Dr. Dieter Schellinger, Chief of Neuroradiology Division, Dr. Homer L. Twigg, Chairman of Radiology Department, Georgetown University Medical Center. We are also most grateful to Dr. Keiji Sano, Chairman and Professor, Department of Neurosurgery, University of Tokyo Faculty of Medicine, and Dr. Hiroshi Hatanaka, Chairman and Professor, Department of Neurosurgery, Teikyo University School of Medicine.

Authors

Contents

Introduction

Methods

At the time of autopsy, in order to identify the canthomeatal line on the brain surface, burr holes were made in the skull parallel to a line drown at a 15° angle from the canthomeatal line as illustrated in Fig. 1.

Four small pins were inserted into the brain through these burr holes for later identification of the line. The brain was kept in formalin for two weeks. Fig. 2 illustrates the angles chosen.

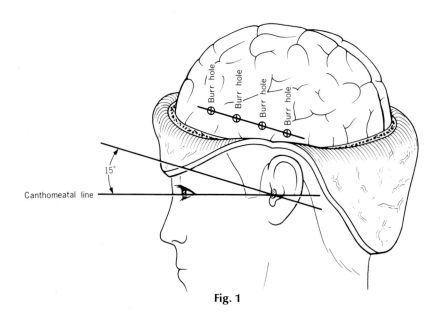

Fig. 1

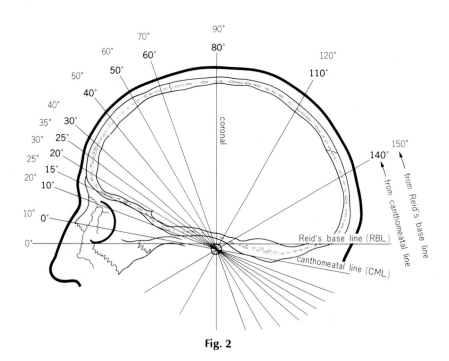

Fig. 2

As shown here, more closely spaced angles between 10° and 30° were chosen due to the frequent use of CT scanning in this region. Once the angle was determined, the following two apparatuses were used to obtain each section (Fig. 3).

(A) The brain *in toto* was placed on the baseboard, and the two horizontal bars were adjusted and secured at the desired angle from the canthomeatal line which was easily idintified due to the presence of the pins. The knife was guided along the horizontal bars resulting in a cut surface at a precisely known angle from the canthomeatal line (Fig. 3A).

(B) Each part of the brain was then placed on the second device with the cut surface down and sliced with the knife guided by peripheral elevations to obtain thin, parallel sections of equal thickness. The sections were numbered from the vertex to the base of the brain (Fig. 3B).

It was established during this process that the line between the preoccipital notch and and a point 6 mm above the Sylvian fissure on the precentral gyrus corresponds to a line 15° from the canthomeatal line. While not used in the preparation of this atlas this line could, in the future, provide a useful guide for practical purposes.

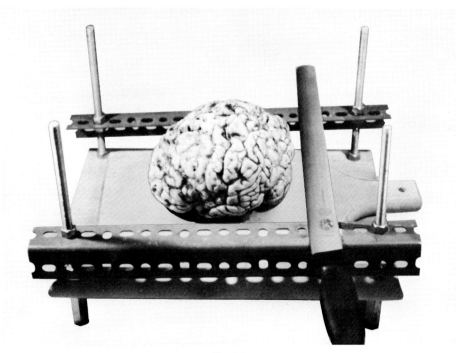

Fig. 3A

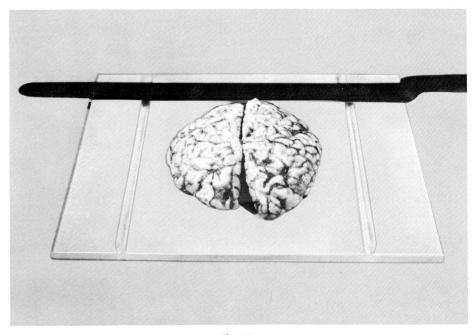

Fig. 3B

Illustrations

15° and 20° from the canthomeatal line (25° and 30° from Reid's line)

Because of the frequent use of 15° and 20° sections we provide extensive illustrations and explanations of each level at these angles. For each level at both angles the text is organized in four pages according to the following scheme:

First page: The illustration is the photograph of the upper surface of the actual brain section. The numbers in the upper left corner indicate the angle and level of the section. For example, 15°-7 indicates that the section was cut at 15° from the canthomeatal line and that it was the 7th from the vertex.

Second page: The illustration is the photograph of the lower surface of the same section as on the previous page. The CT scanning image of the structures between these two surfaces is provided at the upper right corner of the page.

Level Index
Brain Level Index

The CT scan at the same level as the section

These numbers indicate the angle and level of the section.
For example, 15°-10 indicates that this section was cut at 15° from the canthomeatal line and is the 10th section from the vertex.

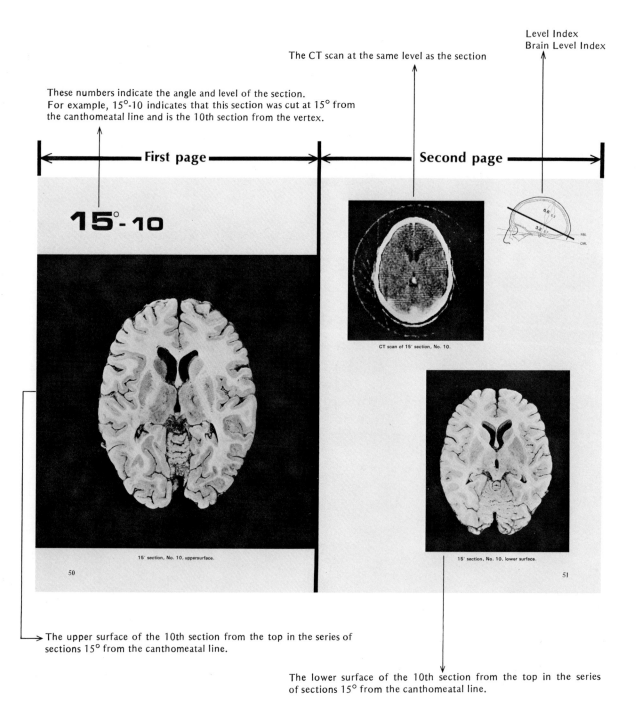

First page ——————

Second page ——————

15°-10

CT scan of 15° section, No. 10.

15° section, No. 10, uppersurface.

15° section, No. 10, lower surface.

50

51

The upper surface of the 10th section from the top in the series of sections 15° from the canthomeatal line.

The lower surface of the 10th section from the top in the series of sections 15° from the canthomeatal line.

Third page: The gyri and lobes are indicated on a photograph identical to that on the first page.

Fourth page: Drawing of the photograph illustrated on the first page shows the various structures other than gyri and lobes.

Level Index
Brain Level Index

The prominent structures of the 10th section from the top in the series of sections 15° from the conthomeatal line.

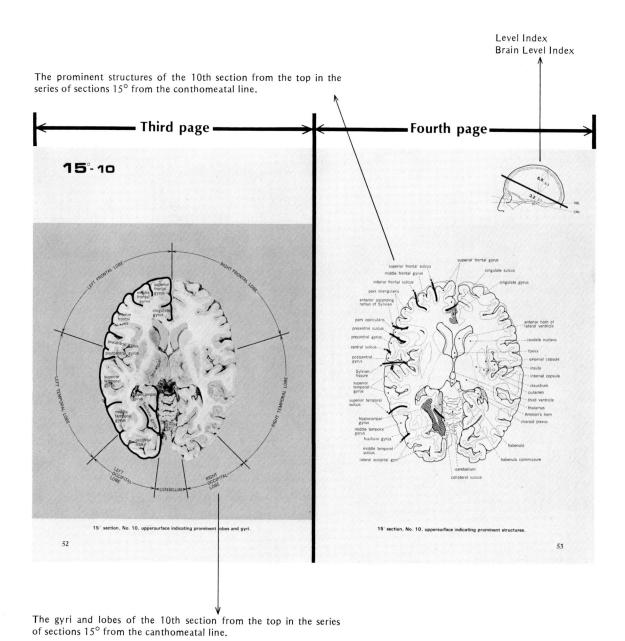

15° section, No. 10, uppersurface indicating prominent lobes and gyri.

15° section, No. 10, uppersurface indicating prominent structures.

52

53

The gyri and lobes of the 10th section from the top in the series of sections 15° from the canthomeatal line.

0°,10°,25°,30°,40°,50°,60°,80°,110° and 140° from the canthomeatal line (10°, 20°, 35°, 40°, 50°, 60°, 70°, 90°, 120° and 150° from Reid's base line)

Each of the levels at 0°, 10°, 25°, 30°, 40°, 60°, 80°, 110° and 140° is illustrated on two pages. The first page is again a photograph of the upper surface of the actual brain section. The second page is the same photograph with the gyri, lobes and other structures labeled.

These numbers indicate the angle and level of the section.
For example, 40°−10 indicates that this section was cut at 40°
from the canthomeatal line and is the 10th section from the vertex.

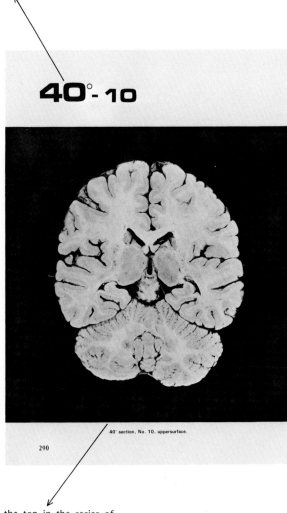

40° section. No. 10. uppersurface.

290

Upper surface of the 10th section from the top in the series of sections 40° from the canthomeatal line.

Level Index
Brain Level Index

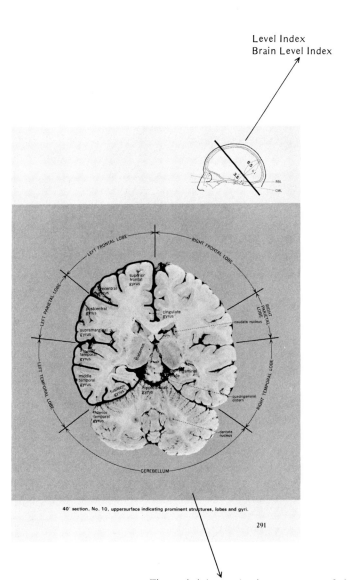

40° section, No. 10, uppersurface indicating prominent structures, lobes and gyri.

291

The gyri, lobes and other structures of the 10th section from the top in the series of sections 25° from the canthomeatal line.

Level index

Because of the difference in size between individual brains it is sometimes difficult to obtain equivalent CT scan levels in different patients. To overcome this difficulty the concept of Level Index has been formulated (Fig. 4). For each patient, the vertical distance Y, between the external auditory canal and a plane passing through the uppermost surface

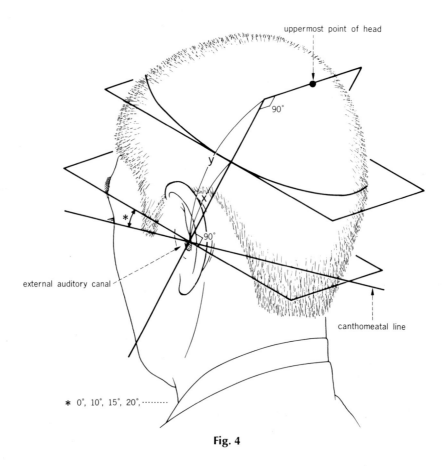

Fig. 4

of the head is measured on a vertical straight line drawn at right angles to the previously selected base line. The Level Index is then calculated as proportion of Y according to the following formula:

$$\frac{X}{Y} = \frac{\text{Level Index}}{10}$$

where X is the distance between the external auditory canal and the level of the scan measured along the same line as Y.

A similar formula for Brain Level Index (Fig. 5) has been generated for use at autopsy. In this case, however, β, the distance between the surface of the brain and the external audiotry canal is first measured on a vertical straight line at right angles to the previously selected base line. The Brain Level Index is then calculated according to the following formula:

$$\frac{\alpha}{\beta} = \frac{\text{Brain Level Index}}{10}$$

in which α is the distance between the external auditory canal and the section along the same line as β (Fig. 5).

It is important to note that all measurements, X, Y, α and B are straight lines between horizontal planes and should not be taken as curves over the surface of the head or brain.

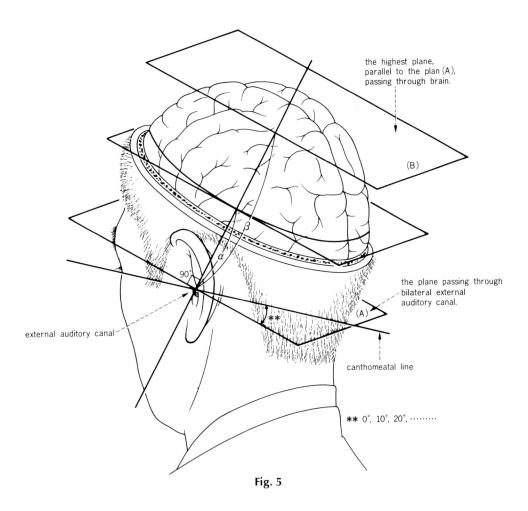

the highest plane, parallel to the plan (A), passing through brain.

(B)

the plane passing through bilateral external auditory canal.

external auditory canal

90°

α

β

(A)

**

canthomeatal line

** 0°, 10°, 20°, ·········

Fig. 5

To Use the Level Index

In order to reproduce the equivalent of, for example, the scan illustrated below and labeled 15°-10 one first notes the Level Index, in this case 3.7. Using the formula:

$$\frac{X}{Y} = \frac{3.7}{10}$$

Y is then measured on the patient's head by measuring the distance between the external auditory canal and the highest surface of the head on a line 105° (15° + 90° = 105°) from the canthomeatal line. X is then calculated and the scan is made at the height above the external auditory canal.

Correlation of level index, brain level index and section index

0° from canthomeatal line

Section no.	Level index	Brain level index
0-1	8.9	10.1
0-2	8.0	9.0
0-3	7.4	8.3
0-4	6.8	7.6
0-5	6.1	6.8
0-6	5.4	6.1
0-7	4.7	5.3
0-8	4.1	4.6
0-9	3.4	3.8
0-10	2.8	3.1
0-11	2.1	2.3
0-12	1.4	1.6
0-13	0.8	0.9
0-14	−0.6	−0.7
0-15	−1.3	−1.5

10° from canthomeatal line

Section no.	Level index	Brain level index
10-1	8.7	10.1
10-2	7.3	8.4
10-3	6.5	7.5
10-4	5.9	6.8
10-5	5.3	6.1
10-6	4.8	5.5
10-7	4.1	4.7
10-8	3.6	4.1
10-9	3.0	3.4
10-10	2.4	2.8
10-11	1.9	2.2
10-12	1.3	1.5
10-13	0.7	0.8
10-14	−0.1	−0.1
10-15	−0.4	−0.5
10-16	−1.0	−1.2

15° from canthomeatal line

Section no.	Level index	Brain level index
15-1	8.7	10.0
15-2	8.1	9.3
15-3	7.2	8.3
15-4	6.7	7.7
15-5	6.1	7.0
15-6	5.6	6.4
15-7	4.9	5.6
15-8	4.4	5.0
15-9	3.8	4.4
15-10	3.2	3.7
15-11	2.7	3.1
15-12	2.1	2.4
15-13	1.6	1.8
15-14	1.0	1.1
15-15	0.3	0.4
15-16	−0.3	−0.3
15-17	−1.0	−1.1

20° from canthomeatal line

Section no.	Level index	Brain level index
20-1	8.7	10.0
20-2	8.0	9.2
20-3	7.2	8.3
20-4	6.5	7.5
20-5	5.8	6.7
20-6	5.0	5.8
20-7	4.4	5.0
20-8	3.7	4.2
20-9	2.9	3.3
20-10	2.2	2.5
20-11	1.5	1.7
20-12	0.7	0.8
20-13	0	0
20-14	−0.7	−0.8

25° from canthomeatal line

Section no.	Level index	Brain level index
25-1	8.7	10.0
25-2	8.1	9.3
25-3	7.5	8.6
25-4	6.9	7.9
25-5	6.3	7.2
25-6	5.7	6.5
25-7	5.1	5.8
25-8	4.4	5.1
25-9	3.8	4.4
25-10	3.2	3.7
25-11	2.6	3.0
25-12	2.0	2.3
25-13	1.4	1.6
25-14	0.8	0.9
25-15	0.2	0.2
25-16	−0.4	−0.5
25-17	−1.0	−1.2

30° from canthomeatal line

Section no.	Level index	Brain level index
30-1	8.7	10.0
30-2	8.1	9.3
30-3	7.6	8.7
30-4	7.0	8.0
30-5	6.4	7.4
30-6	5.8	6.7
30-7	5.2	6.0
30-8	4.7	5.4
30-9	4.1	4.7
30-10	3.6	4.1
30-11	3.0	3.4
30-12	2.4	2.7
30-13	1.8	2.1
30-14	1.2	1.4
30-15	0.7	0.8
30-16	0.1	0.1
30-17	−0.6	−0.7
30-18	−1.4	−1.6
30-19	−2.2	−2.5

40° from canthomeatal line

Section no.	Level index	Brain level index
40-1	9.1	10.0
40-2	7.8	8.5
40-3	7.1	7.8
40-4	6.6	7.2
40-5	6.1	6.7
40-6	5.6	6.2
40-7	5.1	5.6
40-8	4.6	5.0
40-9	4.1	4.5
40-10	3.5	3.9
40-11	2.9	3.2
40-12	2.4	2.7
40-13	1.8	2.1
40-14	1.2	1.4
40-15	0.7	0.7
40-16	0.2	0.2
40-17	−0.4	−0.4
40-18	−1.0	−1.0
40-19	−1.6	−1.7
40-20	−2.2	−2.4
40-21	−2.8	−3.1

50° from canthomeatal line

Section no.	Level index	Brain level index
50-1	9.2	10.0
50-2	7.9	8.6
50-3	7.3	8.0
50-4	6.7	7.3
50-5	6.1	6.7
50-6	5.5	6.0
50-7	4.9	5.4
50-8	4.4	4.7
50-9	3.8	4.1
50-10	3.2	3.4
50-11	2.6	2.8
50-12	2.0	2.2
50-13	1.4	1.5
50-14	0.8	0.9
50-15	0.2	0.2
50-16	−0.4	−0.4
50-17	−0.9	−1.0
50-18	−1.5	−1.6
50-19	−2.1	−2.3
50-20	−2.7	−2.9
50-21	−3.3	−3.6
50-22	−3.9	−4.2

60° from canthomeatal line

Section no.	Level index	Brain level index
60-1	9.3	10.0
60-2	8.0	8.6
60-3	7.3	7.9
60-4	6.7	7.2
60-5	6.0	6.5
60-6	5.3	5.8
60-7	4.8	5.2
60-8	4.1	4.5
60-9	3.4	3.8
60-10	2.8	3.1
60-11	2.2	2.4
60-12	1.5	1.7
60-13	0.9	1.0
60-14	0.2	0.2
60-15	−0.3	−0.4
60-16	−1.0	−1.1
60-17	−1.6	−1.8
60-18	−2.3	−2.5
60-19	−3.0	−3.2
60-20	−3.6	−3.9
60-21	−4.3	−4.6

80° from canthomeatal line

Section no.	Level index	Brain level index
80-1	7.6	10.0
80-2	7.1	9.3
80-3	6.5	8.5
80-4	6.0	7.8
80-5	5.4	7.1
80-6	4.8	6.3
80-7	4.2	5.6
80-8	3.6	4.7
80-9	2.9	3.8
80-10	2.2	2.9
80-11	1.6	2.1
80-12	1.0	1.3
80-13	0.5	0.6
80-14	−0.1	−0.1
80-15	−0.7	−0.9
80-16	−1.2	−1.6
80-17	−1.8	−2.4
80-18	−2.4	−3.1
80-19	−2.9	−3.8
80-20	−3.5	−4.6
80-21	−4.0	−5.3
80-22	−4.6	−6.0
80-23	−5.2	−6.8
80-24	−5.7	−7.5
80-25	−6.3	−8.2
80-26	−6.9	−9.0

110° from canthomeatal line

Section no.	Level index	Brain level index
110-1	9.4	10.0
110-2	8.4	8.9
110-3	7.9	8.3
110-4	7.3	7.7
110-5	6.7	7.1
110-6	6.2	6.5
110-7	5.6	6.0
110-8	5.1	5.4
110-9	4.3	4.8
110-10	3.9	4.2
110-11	3.4	3.6
110-12	2.9	3.1
110-13	2.5	2.6
110-14	2.0	2.1
110-15	1.5	1.5
110-16	0.9	1.0
110-17	0.3	0.4
110-18	−0.2	−0.2
110-19	−1.0	−1.1
110-20	−1.8	−1.9
110-21	−2.6	−2.7
110-22	−3.4	−3.6
110-23	−4.2	−4.4
110-24	−4.9	−5.2
110-25	−5.7	−6.1

140° from canthomeatal line

Section no.	Level index	Brain level index
140-1	9.1	10.0
140-2	8.6	9.4
140-3	8.1	8.9
140-4	7.6	8.3
140-5	7.0	7.8
140-6	6.5	7.2
140-7	6.0	6.6
140-8	5.4	6.0
140-9	4.9	5.4
140-10	4.4	4.8
140-11	3.9	4.3
140-12	3.4	3.7
140-13	2.9	3.1
140-14	2.3	2.6
140-15	1.9	2.1
140-16	1.5	1.7
140-17	0.9	1.0
140-18	0.3	0.3
140-19	−0.3	−0.3
140-20	−1.0	−1.1
140-21	−1.7	−1.9
140-22	−2.4	−2.7
140-23	−3.2	−3.5

11

Anatomical Atlas of Brain

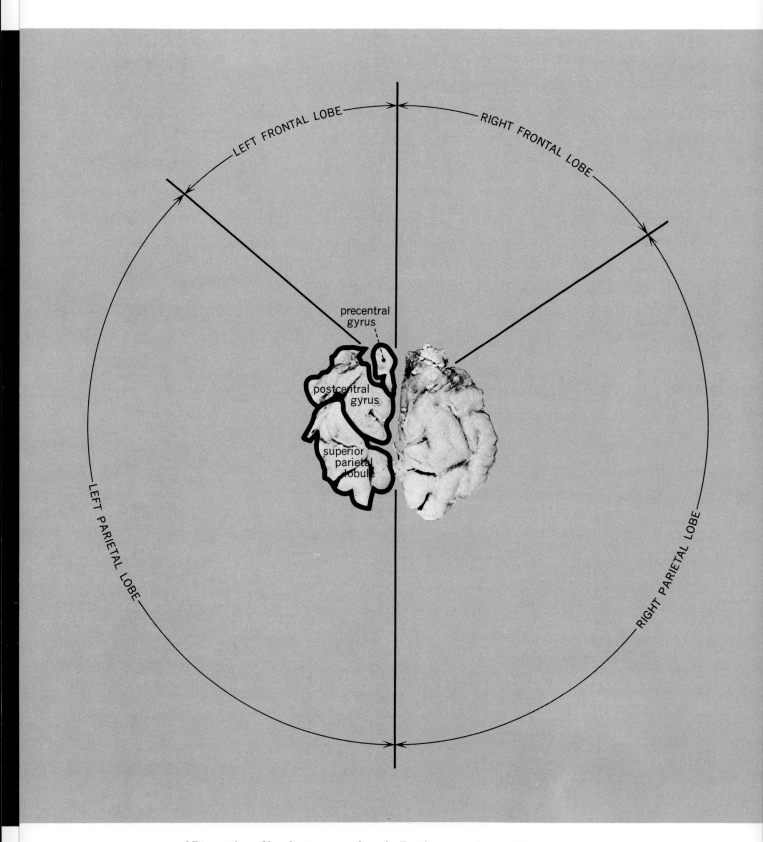

15° section, No. 1, uppersurface indicating prominent lobes and gyri.

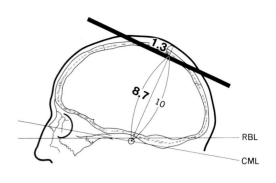

RBL

CML

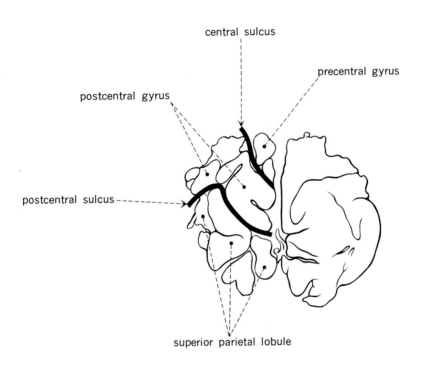

central sulcus

precentral gyrus

postcentral gyrus

postcentral sulcus

superior parietal lobule

15° section, No. 1, uppersurface indicating prominent structures.

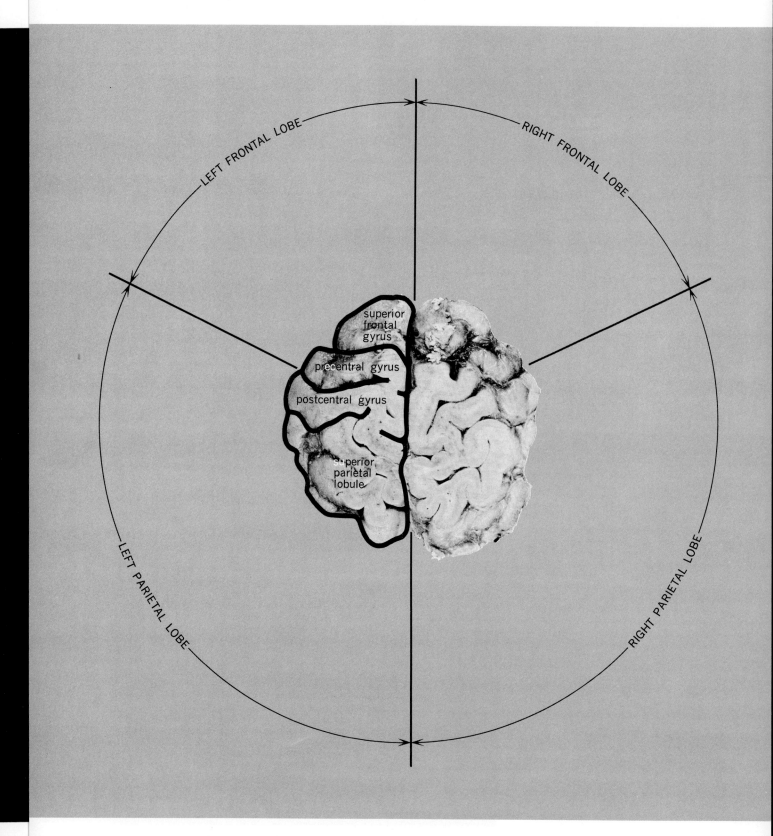

15° section, No. 2, uppersurface indicating prominent lobes and gyri.

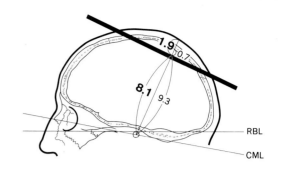

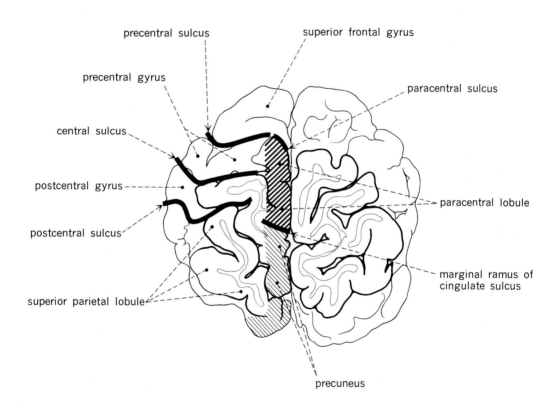

precentral sulcus

superior frontal gyrus

precentral gyrus

paracentral sulcus

central sulcus

postcentral gyrus

paracentral lobule

postcentral sulcus

marginal ramus of
cingulate sulcus

superior parietal lobule

precuneus

15° section, No. 2, uppersurface indicating prominent structures.

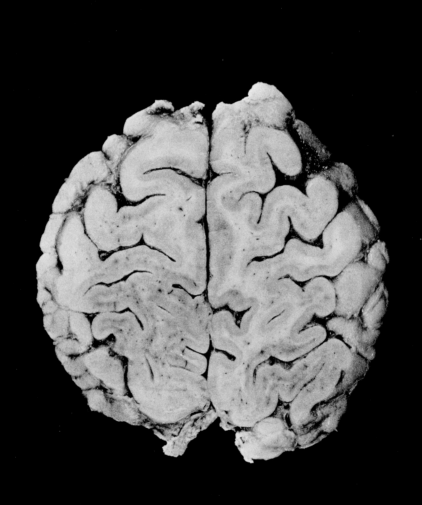

15° section, No. 3, uppersurface.

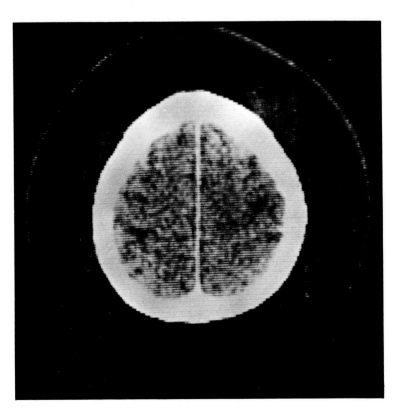
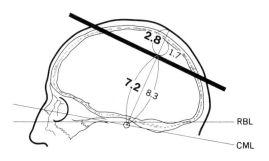

CT scan of 15° section, No. 3.

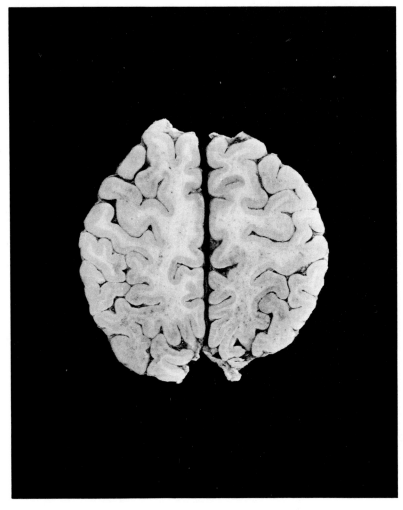

15° section, No. 3, lower surface.

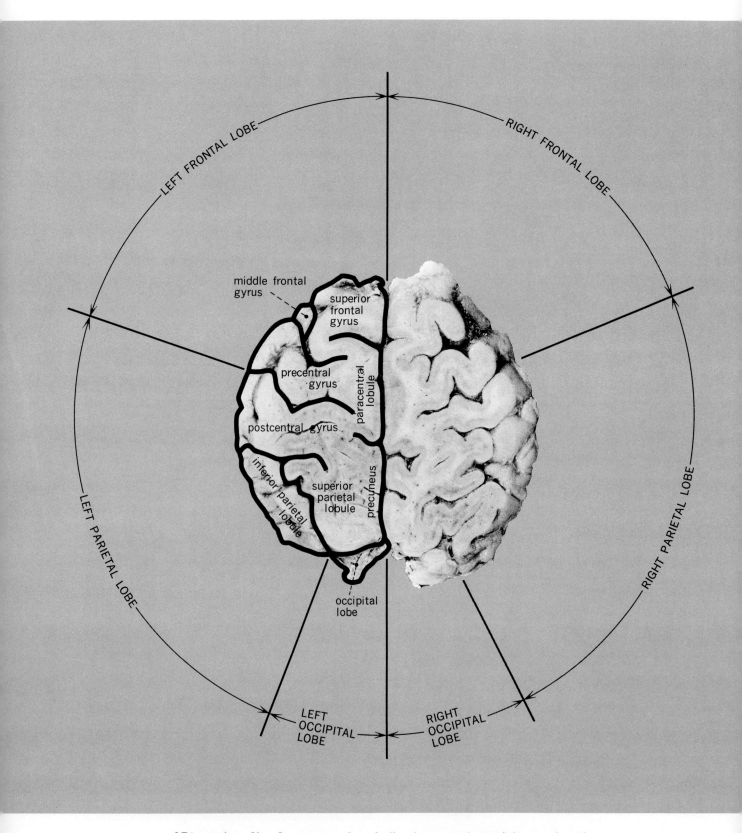

LEFT FRONTAL LOBE

RIGHT FRONTAL LOBE

middle frontal gyrus

superior frontal gyrus

precentral gyrus

paracentral lobule

postcentral gyrus

inferior parietal lobule

superior parietal lobule

precuneus

occipital lobe

LEFT PARIETAL LOBE

RIGHT PARIETAL LOBE

LEFT OCCIPITAL LOBE

RIGHT OCCIPITAL LOBE

15° section, No. 3, uppersurface indicating prominent lobes and gyri.

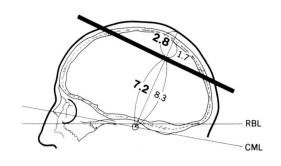

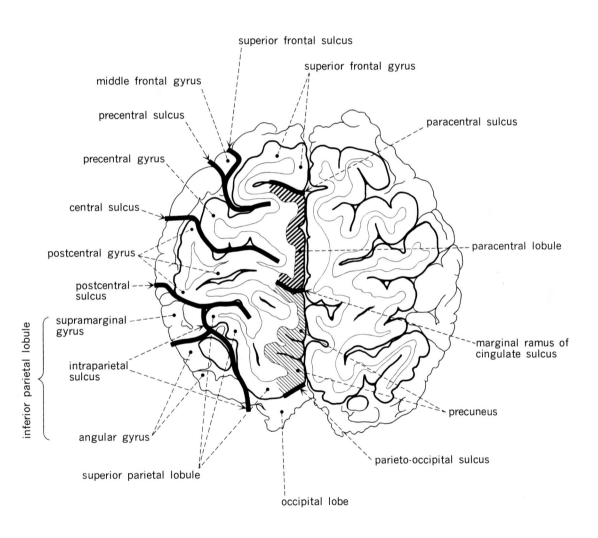

superior frontal sulcus

superior frontal gyrus

middle frontal gyrus

precentral sulcus

paracentral sulcus

precentral gyrus

central sulcus

postcentral gyrus

paracentral lobule

postcentral sulcus

supramarginal gyrus

marginal ramus of cingulate sulcus

intraparietal sulcus

inferior parietal lobule

angular gyrus

precuneus

superior parietal lobule

parieto-occipital sulcus

occipital lobe

15° section, No. 3, uppersurface indicating prominent structures.

15°-4

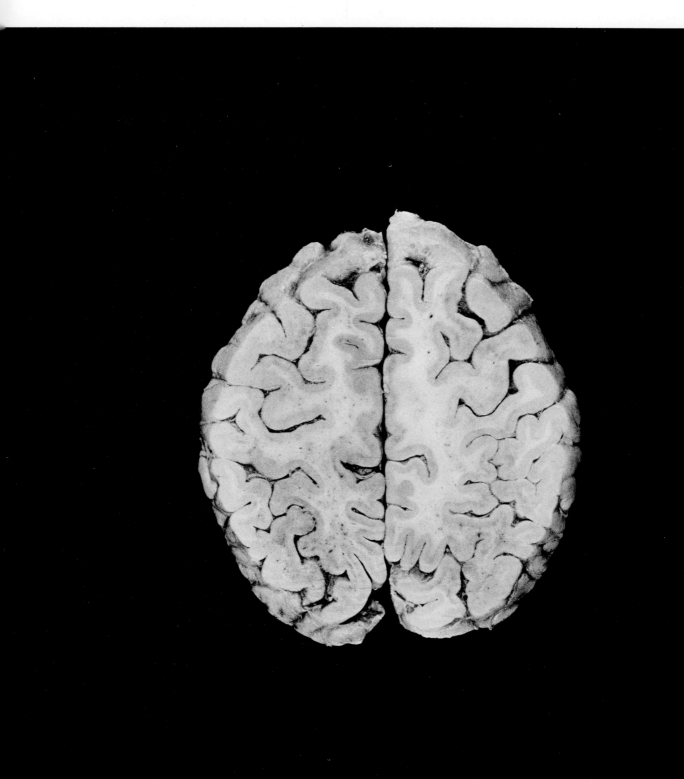

15° section, No. 4, uppersurface.

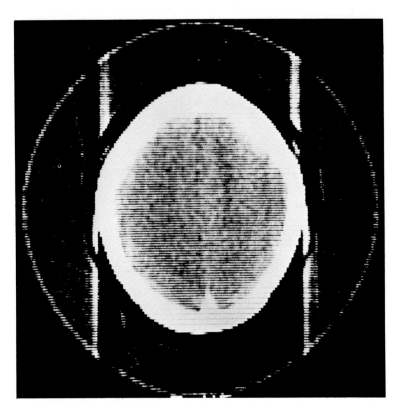
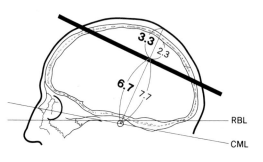

CT scan of 15° section, No. 4.

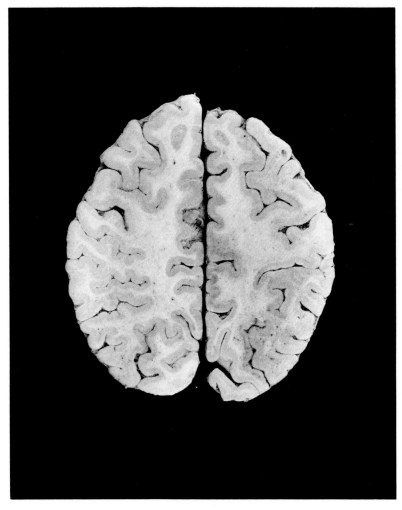

15° section, No. 4, lower surface.

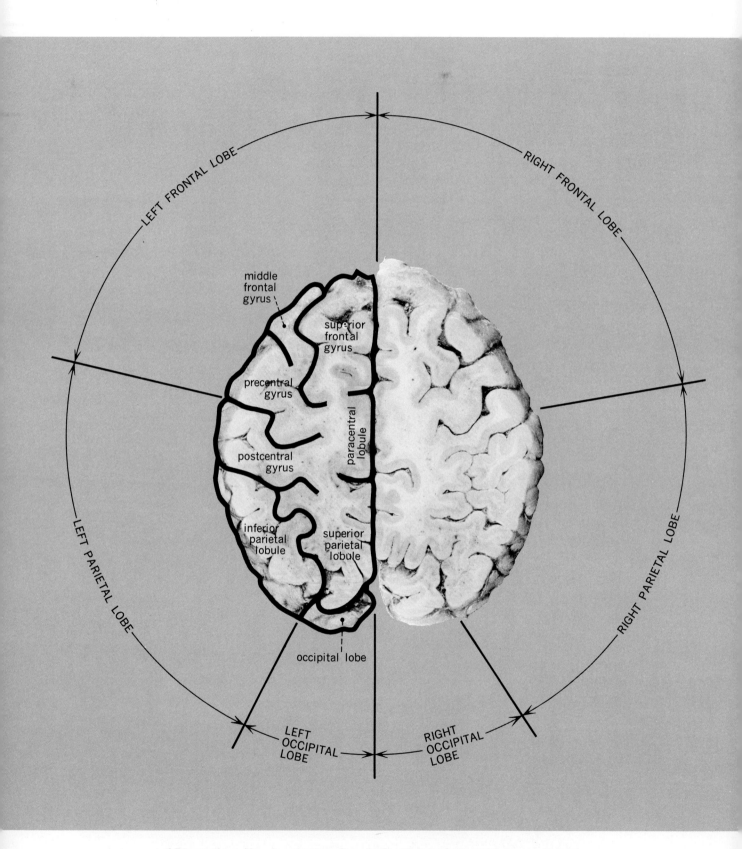

LEFT FRONTAL LOBE

RIGHT FRONTAL LOBE

middle
frontal
gyrus

superior
frontal
gyrus

precentral
gyrus

paracentral
lobule

postcentral
gyrus

LEFT PARIETAL LOBE

RIGHT PARIETAL LOBE

inferior
parietal
lobule

superior
parietal
lobule

occipital lobe

LEFT
OCCIPITAL
LOBE

RIGHT
OCCIPITAL
LOBE

15° section, No. 4, uppersurface indicating prominent lobes and gyri.

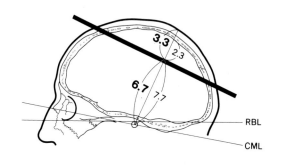

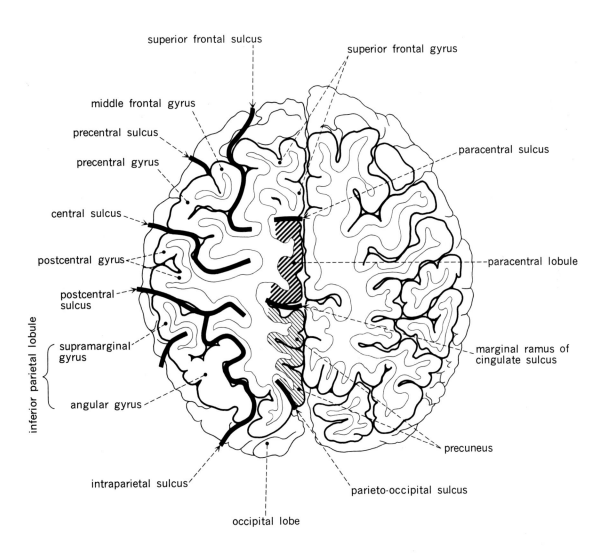

superior frontal sulcus

superior frontal gyrus

middle frontal gyrus

precentral sulcus

precentral gyrus

paracentral sulcus

central sulcus

postcentral gyrus

postcentral sulcus

paracentral lobule

inferior parietal lobule

supramarginal gyrus

marginal ramus of cingulate sulcus

angular gyrus

precuneus

intraparietal sulcus

parieto-occipital sulcus

occipital lobe

15° section, No. 4, uppersurface indicating prominent structures.

15°-5

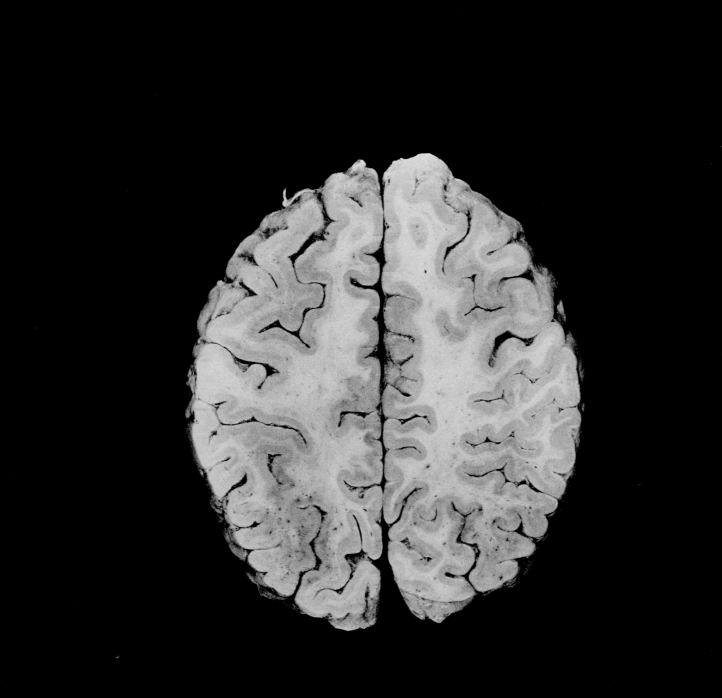

15° section, No. 5, uppersurface.

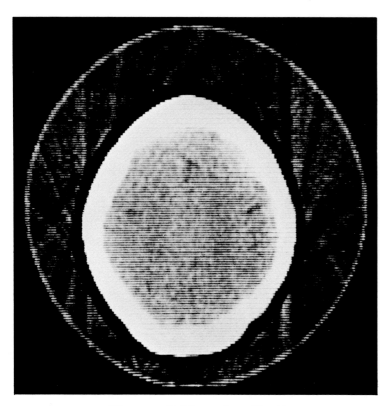

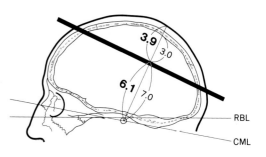

CT scan of 15° section, No. 5.

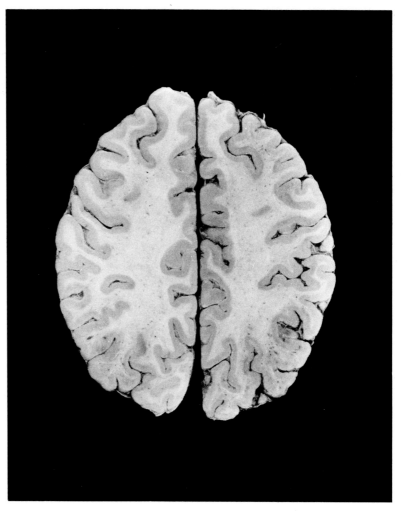

15° section, No. 5, lower surface.

31

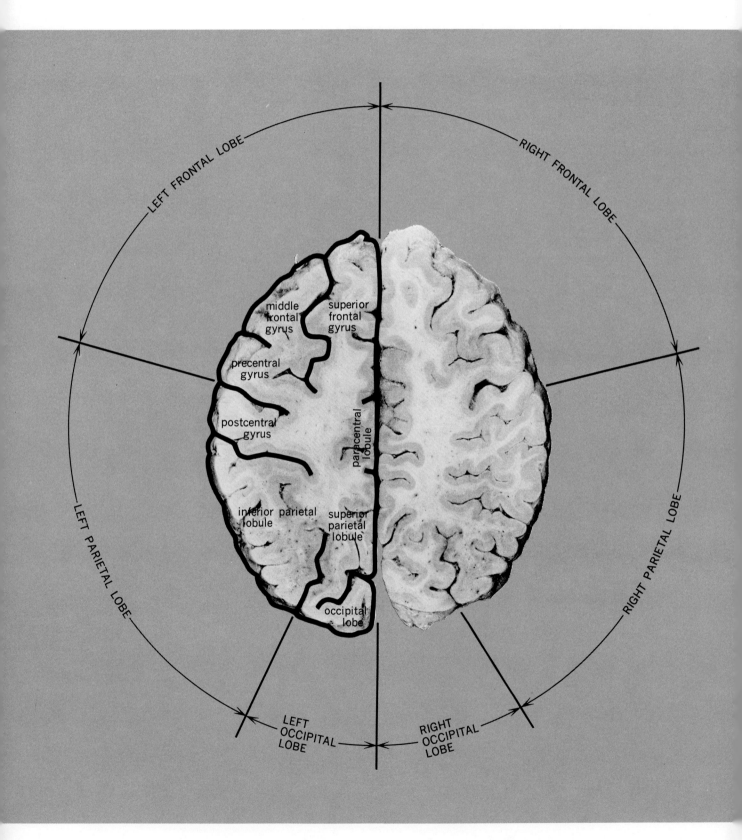

15° section, No. 5, uppersurface indicating prominent lobes and gyri.

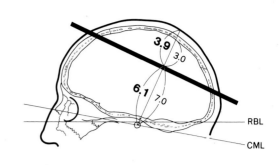

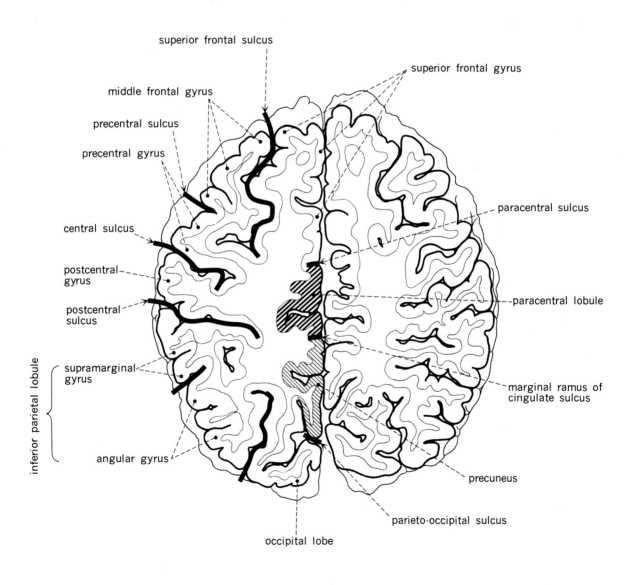

superior frontal sulcus

superior frontal gyrus

middle frontal gyrus

precentral sulcus

precentral gyrus

paracentral sulcus

central sulcus

postcentral gyrus

paracentral lobule

postcentral sulcus

inferior parietal lobule

supramarginal gyrus

marginal ramus of cingulate sulcus

angular gyrus

precuneus

parieto-occipital sulcus

occipital lobe

15° section, No. 5, uppersurface indicating prominent structures.

15°-6

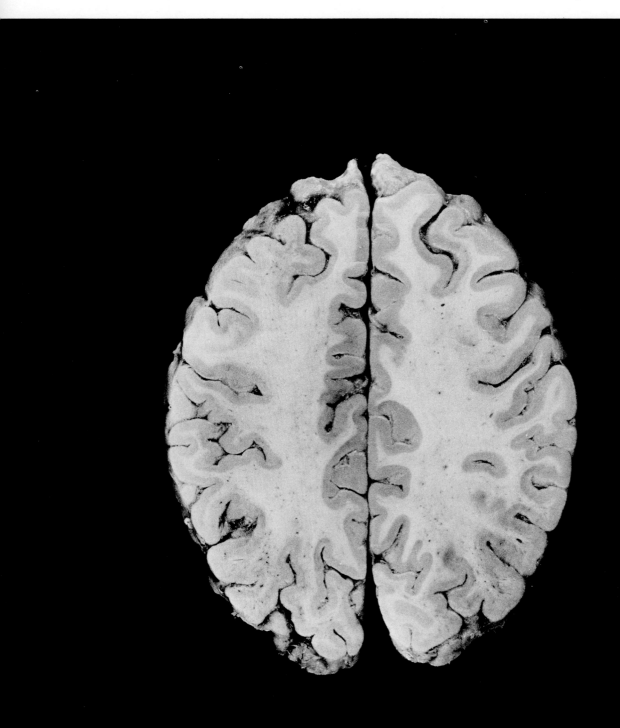

15° section, No. 6, uppersurface.

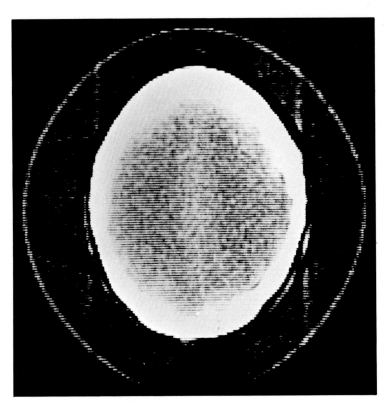
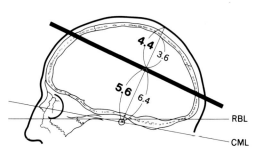

CT scan of 15° section, No. 6.

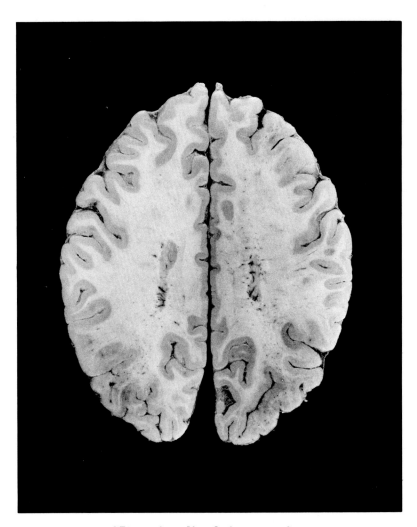

15° section, No. 6, lower surface.

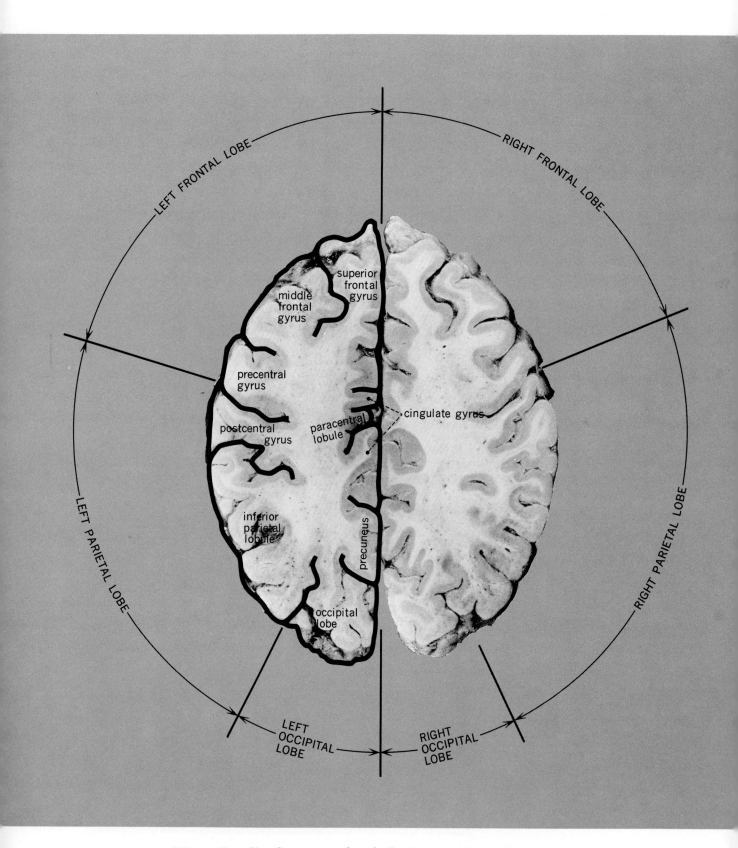

LEFT FRONTAL LOBE

RIGHT FRONTAL LOBE

superior
frontal
gyrus

middle
frontal
gyrus

precentral
gyrus

cingulate gyrus

postcentral
gyrus

paracentral
lobule

LEFT PARIETAL LOBE

RIGHT PARIETAL LOBE

inferior
parietal
lobule

precuneus

occipital
lobe

**LEFT
OCCIPITAL
LOBE**

**RIGHT
OCCIPITAL
LOBE**

15° section, No. 6, uppersurface indicating prominent lobes and gyri.

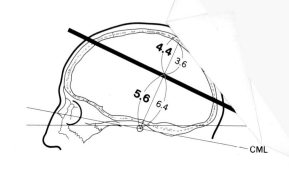

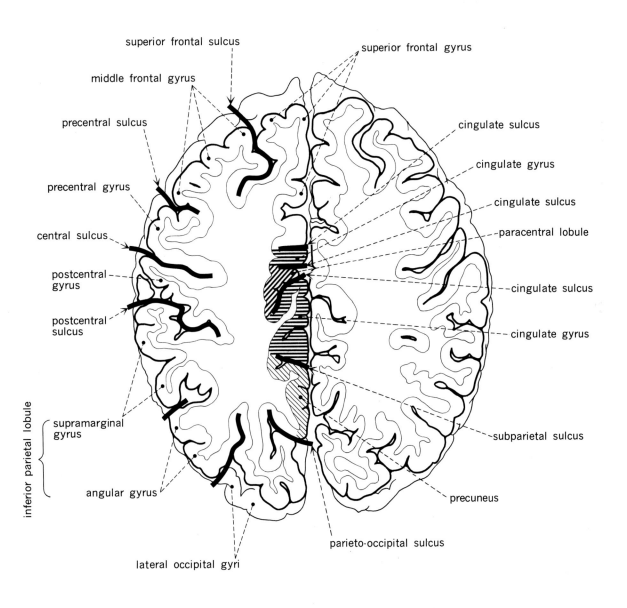

superior frontal sulcus

middle frontal gyrus

precentral sulcus

precentral gyrus

central sulcus

postcentral gyrus

postcentral sulcus

inferior parietal lobule

supramarginal gyrus

angular gyrus

lateral occipital gyri

superior frontal gyrus

cingulate sulcus

cingulate gyrus

cingulate sulcus

paracentral lobule

cingulate sulcus

cingulate gyrus

subparietal sulcus

precuneus

parieto-occipital sulcus

15° section, No. 6, uppersurface indicating prominent structures.

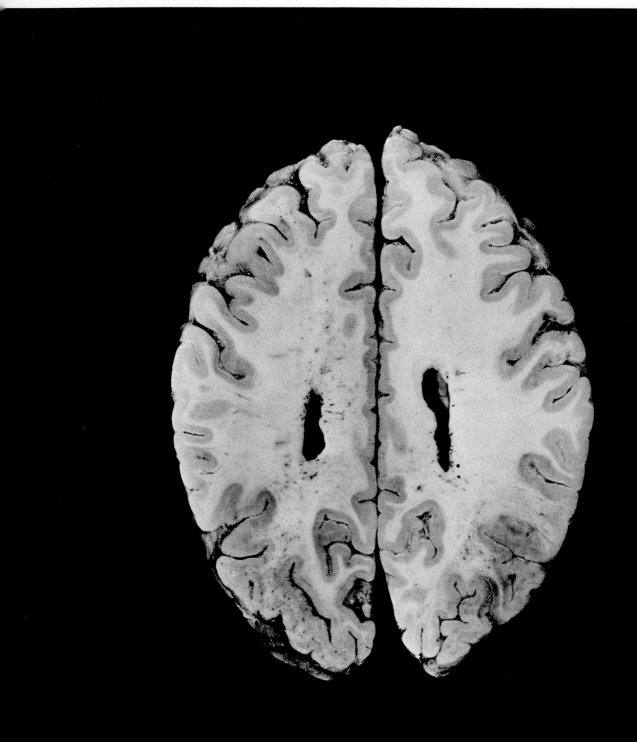

15° section, No. 7, uppersurface.

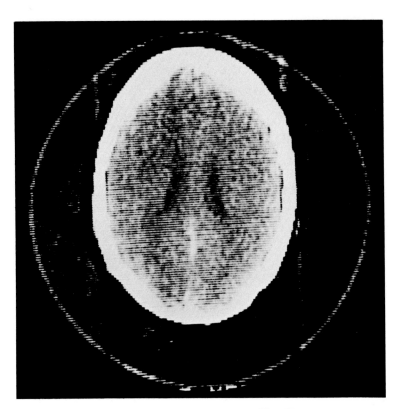
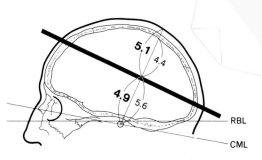

CT scan of 15° section, No. 7.

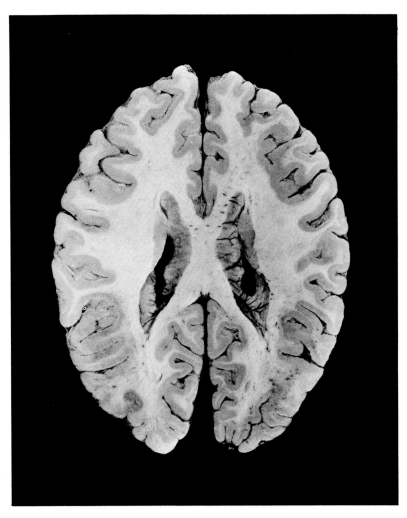

15° section, No. 7, lower surface.

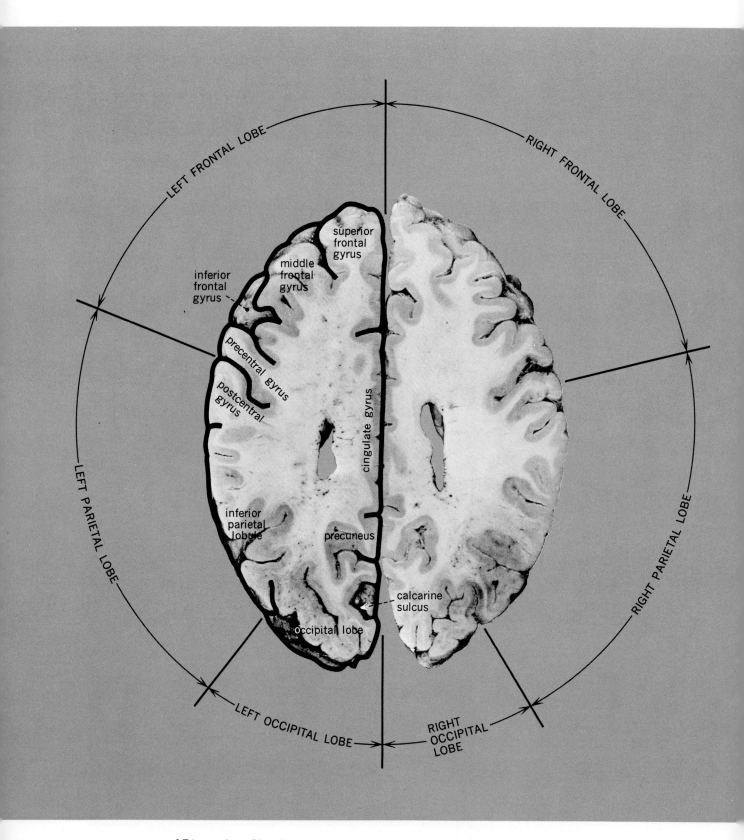

15° section, No. 7, uppersurface indicating prominent lobes and gyri.

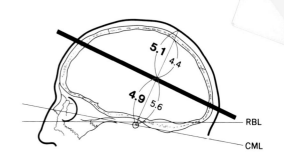

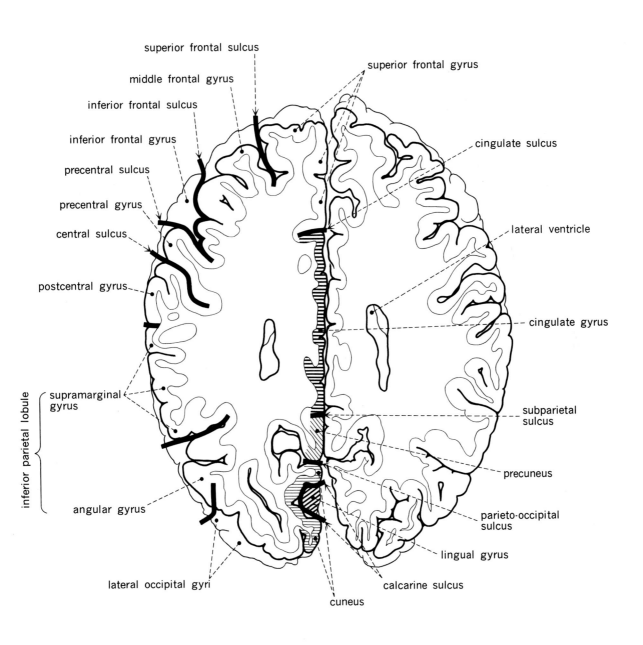

superior frontal sulcus

middle frontal gyrus

inferior frontal sulcus

inferior frontal gyrus

precentral sulcus

precentral gyrus

central sulcus

postcentral gyrus

inferior parietal lobule

supramarginal gyrus

angular gyrus

lateral occipital gyri

cuneus

superior frontal gyrus

cingulate sulcus

lateral ventricle

cingulate gyrus

subparietal sulcus

precuneus

parieto-occipital sulcus

lingual gyrus

calcarine sulcus

RBL

CML

15° section, No. 7, uppersurface indicating prominent structures.

41

15°-8

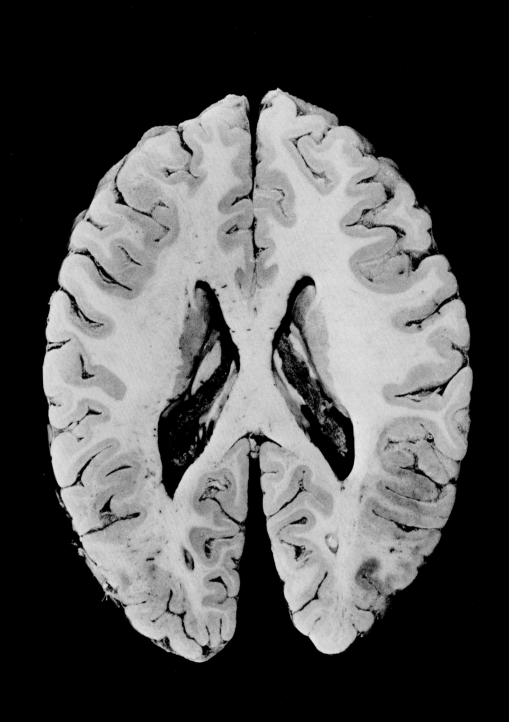

15° section, No. 8, uppersurface.

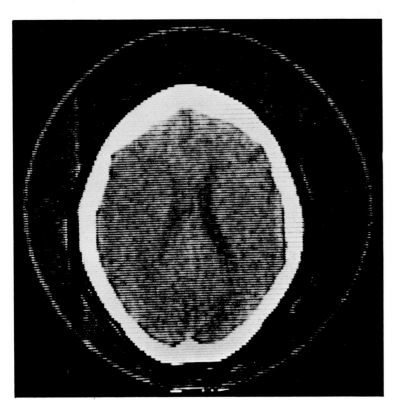
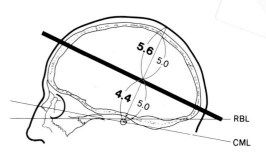

CT scan of 15° section, No. 8.

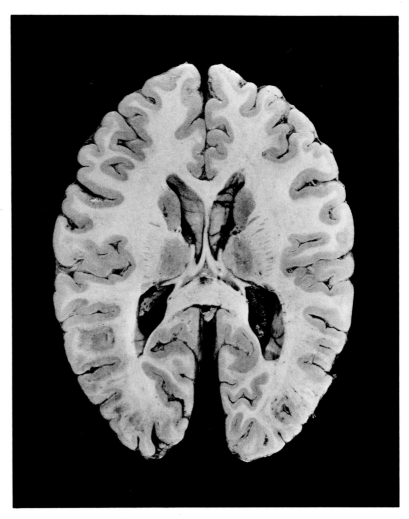

15° section, No. 8, lower surface.

15°-8

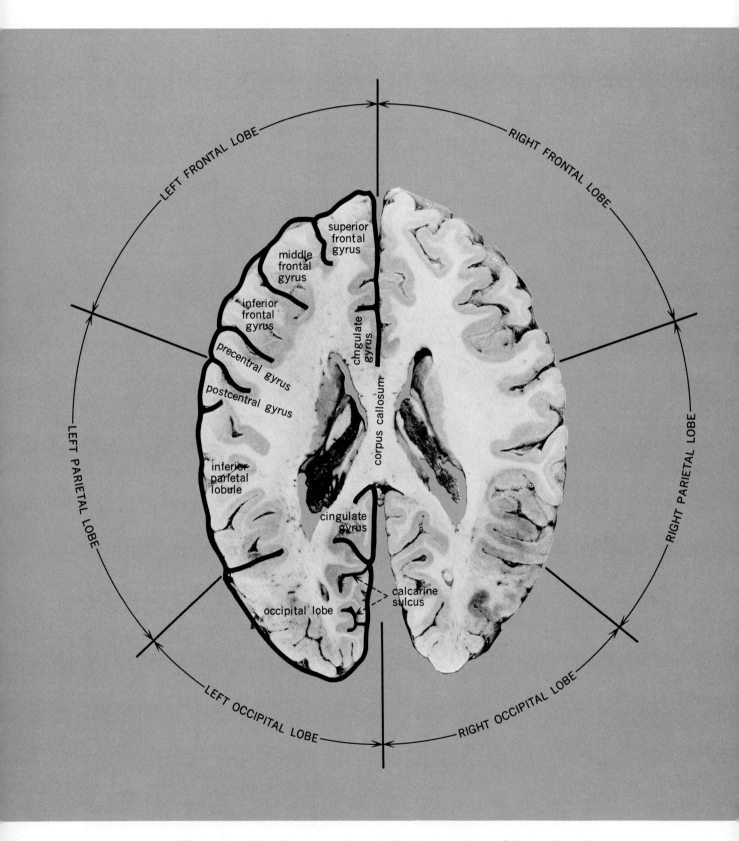

15° section, No. 8, uppersurface indicating prominent lobes and gyri.

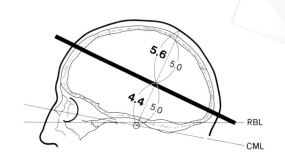

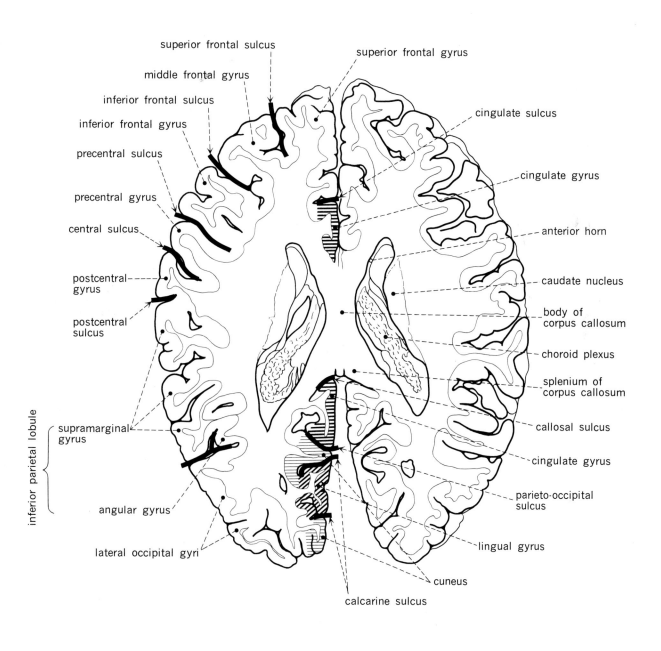

superior frontal sulcus

middle frontal gyrus

inferior frontal sulcus

inferior frontal gyrus

precentral sulcus

precentral gyrus

central sulcus

postcentral gyrus

postcentral sulcus

inferior parietal lobule

supramarginal gyrus

angular gyrus

lateral occipital gyri

calcarine sulcus

superior frontal gyrus

cingulate sulcus

cingulate gyrus

anterior horn

caudate nucleus

body of corpus callosum

choroid plexus

splenium of corpus callosum

callosal sulcus

cingulate gyrus

parieto-occipital sulcus

lingual gyrus

cuneus

15° section, No. 8, uppersurface indicating prominent structures.

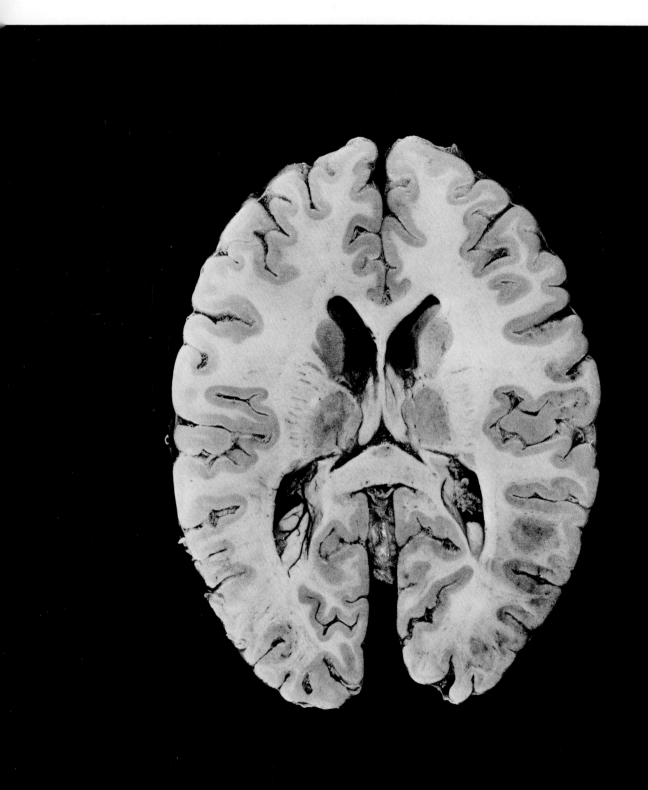

15° section, No. 9, uppersurface.

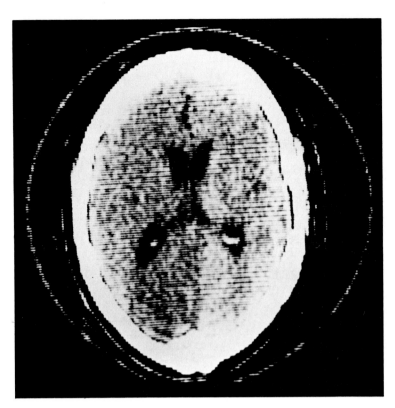

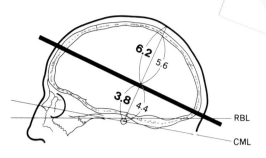

CT scan of 15° section, No. 9.

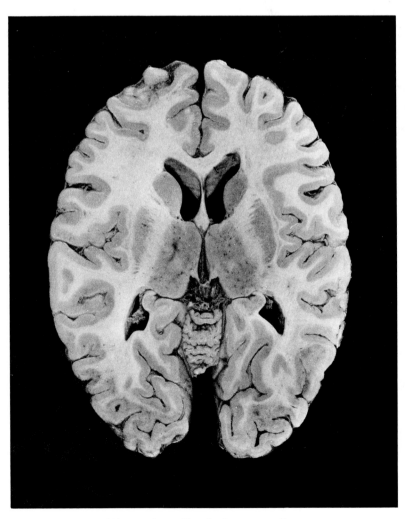

15° section, No. 9, lower surface.

47

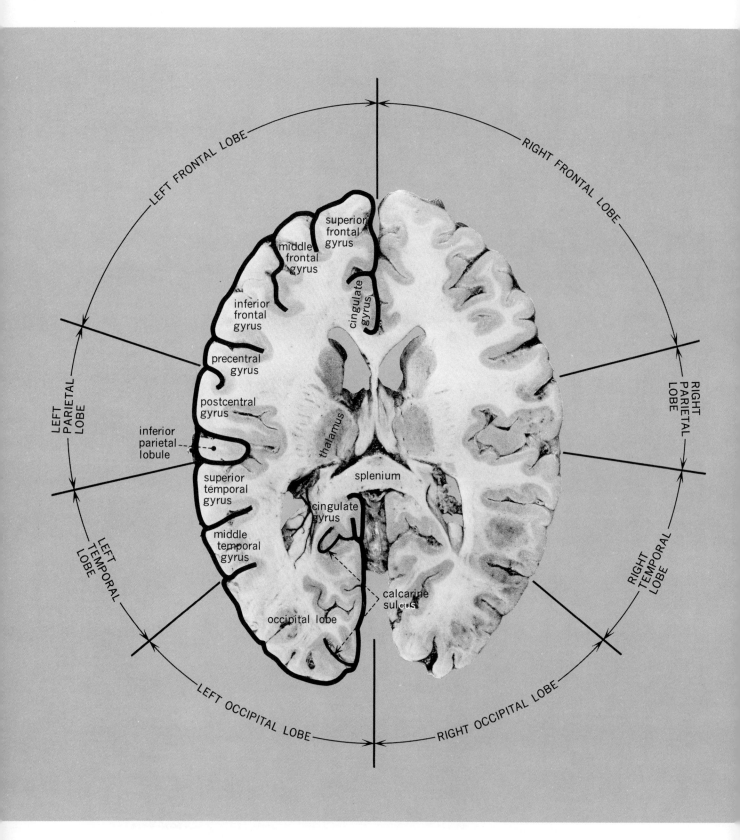

15° section, No. 9, uppersurface indicating prominent lobes and gyri.

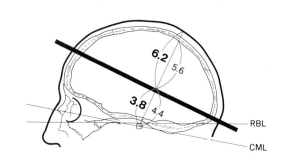

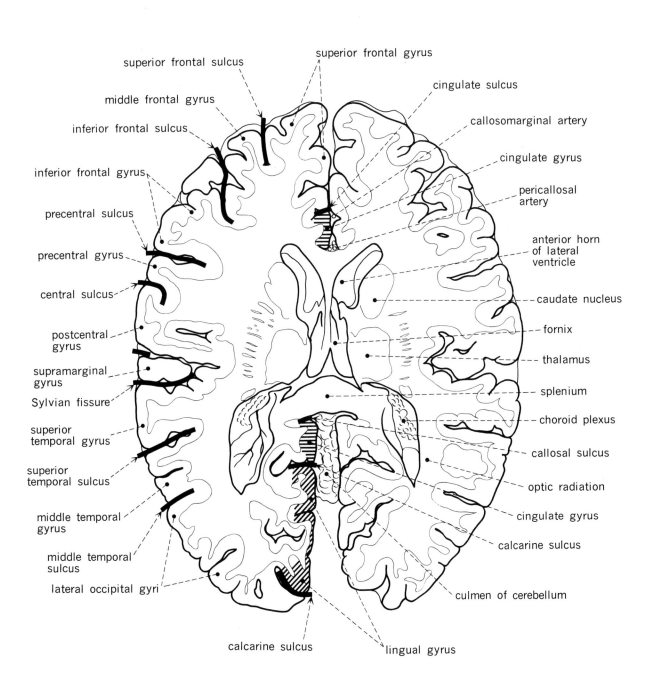

superior frontal sulcus

superior frontal gyrus

middle frontal gyrus

cingulate sulcus

inferior frontal sulcus

callosomarginal artery

inferior frontal gyrus

cingulate gyrus

precentral sulcus

pericallosal artery

precentral gyrus

anterior horn of lateral ventricle

central sulcus

caudate nucleus

postcentral gyrus

fornix

supramarginal gyrus

thalamus

Sylvian fissure

splenium

superior temporal gyrus

choroid plexus

superior temporal sulcus

callosal sulcus

middle temporal gyrus

optic radiation

middle temporal sulcus

cingulate gyrus

lateral occipital gyri

calcarine sulcus

culmen of cerebellum

calcarine sulcus

lingual gyrus

15° section, No. 9, uppersurface indicating prominent structures.

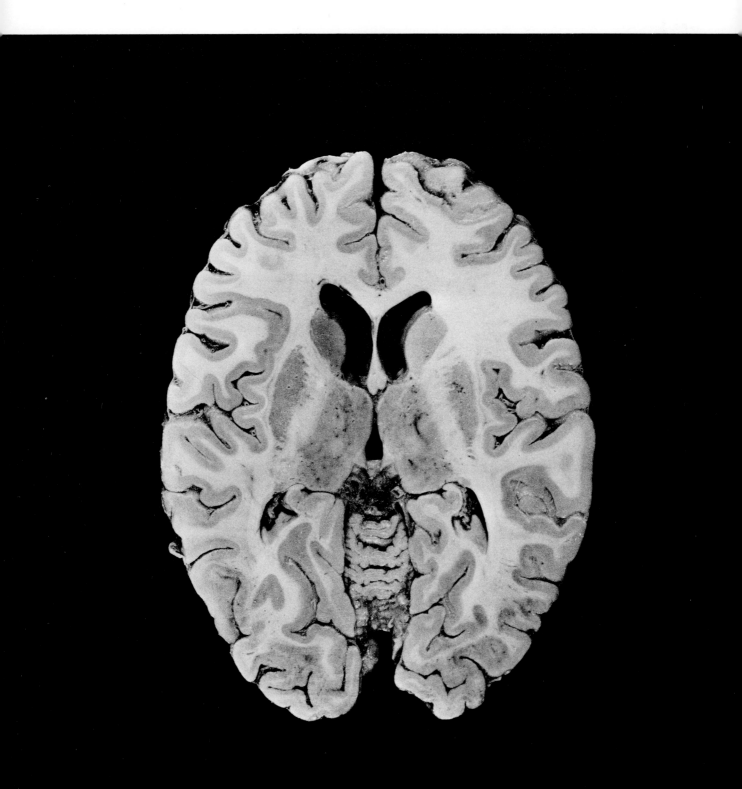

15° section, No. 10, uppersurface.

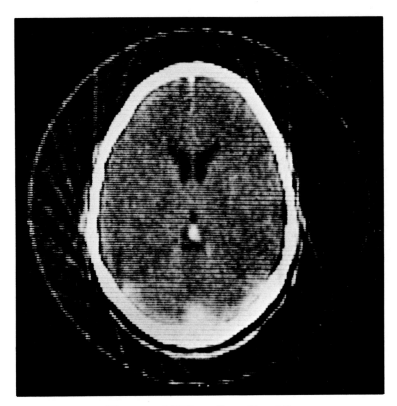
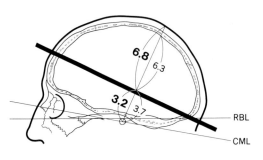

CT scan of 15° section, No. 10.

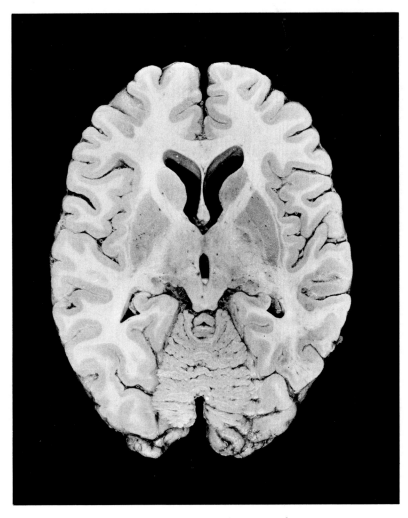

15° section, No. 10, lower surface.

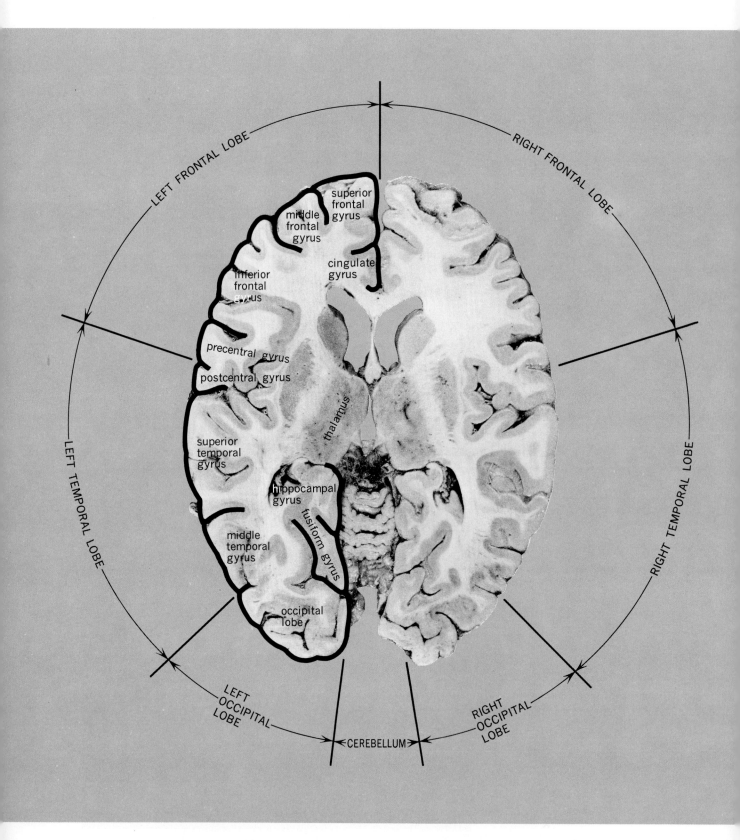

15° section, No. 10, uppersurface indicating prominent lobes and gyri.

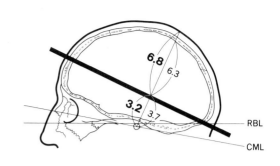

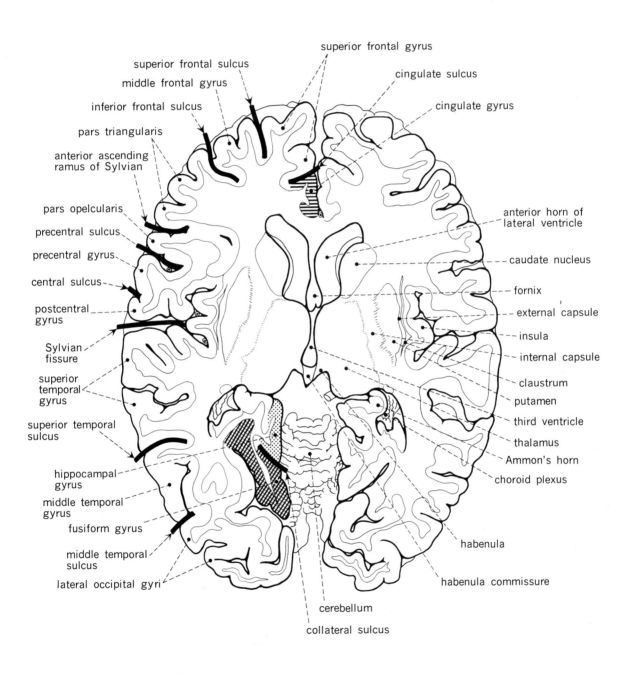

superior frontal gyrus

superior frontal sulcus

cingulate sulcus

middle frontal gyrus

inferior frontal sulcus

cingulate gyrus

pars triangularis

anterior ascending
ramus of Sylvian

anterior horn of
lateral ventricle

pars opelcularis

precentral sulcus

caudate nucleus

precentral gyrus

fornix

central sulcus

external capsule

postcentral
gyrus

insula

Sylvian
fissure

internal capsule

superior
temporal
gyrus

claustrum

putamen

superior temporal
sulcus

third ventricle

thalamus

Ammon's horn

hippocampal
gyrus

choroid plexus

middle temporal
gyrus

fusiform gyrus

middle temporal
sulcus

habenula

lateral occipital gyri

habenula commissure

cerebellum

collateral sulcus

15° section, No. 10, uppersurface indicating prominent structures.

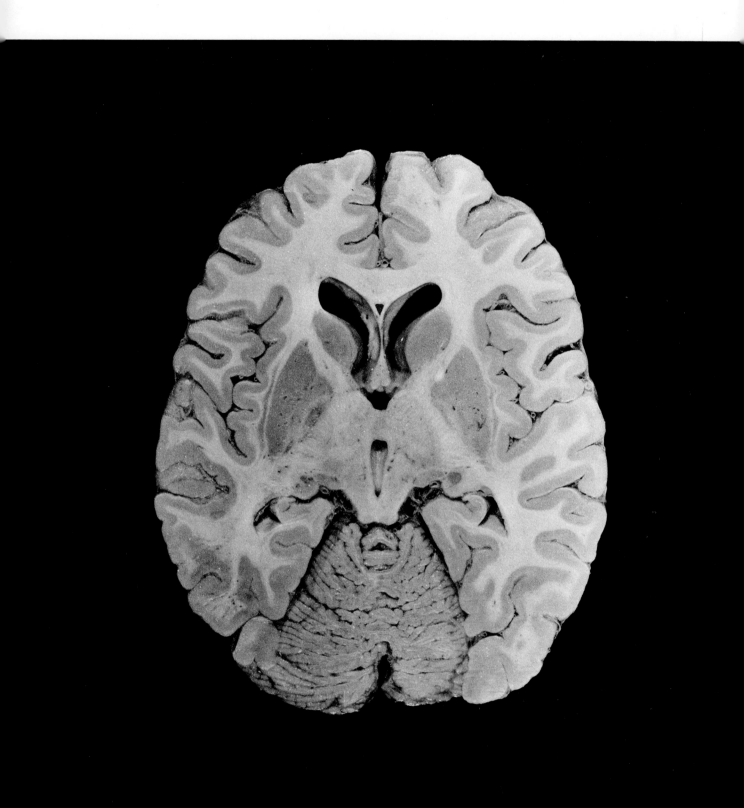

15° section, No. 11, uppersurface.

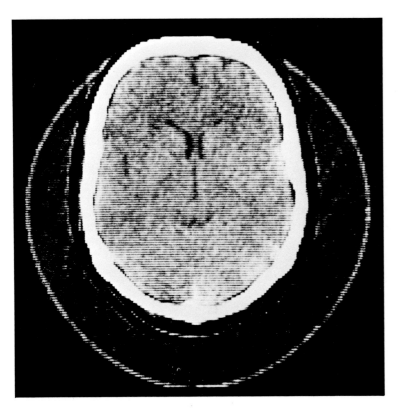
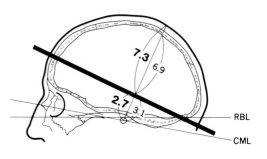

CT scan of 15° section, No. 11.

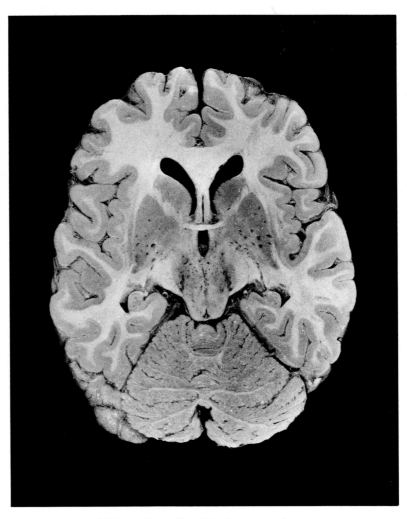

15° section, No. 11, lower surface.

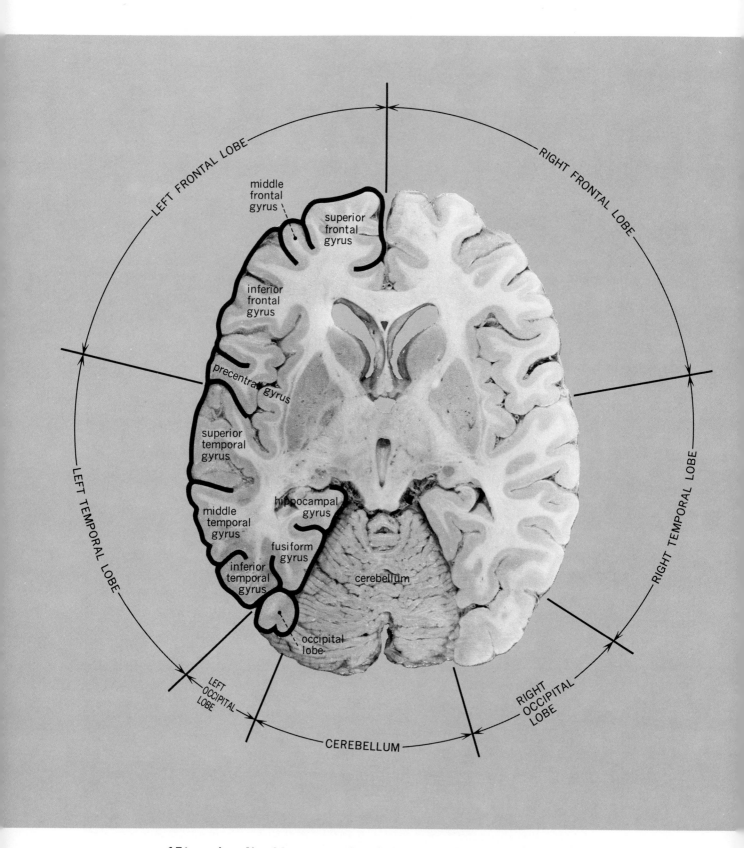

15° section, No. 11, uppersurface indicating prominent lobes and gyri.

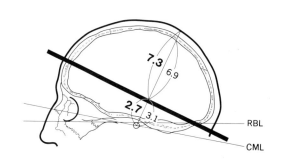

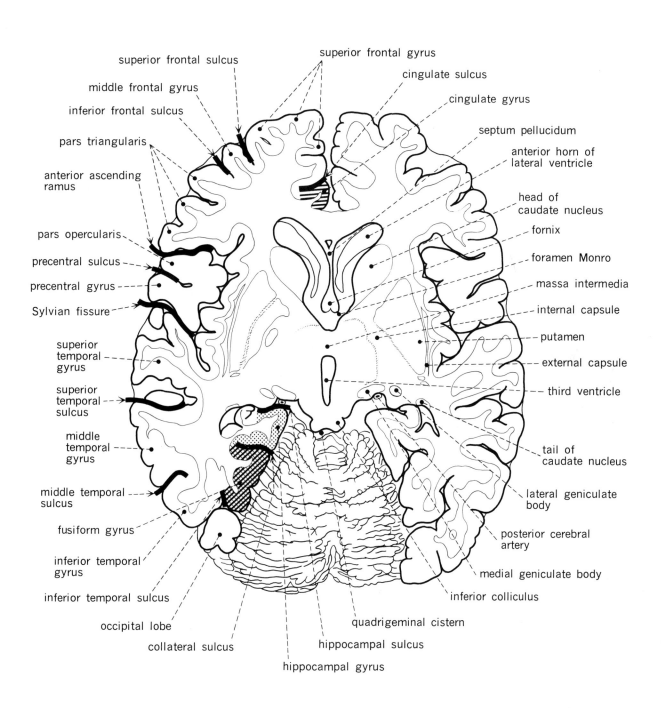

superior frontal sulcus

middle frontal gyrus

inferior frontal sulcus

pars triangularis

anterior ascending ramus

pars opercularis

precentral sulcus

precentral gyrus

Sylvian fissure

superior temporal gyrus

superior temporal sulcus

middle temporal gyrus

middle temporal sulcus

fusiform gyrus

inferior temporal gyrus

inferior temporal sulcus

occipital lobe

collateral sulcus

hippocampal gyrus

hippocampal sulcus

quadrigeminal cistern

inferior colliculus

medial geniculate body

posterior cerebral artery

lateral geniculate body

tail of caudate nucleus

third ventricle

external capsule

putamen

internal capsule

massa intermedia

foramen Monro

fornix

head of caudate nucleus

anterior horn of lateral ventricle

septum pellucidum

cingulate gyrus

cingulate sulcus

superior frontal gyrus

15° section, No. 11, uppersurface indicating prominent structures.

15°- 12

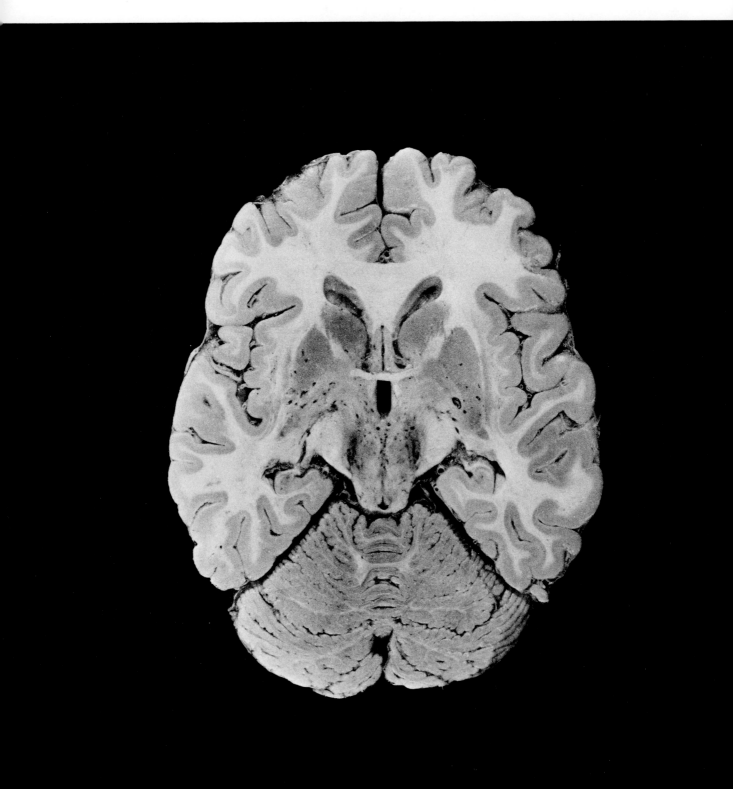

15° section, No. 12, uppersurface.

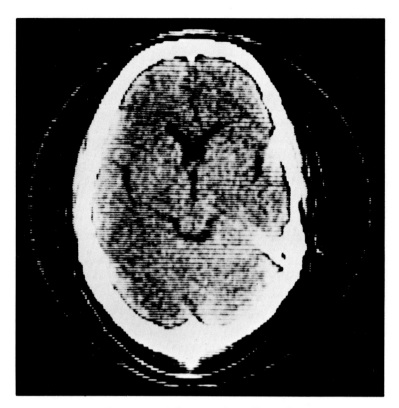

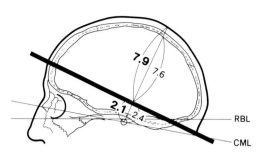

CT scan of 15° section, No. 12.

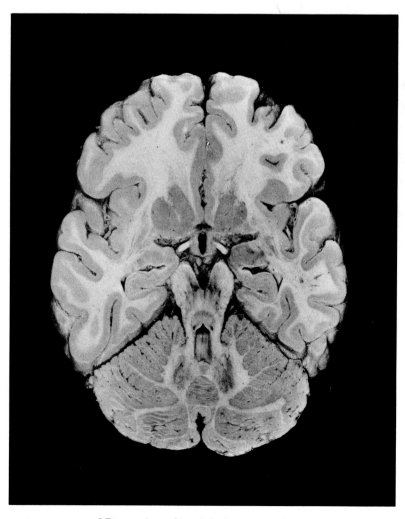

15° section, No. 12, lower surface.

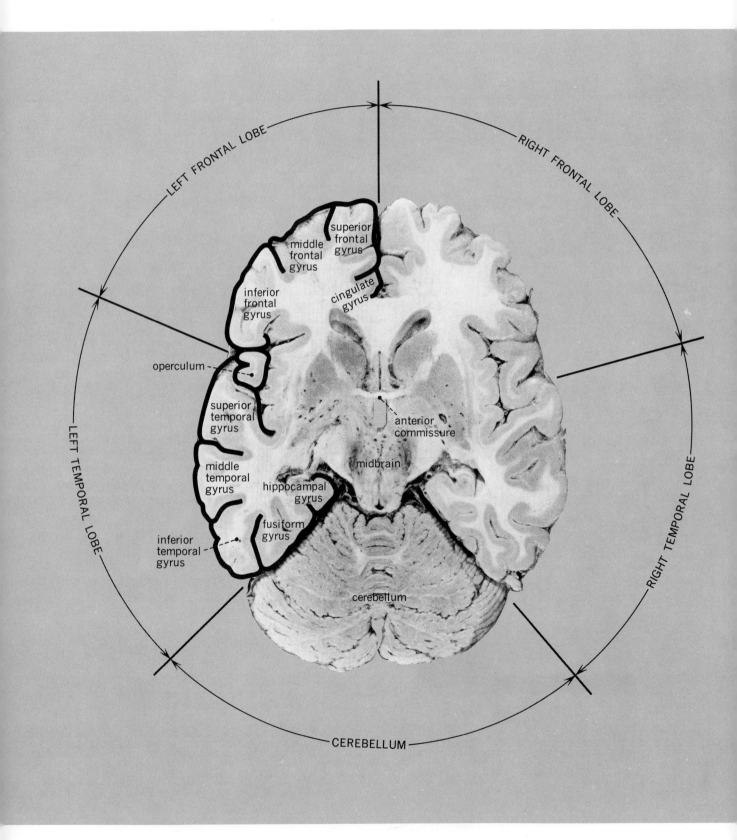

15° section, No. 12, uppersurface indicating prominent lobes and gyri.

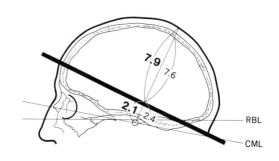

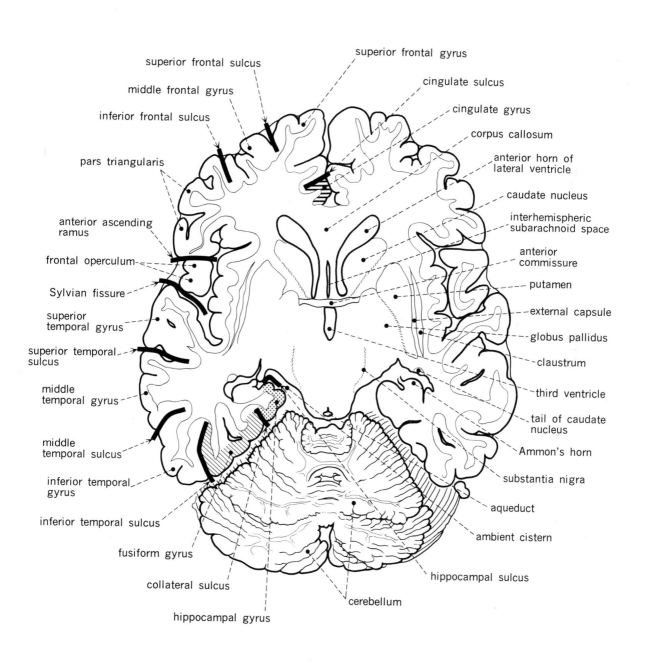

superior frontal sulcus

middle frontal gyrus

inferior frontal sulcus

pars triangularis

anterior ascending ramus

frontal operculum

Sylvian fissure

superior temporal gyrus

superior temporal sulcus

middle temporal gyrus

middle temporal sulcus

inferior temporal gyrus

inferior temporal sulcus

fusiform gyrus

collateral sulcus

hippocampal gyrus

superior frontal gyrus

cingulate sulcus

cingulate gyrus

corpus callosum

anterior horn of lateral ventricle

caudate nucleus

interhemispheric subarachnoid space

anterior commissure

putamen

external capsule

globus pallidus

claustrum

third ventricle

tail of caudate nucleus

Ammon's horn

substantia nigra

aqueduct

ambient cistern

hippocampal sulcus

cerebellum

15° section, No. 12, uppersurface indicating prominent structures.

15°-13

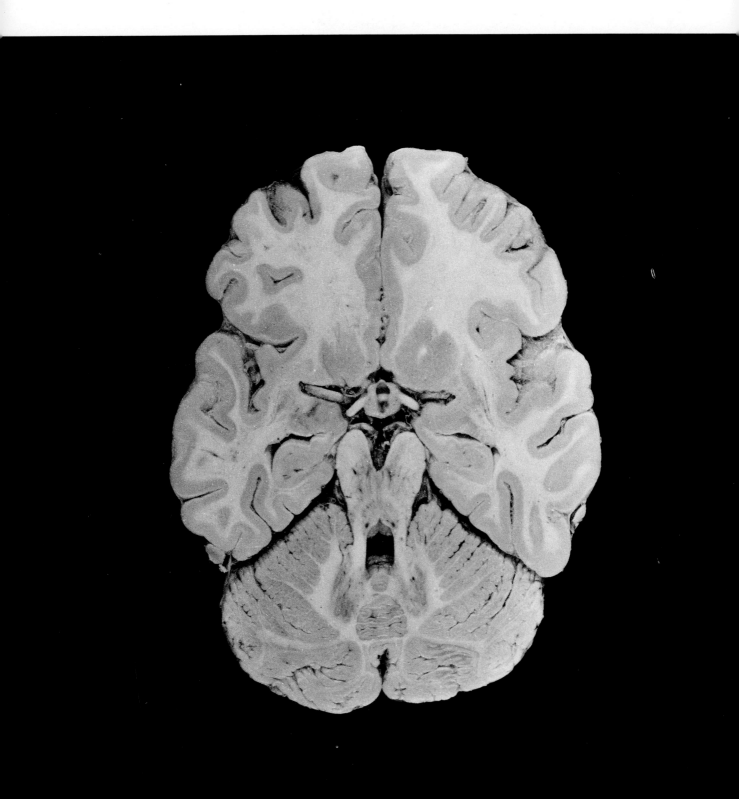

15° section, No. 13, uppersurface.

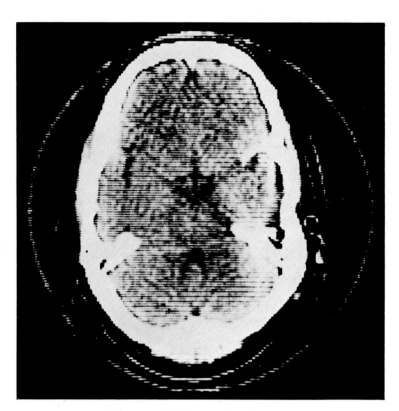

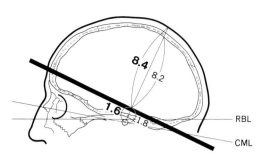

CT scan of 15° section, No. 13.

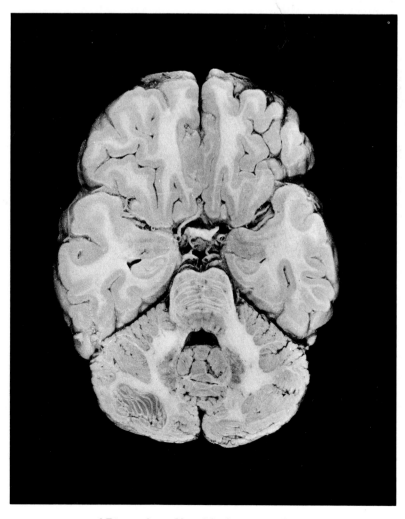

15° section, No. 13, lower surface.

63

15°·13

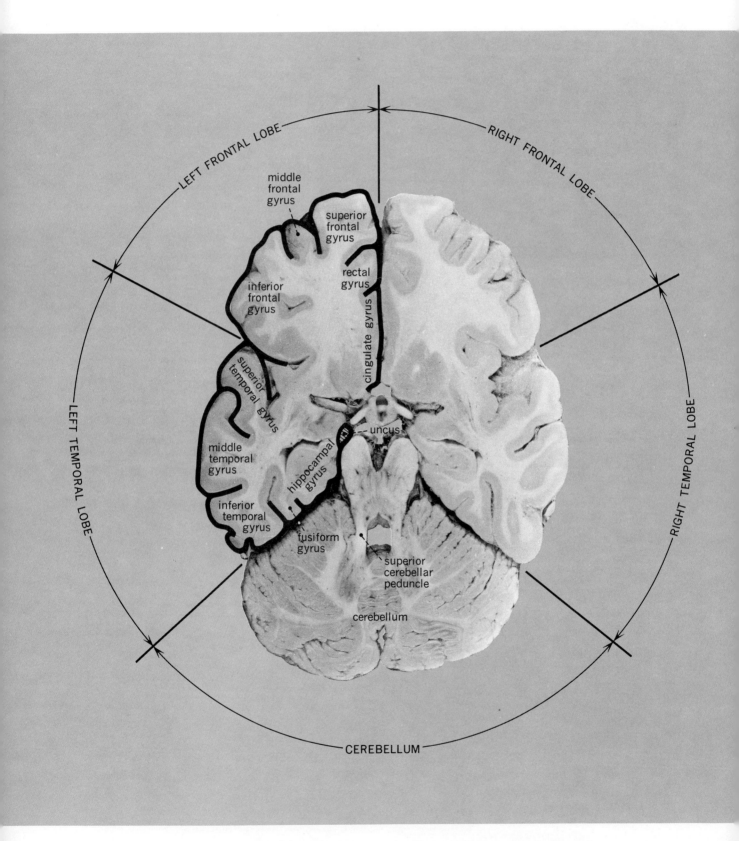

LEFT FRONTAL LOBE

RIGHT FRONTAL LOBE

middle frontal gyrus

superior frontal gyrus

rectal gyrus

inferior frontal gyrus

cingulate gyrus

superior temporal gyrus

uncus

LEFT TEMPORAL LOBE

RIGHT TEMPORAL LOBE

middle temporal gyrus

hippocampal gyrus

inferior temporal gyrus

fusiform gyrus

superior cerebellar peduncle

cerebellum

CEREBELLUM

15° section, No. 13, uppersurface indicating prominent lobes and gyri.

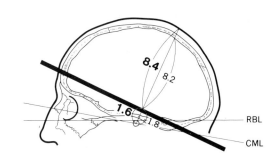

superior frontal sulcus

middle frontal gyrus

inferior frontal sulcus

inferior frontal gyrus

Sylvian fissure

superior temporal gyrus

superior temporal sulcus

amygdaloid nucleus

middle temporal gyrus

middle temporal sulcus

inferior temporal gyrus

inferior temporal sulcus

fusiform gyrus

collateral sulcus

hippocampal gyrus

superior cerebellar peduncle

fourth ventricle

superior frontal gyrus

rectal gyrus

cingulate gyrus

caudate nucleus

putamen

infundibular recess

middle cerebral artery

optic tract

inferior horn of lateral ventricle

posterior cerebral artery

uncus

locus ceruleus

dentate nucleus

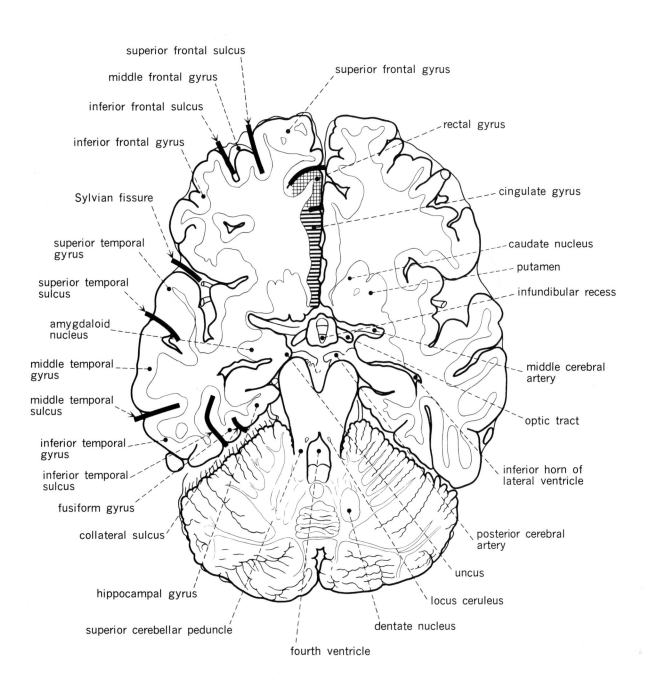

15° section, No. 13, uppersurface indicating prominent structures.

65

15°- 14

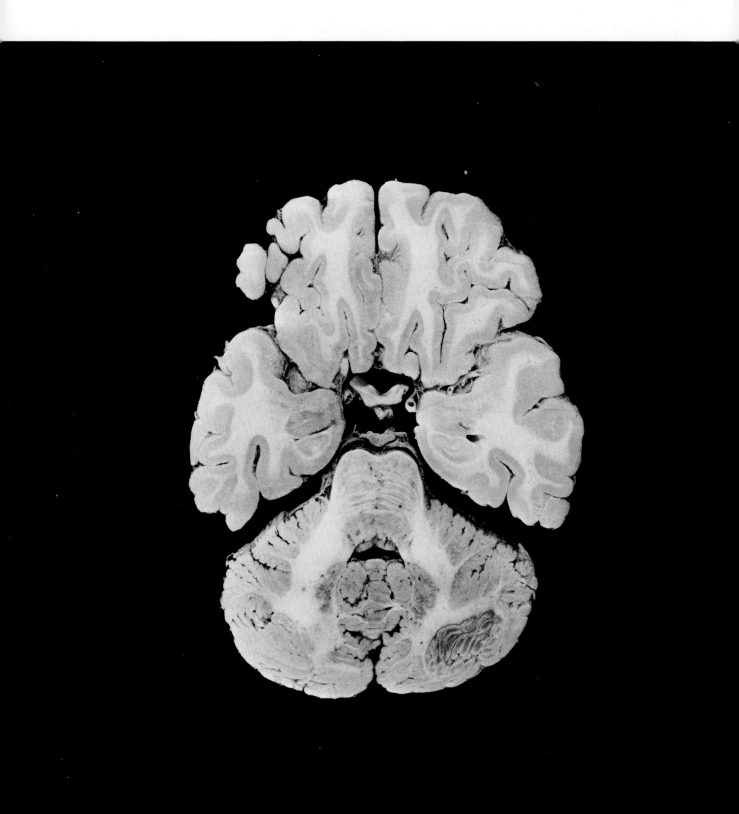

15° section, No. 14, uppersurface.

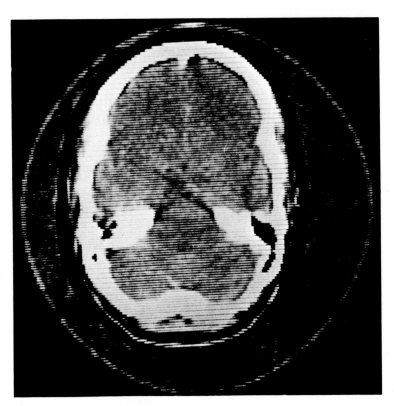

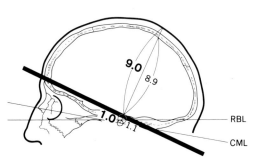

CT scan of 15° section, No. 14.

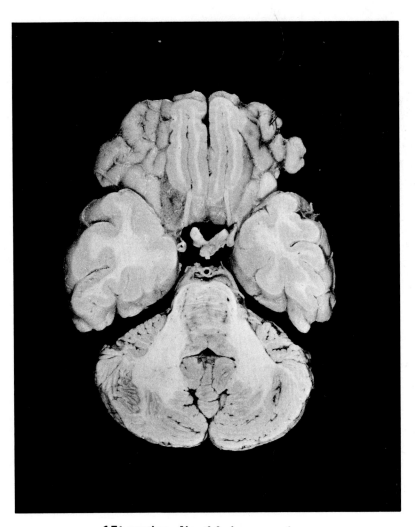

15° section, No. 14, lower surface.

67

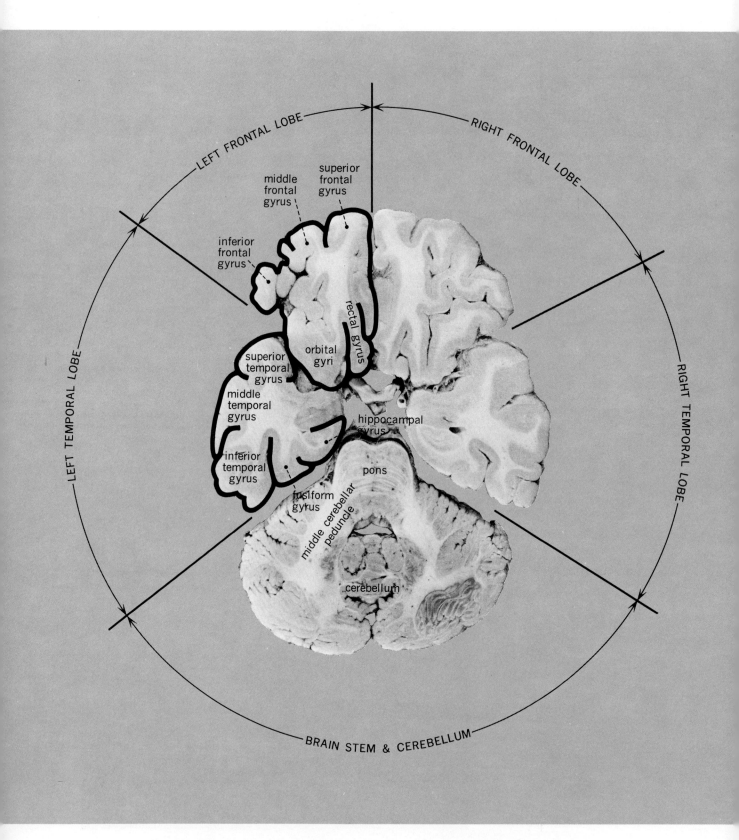

LEFT FRONTAL LOBE

RIGHT FRONTAL LOBE

middle frontal gyrus

superior frontal gyrus

inferior frontal gyrus

rectal gyrus

orbital gyri

superior temporal gyrus

middle temporal gyrus

hippocampal gyrus

inferior temporal gyrus

fusiform gyrus

pons

middle cerebellar peduncle

cerebellum

LEFT TEMPORAL LOBE

RIGHT TEMPORAL LOBE

BRAIN STEM & CEREBELLUM

15° section, No. 14, uppersurface indicating prominent lobes and gyri.

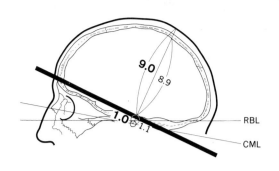

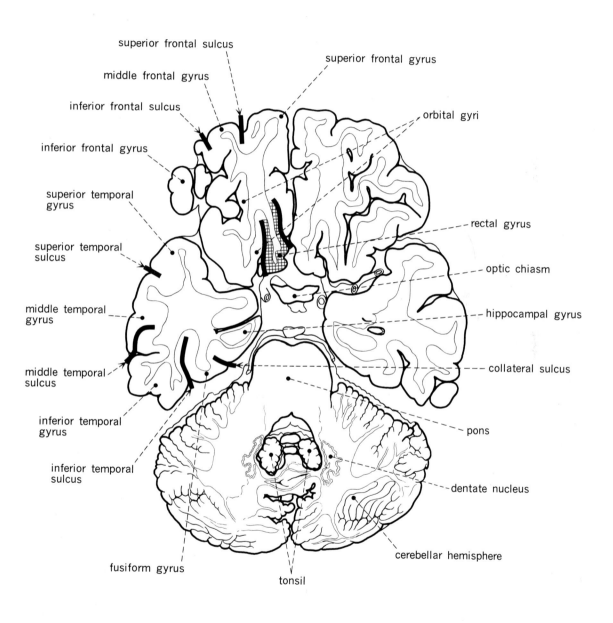

superior frontal sulcus

middle frontal gyrus

inferior frontal sulcus

inferior frontal gyrus

superior temporal gyrus

superior temporal sulcus

middle temporal gyrus

middle temporal sulcus

inferior temporal gyrus

inferior temporal sulcus

fusiform gyrus

tonsil

superior frontal gyrus

orbital gyri

rectal gyrus

optic chiasm

hippocampal gyrus

collateral sulcus

pons

dentate nucleus

cerebellar hemisphere

15° section, No. 14, uppersurface indicating prominent structures.

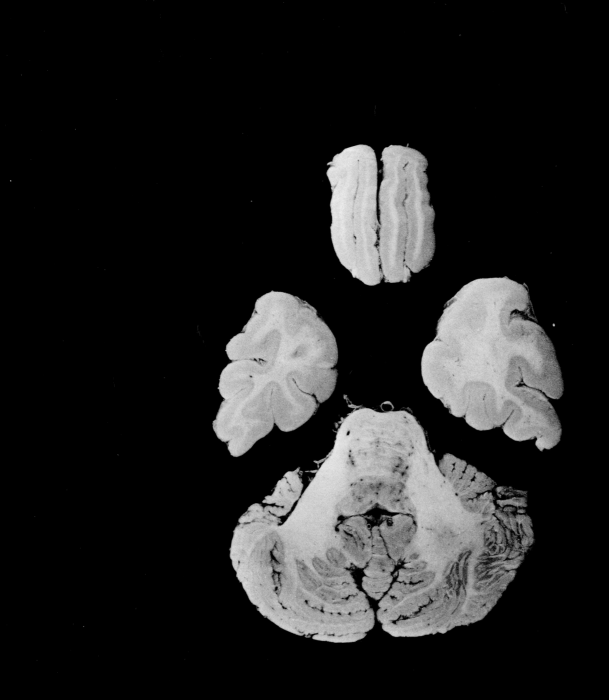

15° section, No. 15, uppersurface.

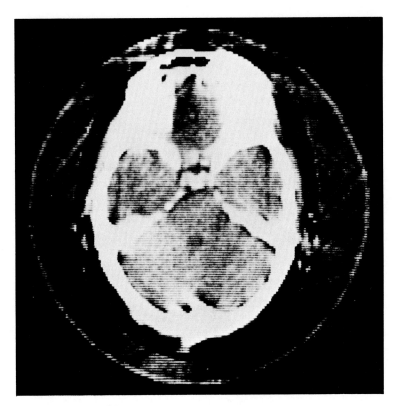
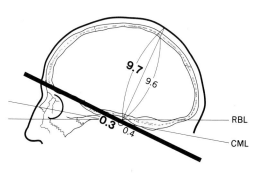

CT scan of 15° section, No. 15.

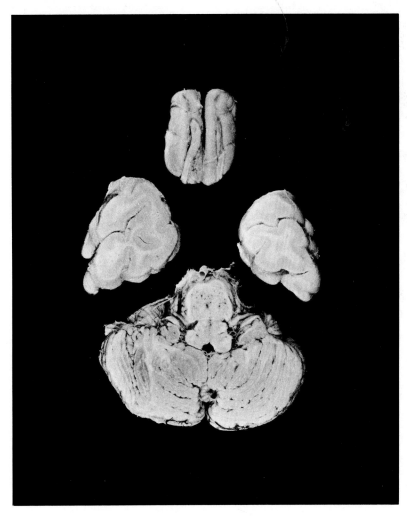

15° section, No. 15, lower surface.

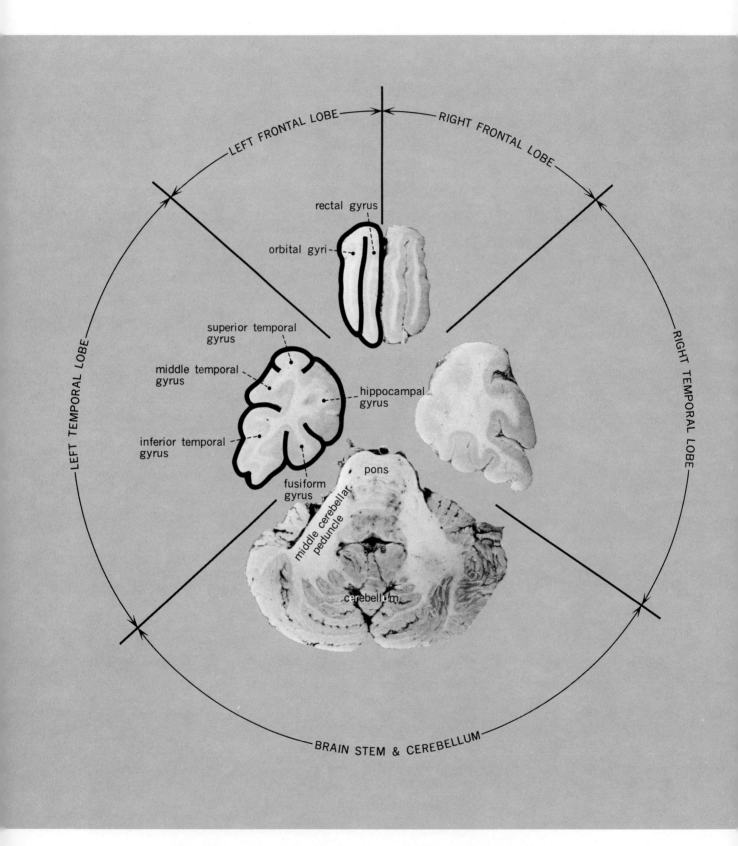

15° section, No. 15, uppersurface indicating prominent lobes and gyri.

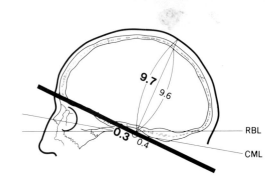

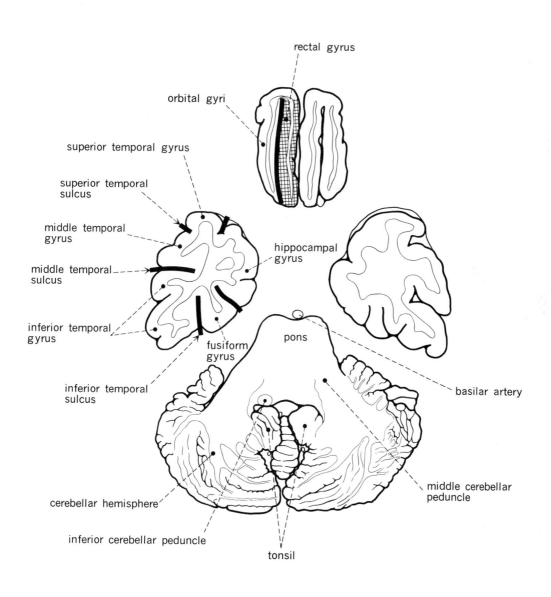

rectal gyrus

orbital gyri

superior temporal gyrus

superior temporal sulcus

middle temporal gyrus

middle temporal sulcus

inferior temporal gyrus

hippocampal gyrus

fusiform gyrus

pons

inferior temporal sulcus

basilar artery

middle cerebellar peduncle

cerebellar hemisphere

inferior cerebellar peduncle

tonsil

15° section, No. 15, uppersurface indicating prominent structures.

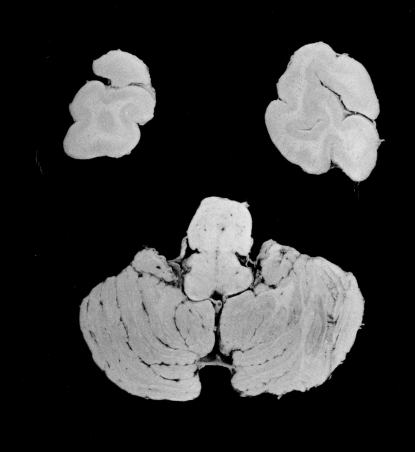

15° section, No. 16, uppersurface.

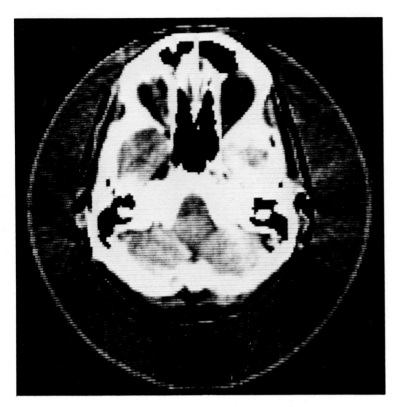
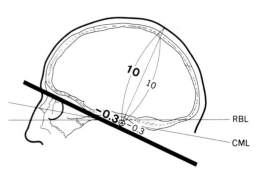

CT scan of 15° section, No. 16.

RBL

CML

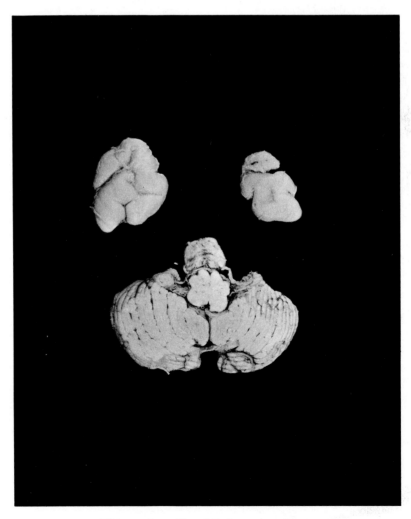

15° section, No. 16, lower surface.

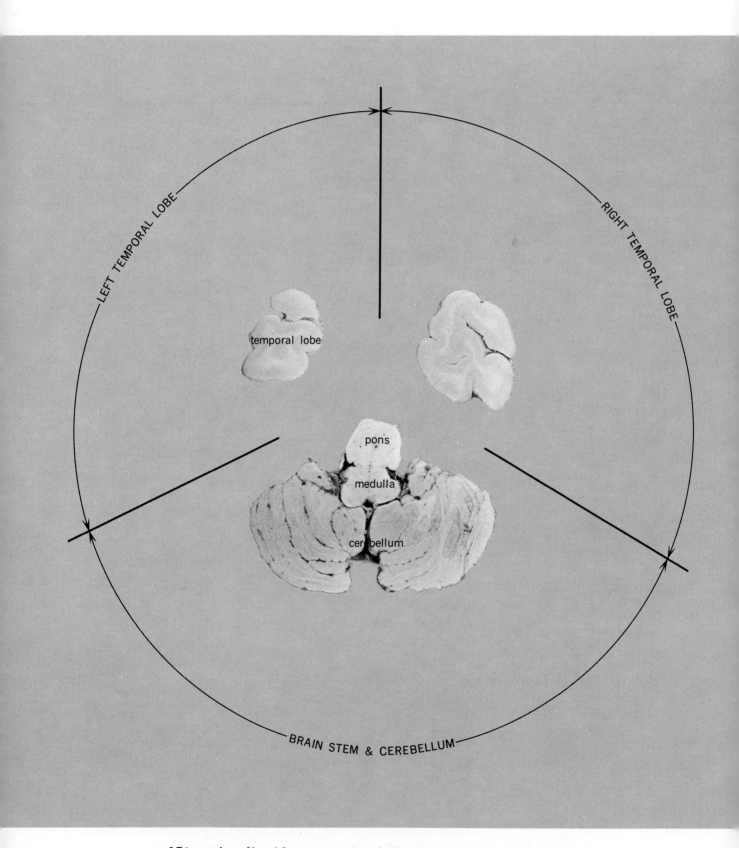

15° section, No. 16, uppersurface indicating prominent lobes and gyri.

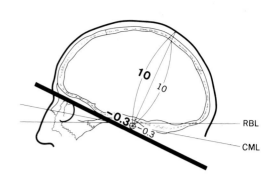

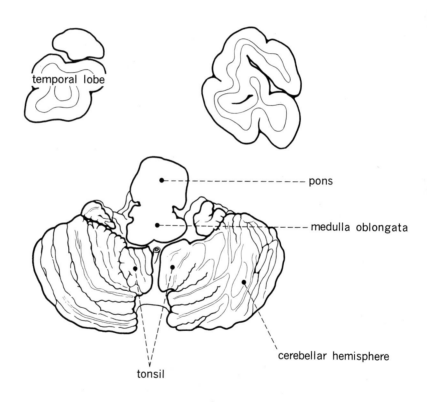

temporal lobe

pons

medulla oblongata

cerebellar hemisphere

tonsil

15° section, No. 16, uppersurface indicating prominent structures.

15°-17

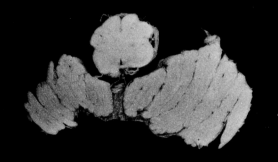

15° section, No. 17, uppersurface.

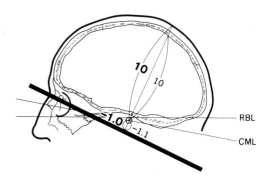

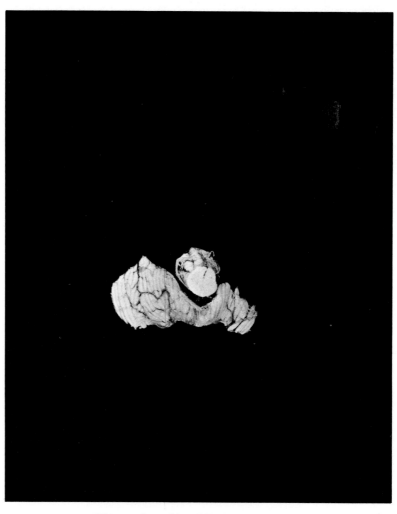

15° section, No. 17, lower surface.

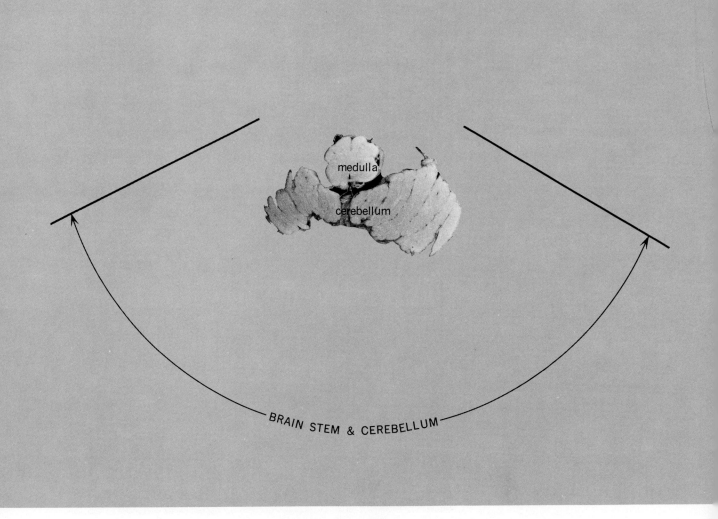

15° section, No. 17, uppersurface indicating prominent lobes and gyri.

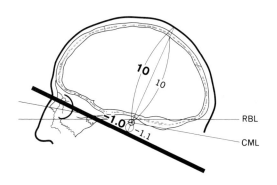

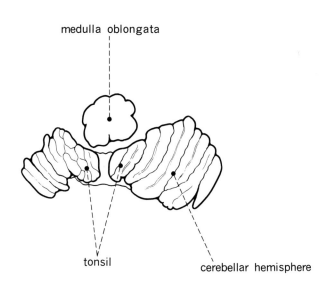

medulla oblongata

tonsil

cerebellar hemisphere

15° section, No. 17, uppersurface indicating prominent structures.

20°-1

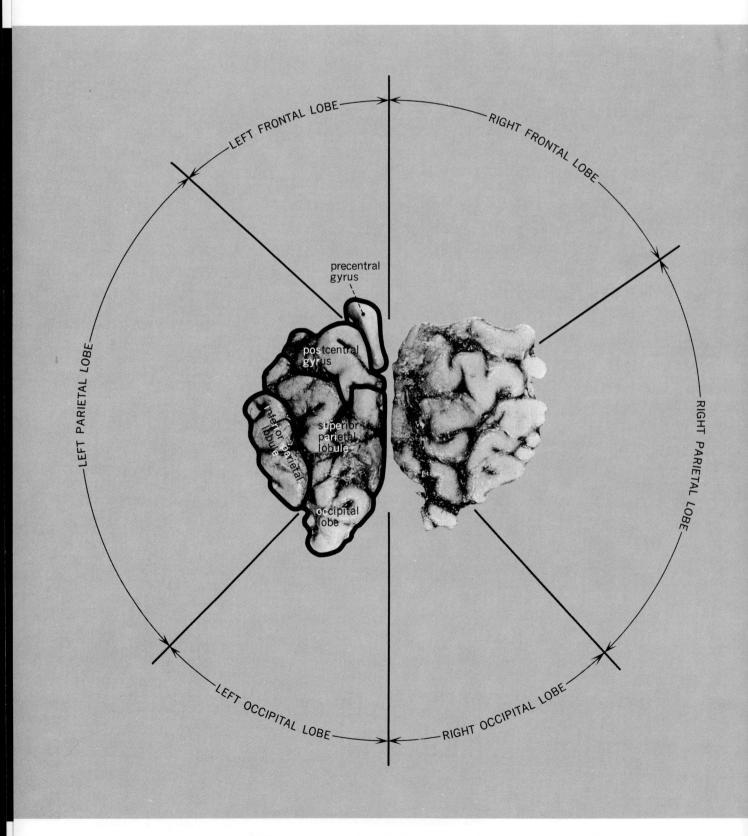

LEFT FRONTAL LOBE

RIGHT FRONTAL LOBE

LEFT PARIETAL LOBE

RIGHT PARIETAL LOBE

precentral
gyrus

postcentral
gyrus

inferior parietal
lobule

superior
parietal
lobule

occipital
lobe

LEFT OCCIPITAL LOBE

RIGHT OCCIPITAL LOBE

20° section, No. 1, uppersurface indicating prominent lobes and gyri.

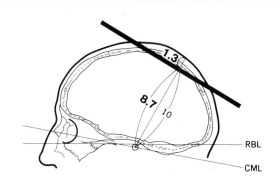

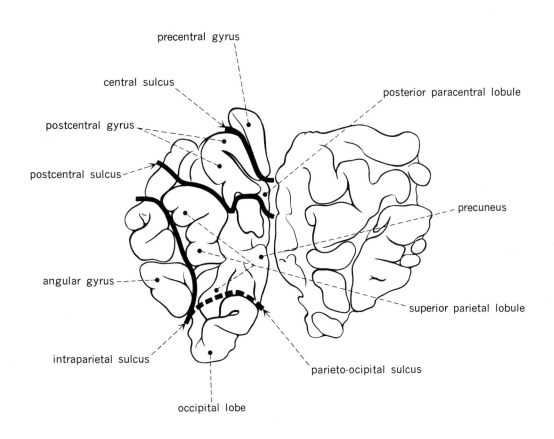

precentral gyrus

central sulcus

postcentral gyrus

postcentral sulcus

posterior paracentral lobule

precuneus

angular gyrus

superior parietal lobule

intraparietal sulcus

parieto-ocipital sulcus

occipital lobe

20° section, No. 1, uppersurface indicating prominent structures.

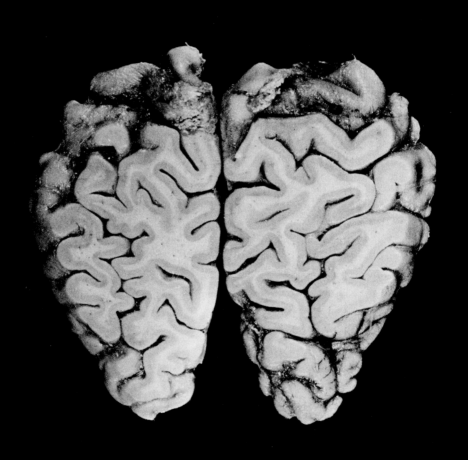

20° section, No. 2, uppersurface.

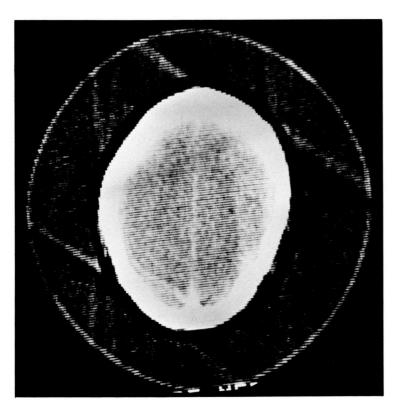

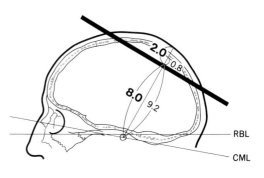

CT scan of 20° section, No. 2.

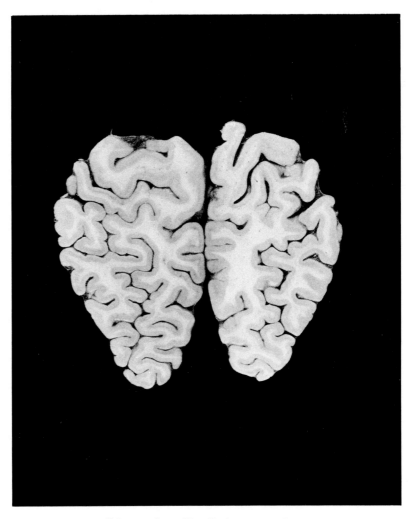

20° section, No. 2, lower surface.

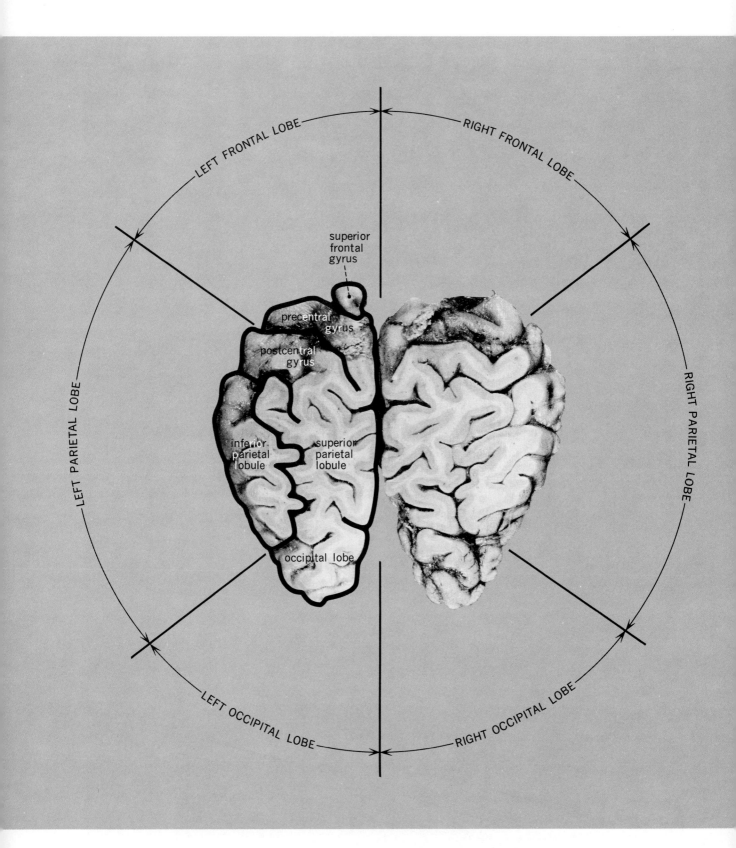

superior
frontal
gyrus

LEFT FRONTAL LOBE

RIGHT FRONTAL LOBE

precentral gyrus

postcentral gyrus

LEFT PARIETAL LOBE

RIGHT PARIETAL LOBE

inferior parietal lobule

superior parietal lobule

occipital lobe

LEFT OCCIPITAL LOBE

RIGHT OCCIPITAL LOBE

20° section, No. 2, uppersurface indicating prominent lobes and gyri.

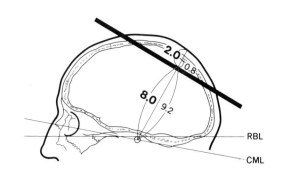

RBL

CML

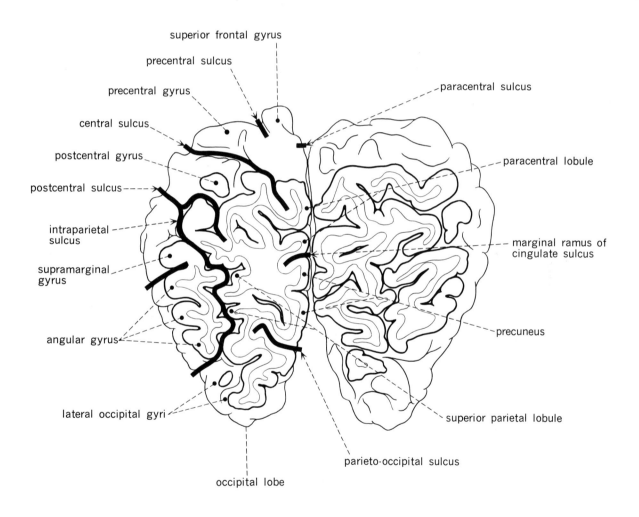

superior frontal gyrus

precentral sulcus

precentral gyrus

central sulcus

postcentral gyrus

postcentral sulcus

intraparietal sulcus

supramarginal gyrus

angular gyrus

lateral occipital gyri

occipital lobe

paracentral sulcus

paracentral lobule

marginal ramus of cingulate sulcus

precuneus

superior parietal lobule

parieto-occipital sulcus

20° section, No. 2, uppersurface indicating prominent structures.

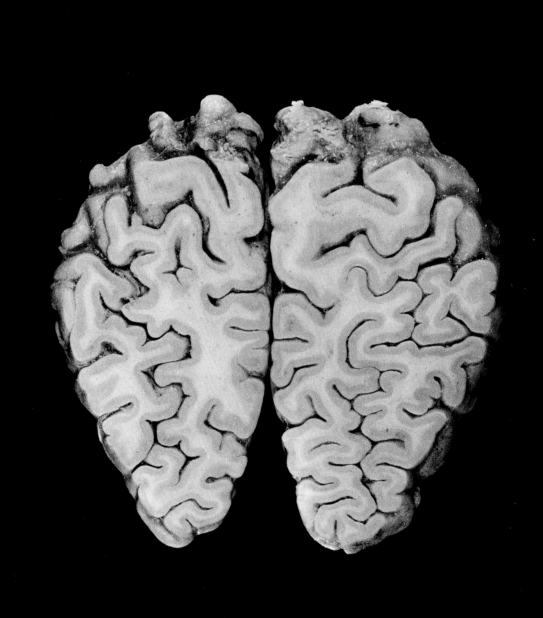

20° section, No. 3, uppersurface.

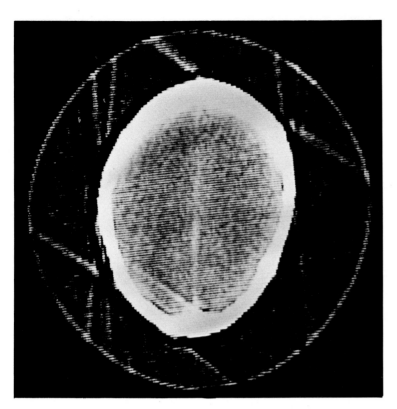
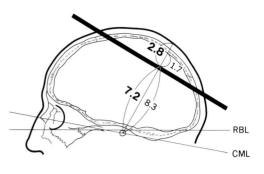

CT scan of 20° section, No. 3.

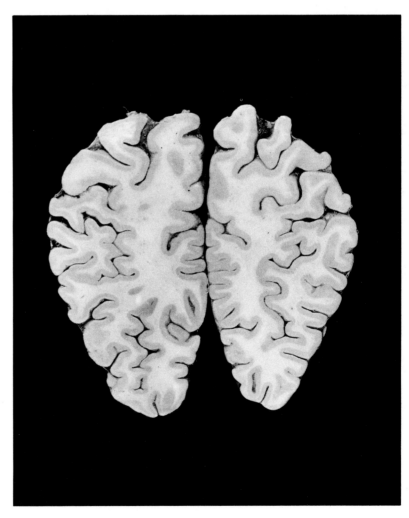

20° section, No. 3, lower surface.

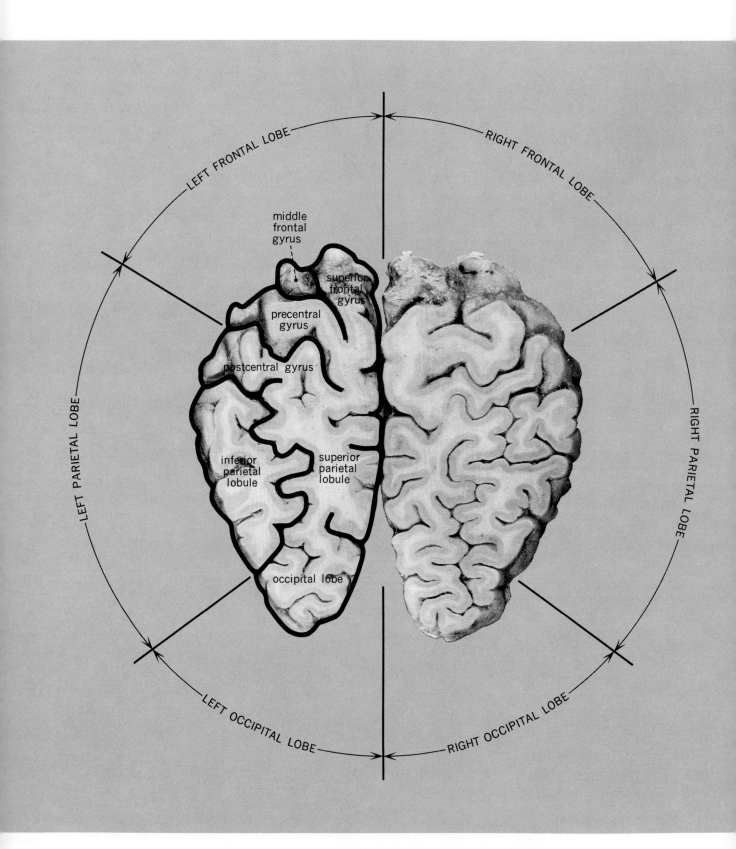

20° section, No. 3, uppersurface indicating prominent lobes and gyri.

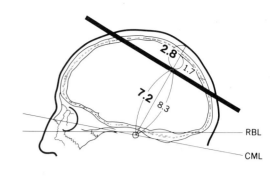

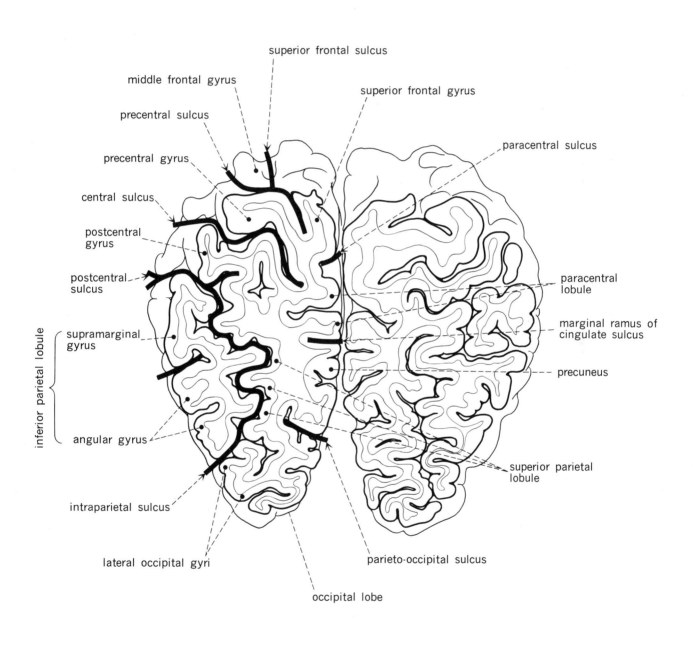

superior frontal sulcus

middle frontal gyrus

precentral sulcus

superior frontal gyrus

precentral gyrus

paracentral sulcus

central sulcus

postcentral gyrus

postcentral sulcus

paracentral lobule

supramarginal gyrus

marginal ramus of cingulate sulcus

precuneus

inferior parietal lobule

angular gyrus

superior parietal lobule

intraparietal sulcus

parieto-occipital sulcus

lateral occipital gyri

occipital lobe

20° section, No. 3, uppersurface indicating prominent structures.

20°-4

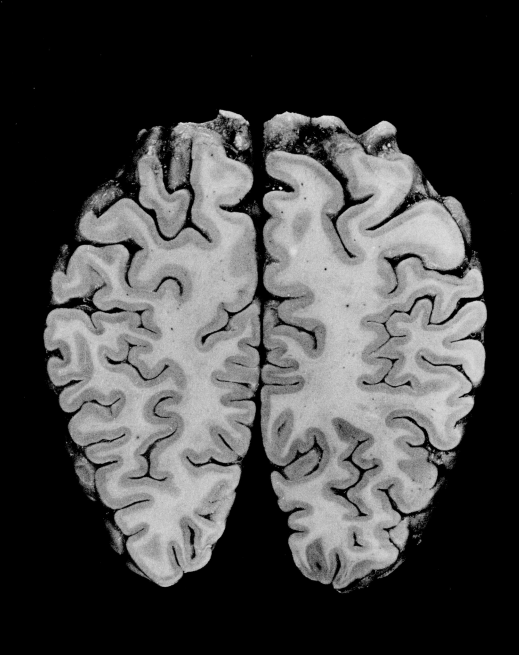

20° section, No. 4, uppersurface.

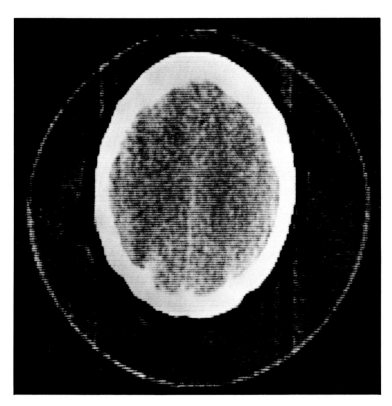

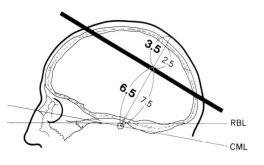

CT scan of 20° section, No. 4.

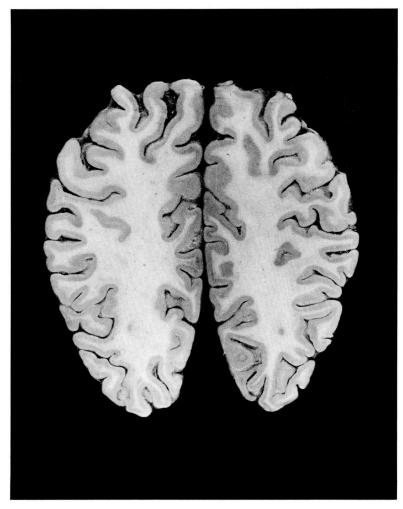

20° section, No. 4, lower surface.

95

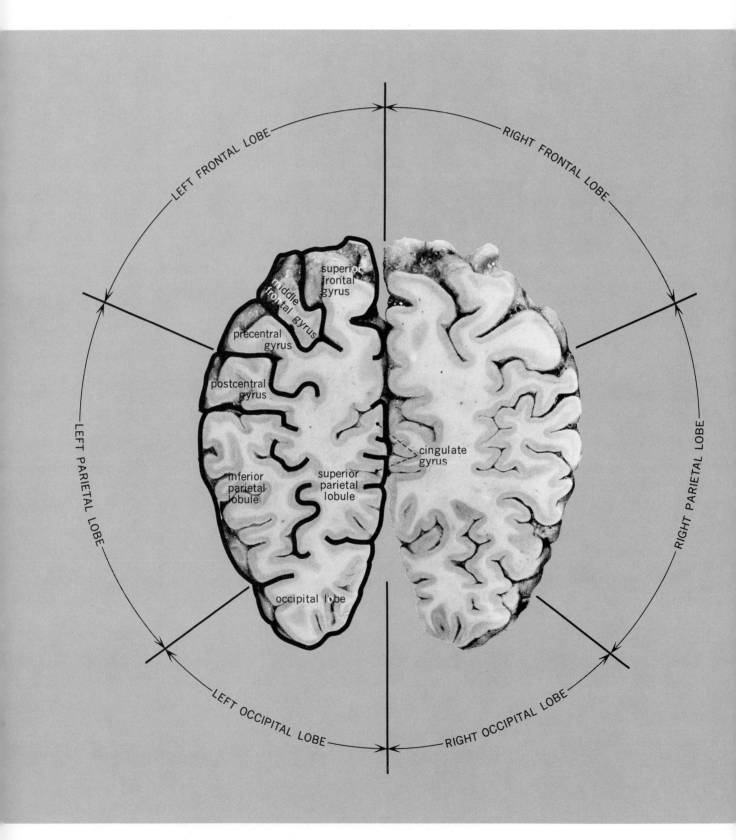

LEFT FRONTAL LOBE

RIGHT FRONTAL LOBE

superior frontal gyrus

middle frontal gyrus

precentral gyrus

postcentral gyrus

cingulate gyrus

inferior parietal lobule

superior parietal lobule

LEFT PARIETAL LOBE

RIGHT PARIETAL LOBE

occipital lobe

LEFT OCCIPITAL LOBE

RIGHT OCCIPITAL LOBE

20° section, No. 4, uppersurface indicating prominent lobes and gyri.

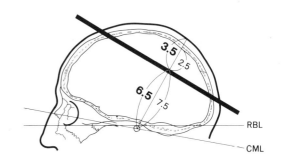

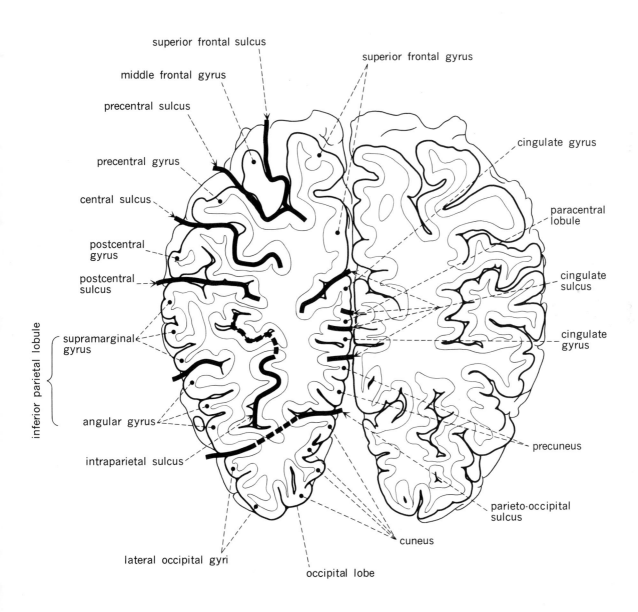

superior frontal sulcus

middle frontal gyrus

precentral sulcus

precentral gyrus

central sulcus

postcentral gyrus

postcentral sulcus

inferior parietal lobule

supramarginal gyrus

angular gyrus

intraparietal sulcus

lateral occipital gyri

occipital lobe

superior frontal gyrus

cingulate gyrus

paracentral lobule

cingulate sulcus

cingulate gyrus

precuneus

parieto-occipital sulcus

cuneus

20° section, No. 4, uppersurface indicating prominent structures.

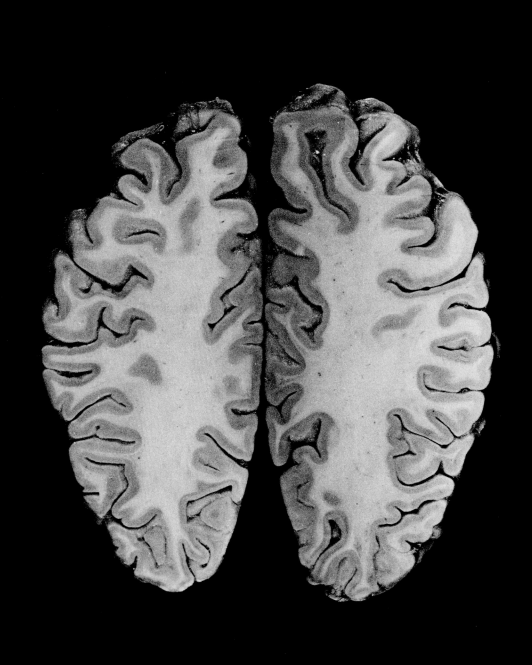

20° section, No. 5, uppersurface.

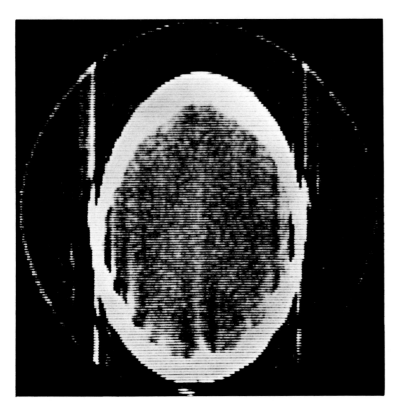

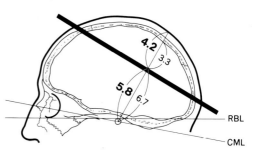

CT scan of 20° section, No. 5.

RBL

CML

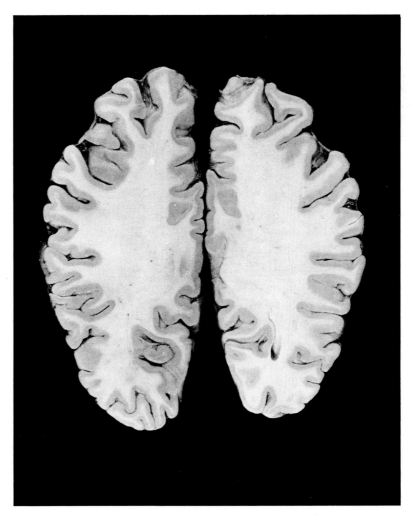

20° section, No. 5, lower surface.

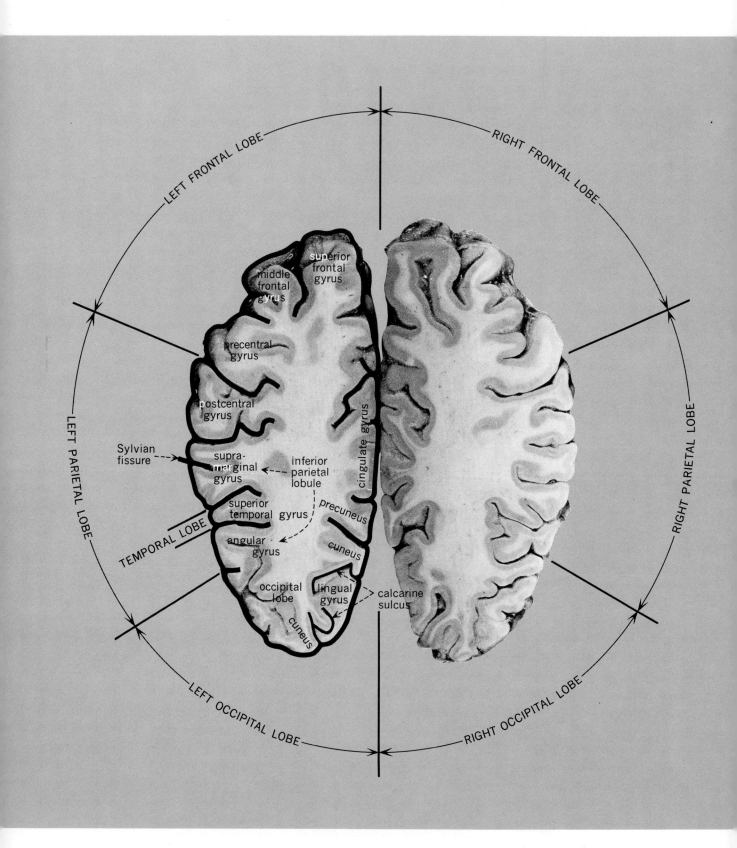

20° section, No. 5, uppersurface indicating prominent lobes and gyri.

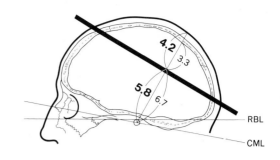

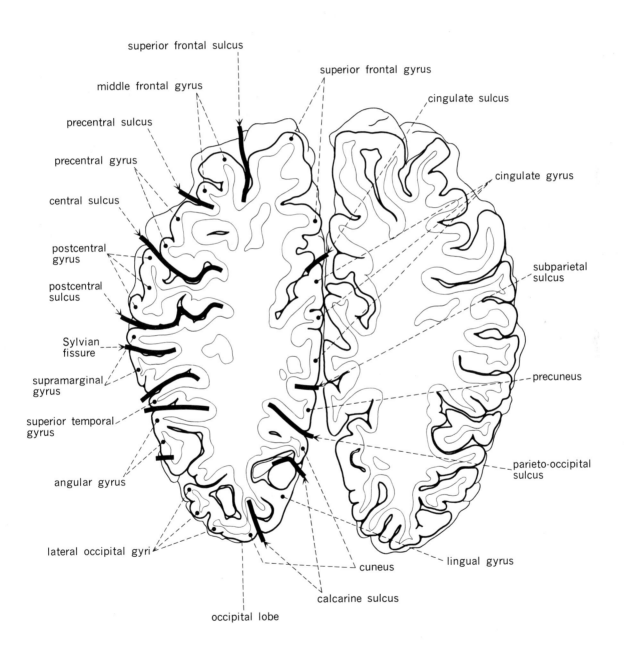

superior frontal sulcus

middle frontal gyrus

precentral sulcus

precentral gyrus

central sulcus

postcentral gyrus

postcentral sulcus

Sylvian fissure

supramarginal gyrus

superior temporal gyrus

angular gyrus

lateral occipital gyri

occipital lobe

calcarine sulcus

cuneus

lingual gyrus

parieto-occipital sulcus

precuneus

subparietal sulcus

cingulate gyrus

cingulate sulcus

superior frontal gyrus

RBL

CML

4.2

3.3

5.8

6.7

20° section, No. 5, uppersurface indicating prominent structures.

20°-6

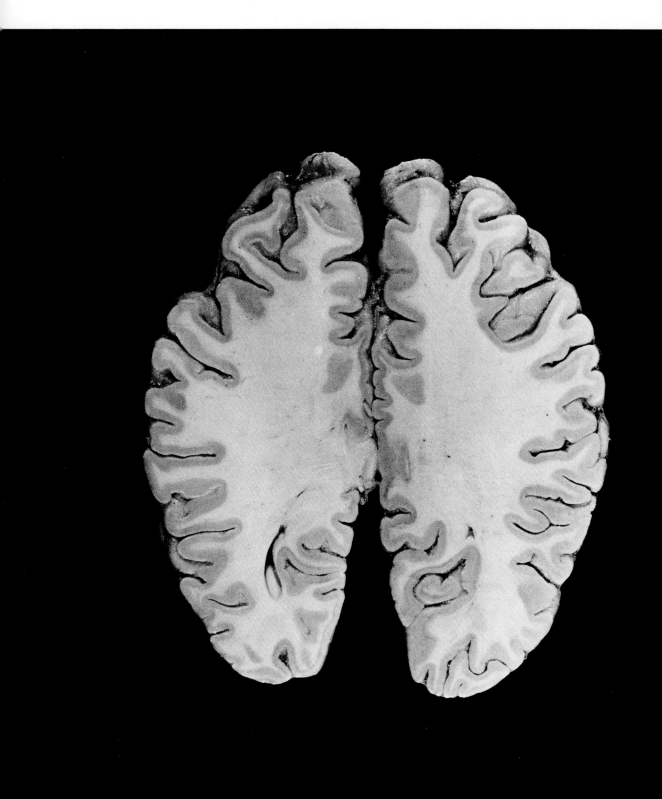

20° section, No. 6, uppersurface.

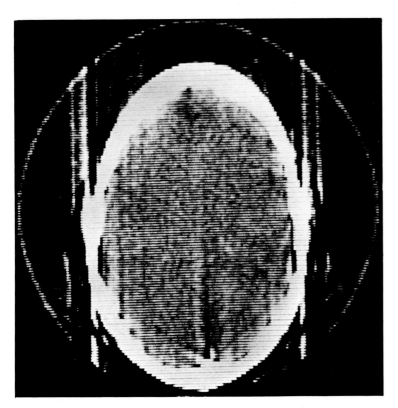

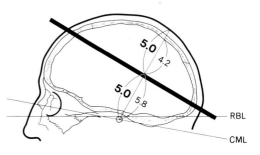

CT scan of 20° section, No. 6.

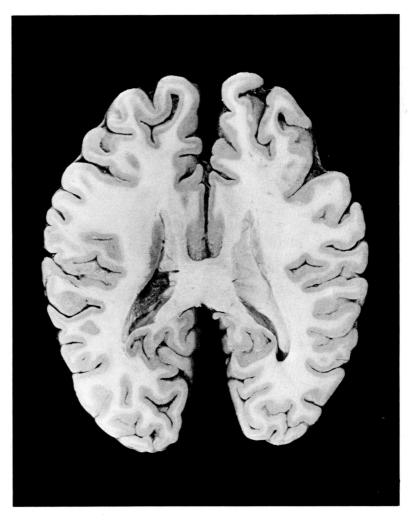

20° section, No. 6, lower surface.

103

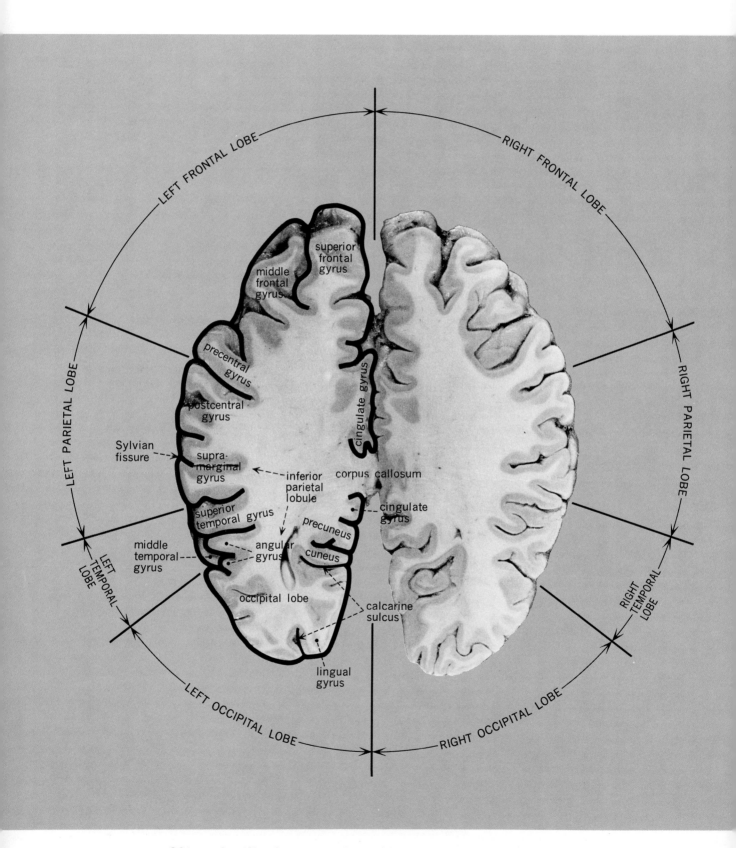

20° section, No. 6, uppersurface indicating prominent lobes and gyri.

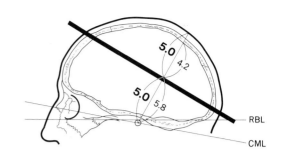

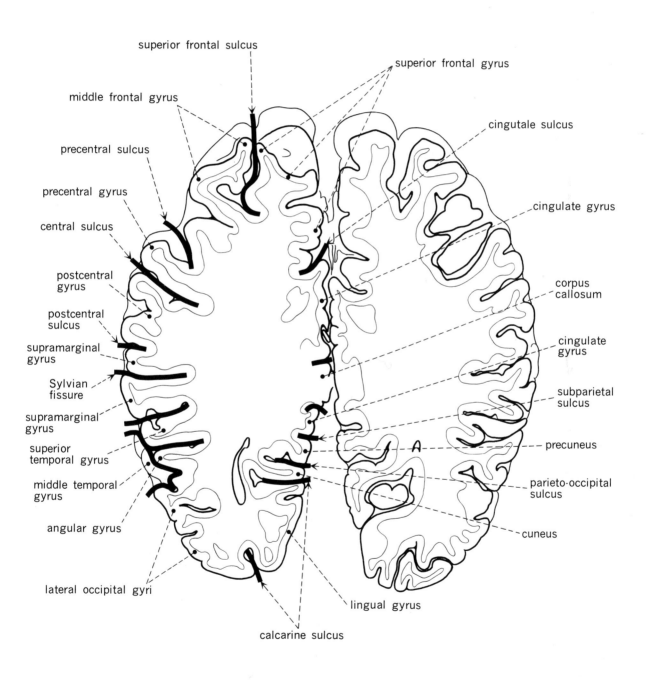

superior frontal sulcus

superior frontal gyrus

middle frontal gyrus

cingutale sulcus

precentral sulcus

precentral gyrus

cingulate gyrus

central sulcus

postcentral gyrus

corpus callosum

postcentral sulcus

cingulate gyrus

supramarginal gyrus

subparietal sulcus

Sylvian fissure

supramarginal gyrus

precuneus

superior temporal gyrus

parieto-occipital sulcus

middle temporal gyrus

angular gyrus

cuneus

lateral occipital gyri

lingual gyrus

calcarine sulcus

20° section, No. 6, uppersurface indicating prominent structures.

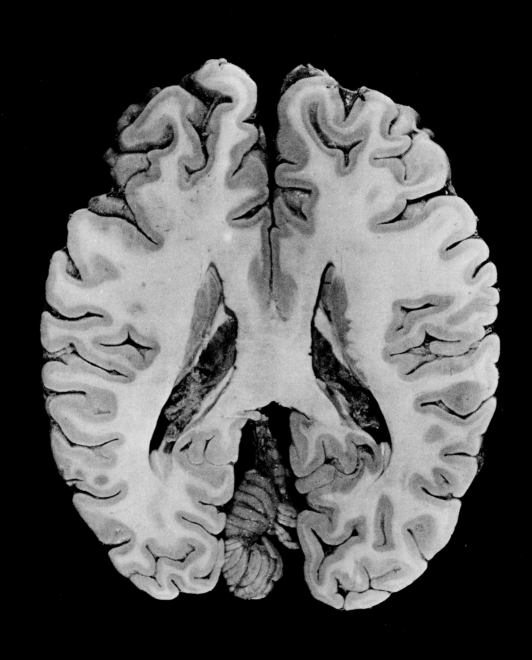

20° section, No. 7, uppersurface.

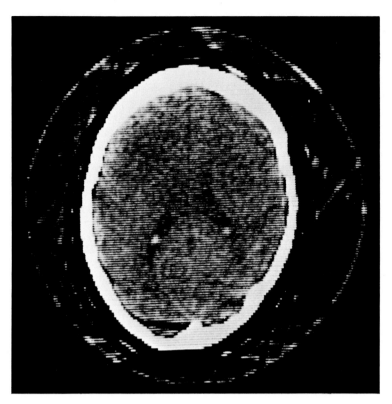

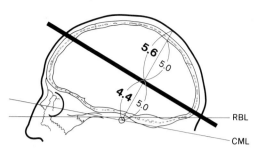

CT scan of 20° section, No. 7.

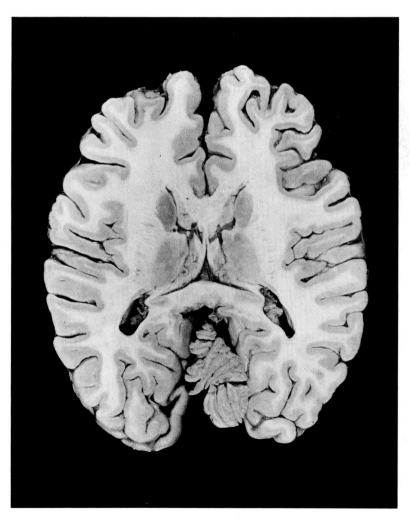

20° section, No. 7, lower surface.

107

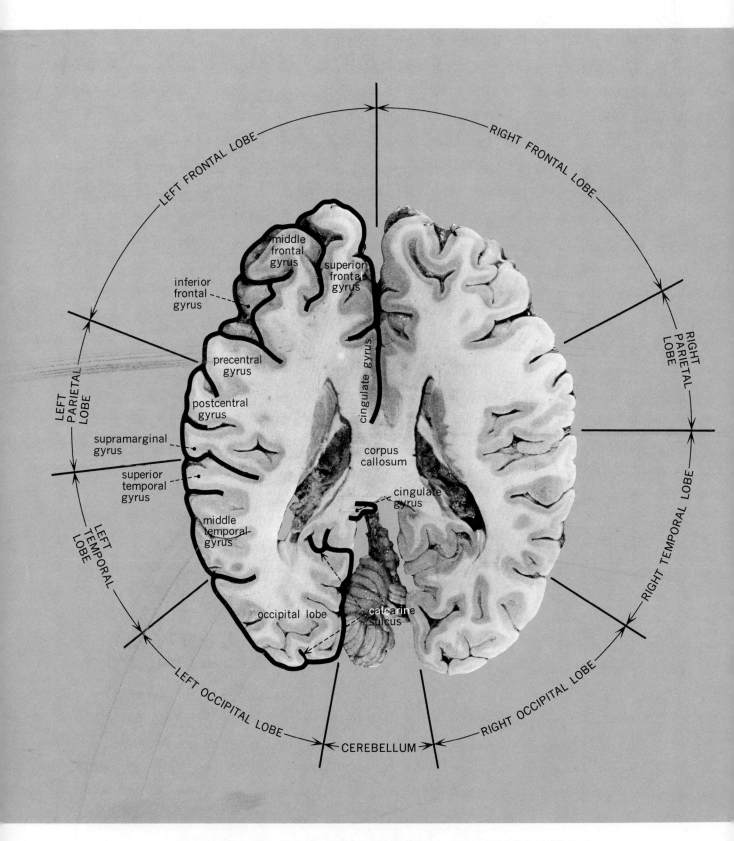

20° section, No. 7, uppersurface indicating prominent lobes and gyri.

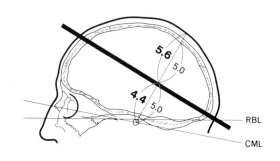

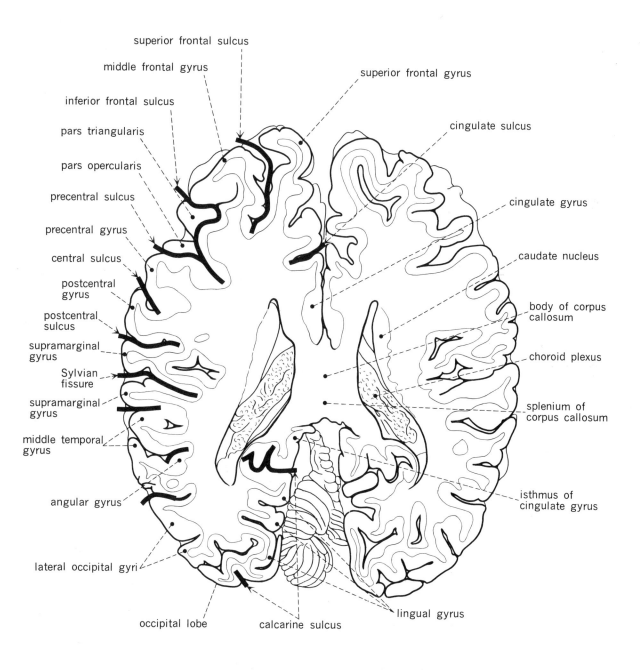

superior frontal sulcus

middle frontal gyrus

inferior frontal sulcus

pars triangularis

pars opercularis

precentral sulcus

precentral gyrus

central sulcus

postcentral gyrus

postcentral sulcus

supramarginal gyrus

Sylvian fissure

supramarginal gyrus

middle temporal gyrus

angular gyrus

lateral occipital gyri

occipital lobe

calcarine sulcus

superior frontal gyrus

cingulate sulcus

cingulate gyrus

caudate nucleus

body of corpus callosum

choroid plexus

splenium of corpus callosum

isthmus of cingulate gyrus

lingual gyrus

5.6 5.0

4.4 5.0

RBL

CML

20° section, No. 7, uppersurface indicating prominent structures.

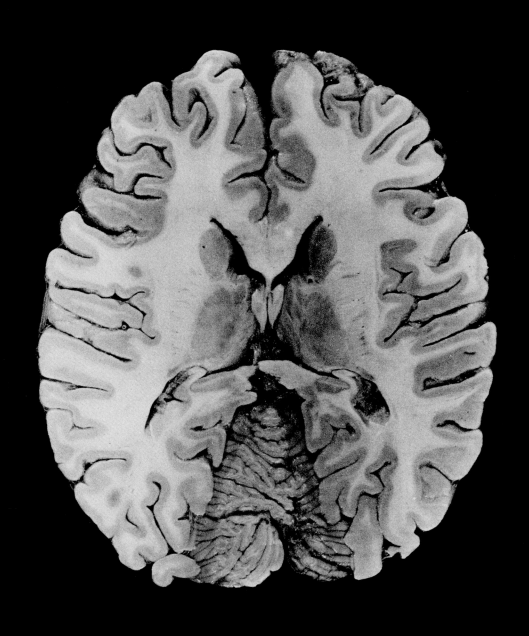

20° section, No. 8, uppersurface.

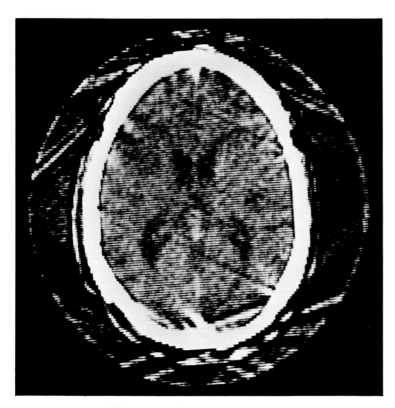

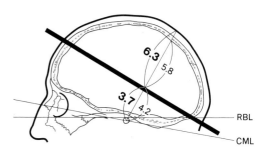

RBL

CML

CT scan of 20° section, No. 8.

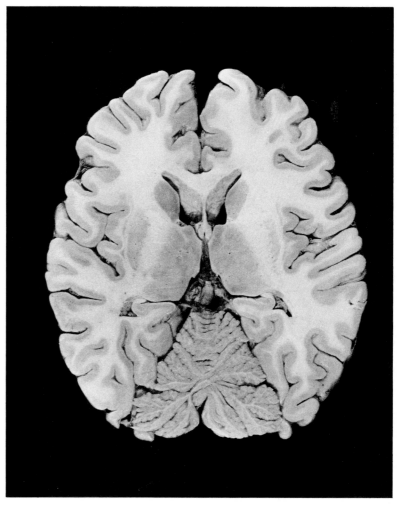

20° section, No. 8, lower surface.

111

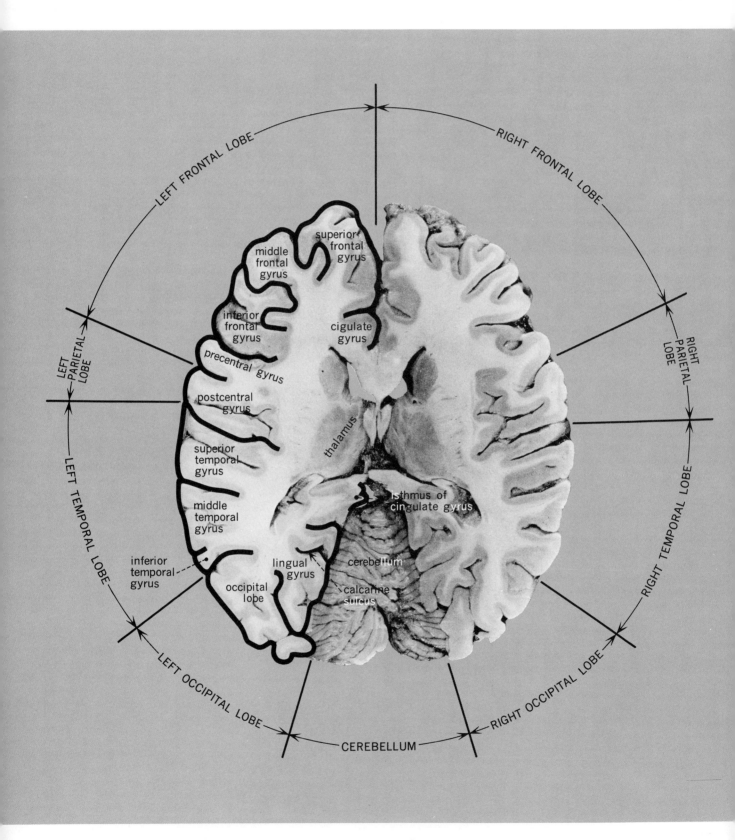

20° section, No. 8, uppersurface indicating prominent lobes and gyri.

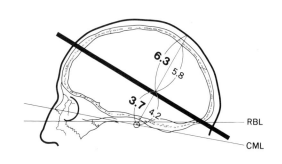

RBL

CML

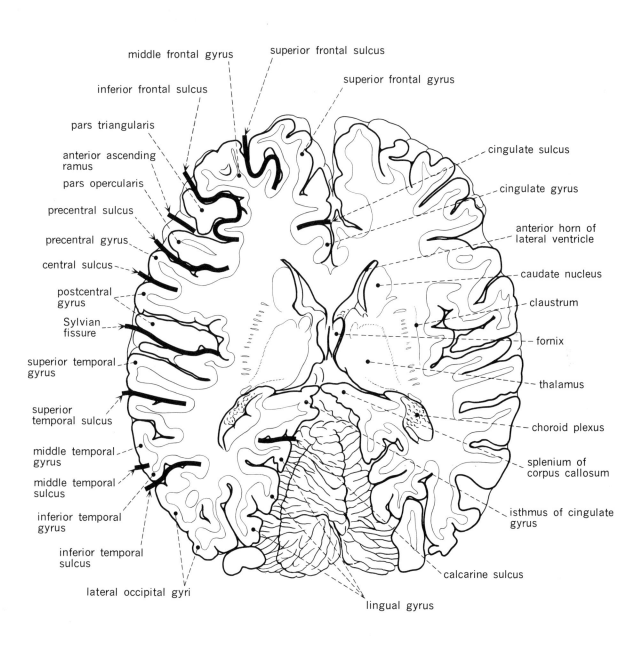

middle frontal gyrus

superior frontal sulcus

superior frontal gyrus

inferior frontal sulcus

pars triangularis

anterior ascending ramus

pars opercularis

precentral sulcus

precentral gyrus

central sulcus

postcentral gyrus

Sylvian fissure

superior temporal gyrus

superior temporal sulcus

middle temporal gyrus

middle temporal sulcus

inferior temporal gyrus

inferior temporal sulcus

lateral occipital gyri

lingual gyrus

cingulate sulcus

cingulate gyrus

anterior horn of lateral ventricle

caudate nucleus

claustrum

fornix

thalamus

choroid plexus

splenium of corpus callosum

isthmus of cingulate gyrus

calcarine sulcus

20° section, No. 8, uppersurface indicating prominent structures.

20°- 9

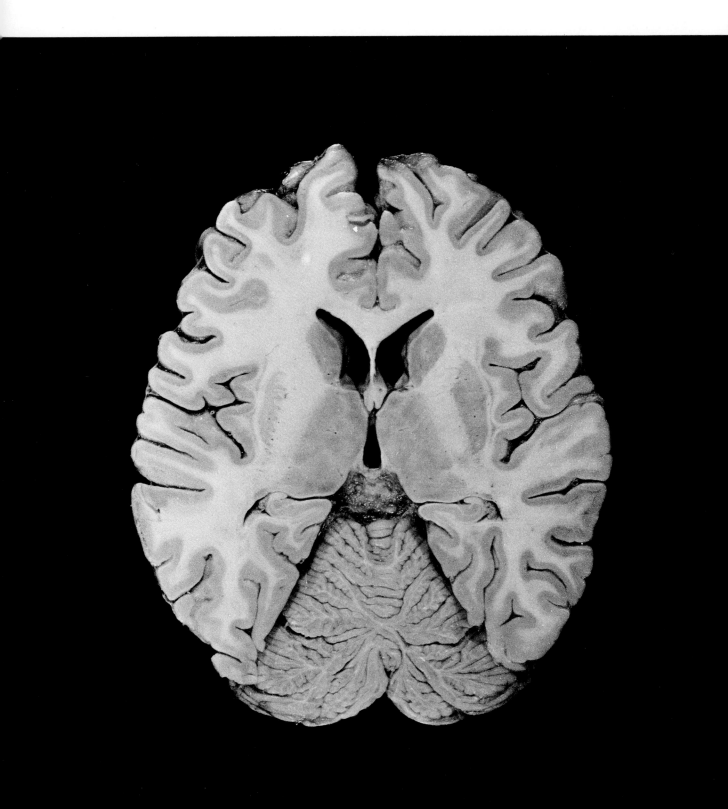

20° section, No. 9 , uppersurface.

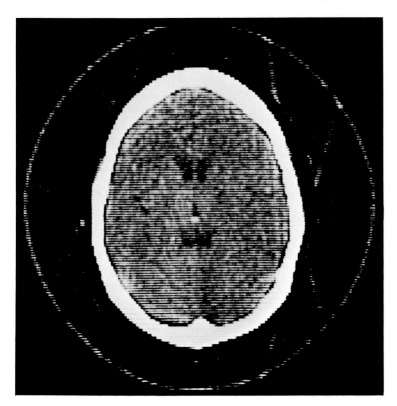
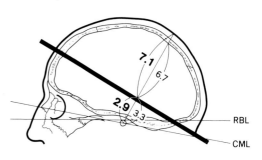

CT scan of 20° section, No. 9.

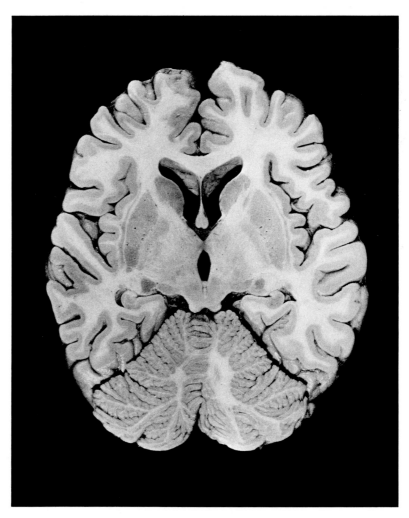

20° section, No. 9, lower surface.

115

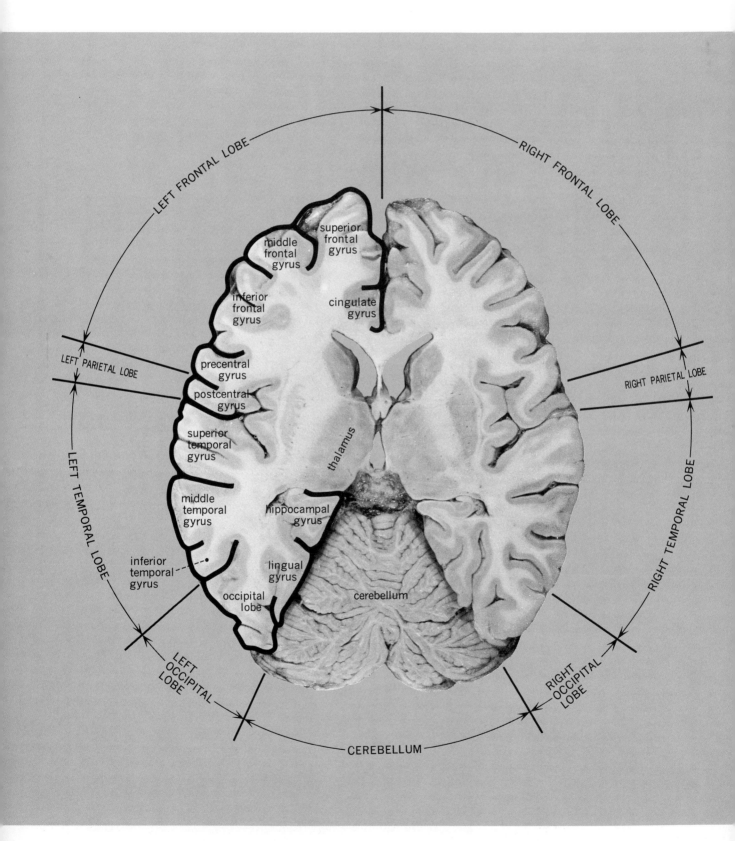

20° section, No. 9, uppersurface indicating prominent lobes and gyri.

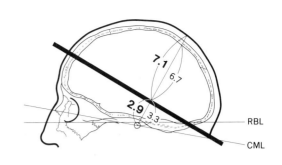

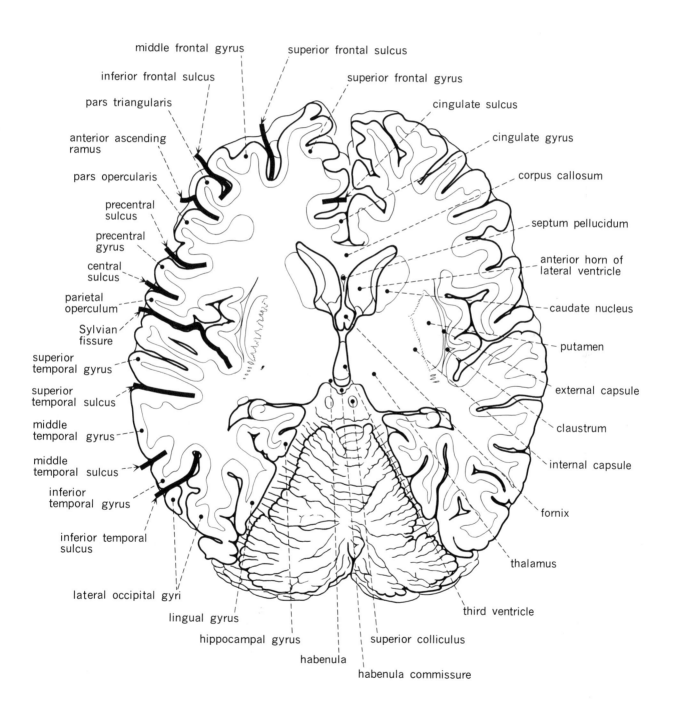

middle frontal gyrus
superior frontal sulcus
inferior frontal sulcus
superior frontal gyrus
pars triangularis
cingulate sulcus
anterior ascending ramus
cingulate gyrus
pars opercularis
corpus callosum
precentral sulcus
septum pellucidum
precentral gyrus
anterior horn of lateral ventricle
central sulcus
caudate nucleus
parietal operculum
putamen
Sylvian fissure
external capsule
superior temporal gyrus
claustrum
superior temporal sulcus
internal capsule
middle temporal gyrus
middle temporal sulcus
fornix
inferior temporal gyrus
thalamus
inferior temporal sulcus
lateral occipital gyri
third ventricle
lingual gyrus
hippocampal gyrus
superior colliculus
habenula
habenula commissure

20° section, No. 9, uppersurface indicating prominent structures.

117

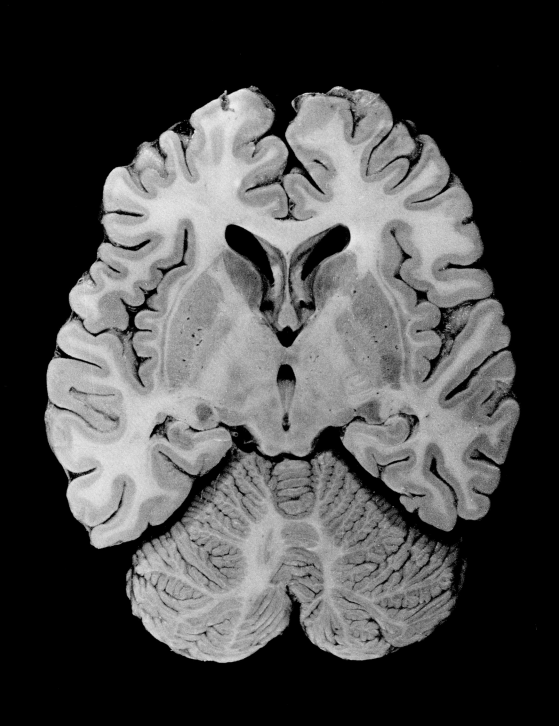

20° section, No. 10, uppersurface.

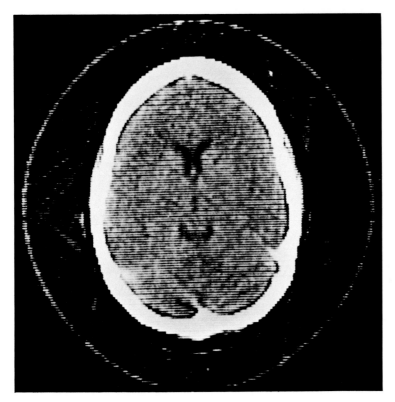
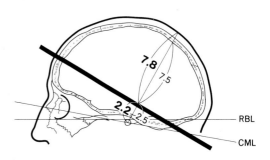

CT scan of 20° section, No. 10.

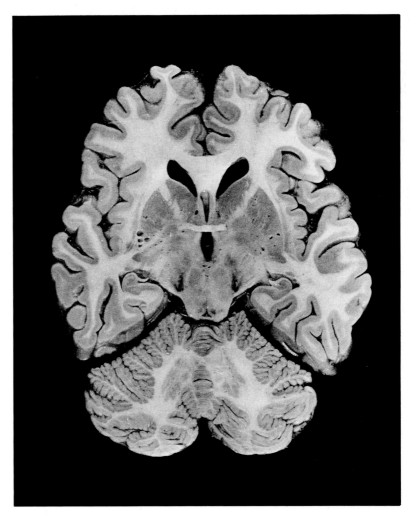

20° section, No. 10, lower surface.

119

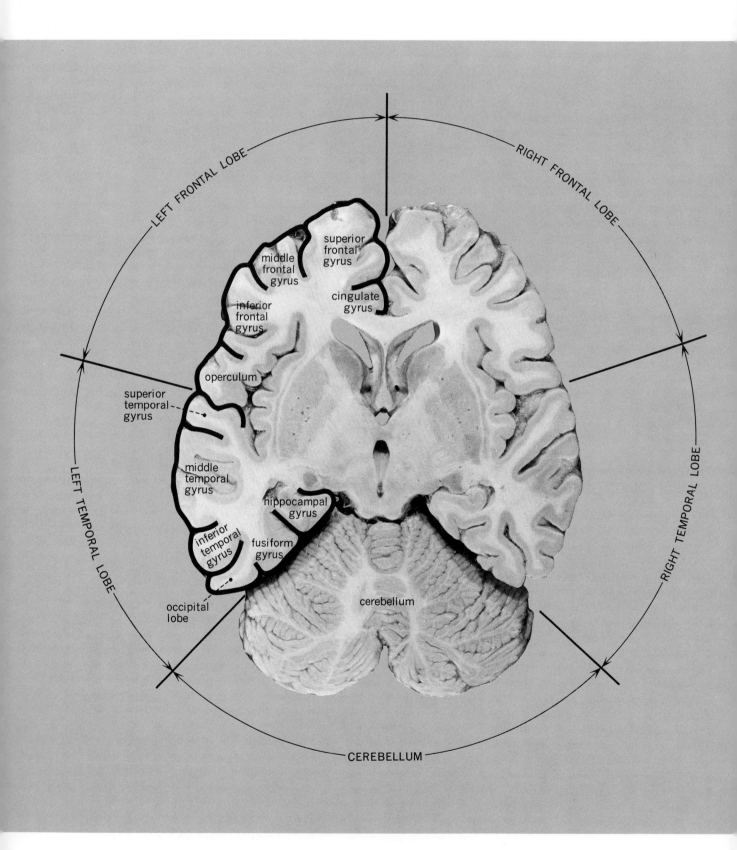

20° section, No. 10, uppersurface indicating prominent lobes and gyri.

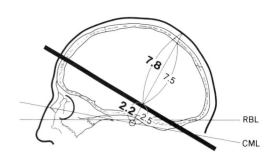

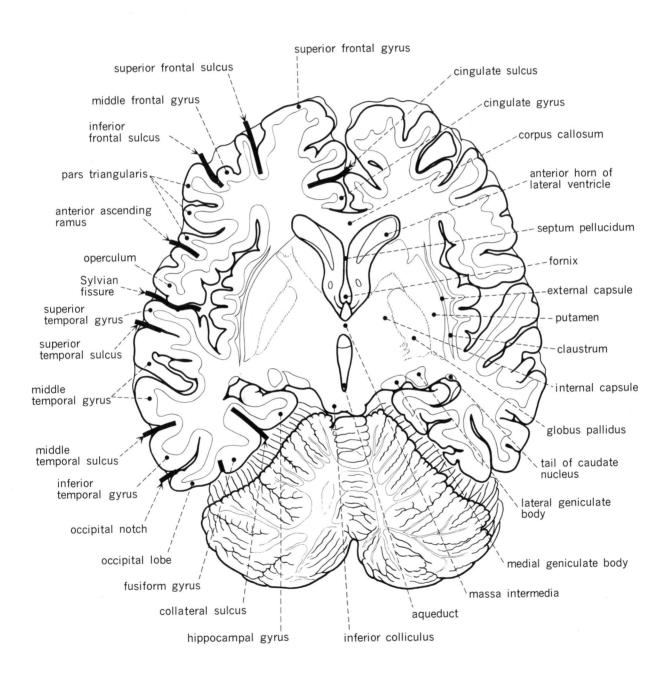

superior frontal gyrus

superior frontal sulcus

cingulate sulcus

middle frontal gyrus

cingulate gyrus

inferior frontal sulcus

corpus callosum

pars triangularis

anterior horn of lateral ventricle

anterior ascending ramus

septum pellucidum

operculum

fornix

Sylvian fissure

external capsule

superior temporal gyrus

putamen

superior temporal sulcus

claustrum

middle temporal gyrus

internal capsule

middle temporal sulcus

globus pallidus

inferior temporal gyrus

tail of caudate nucleus

occipital notch

lateral geniculate body

occipital lobe

medial geniculate body

fusiform gyrus

massa intermedia

collateral sulcus

aqueduct

hippocampal gyrus

inferior colliculus

20° section, No. 10, uppersurface indicating prominent structures.

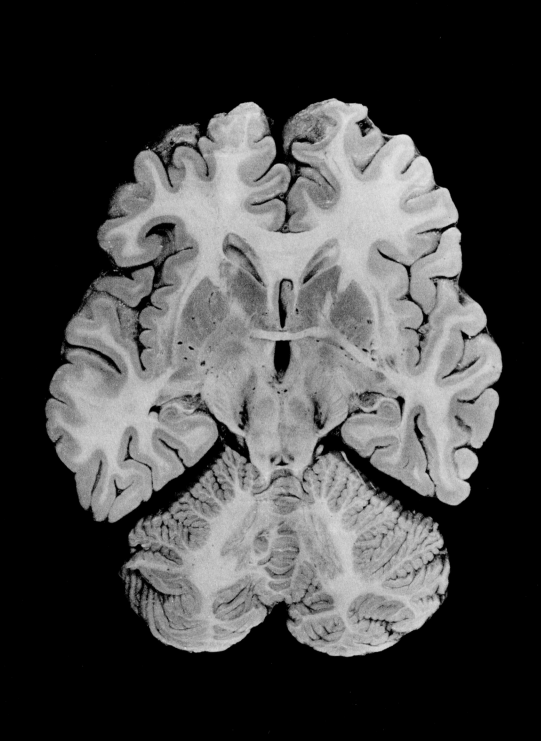

20° section, No. 11, uppersurface.

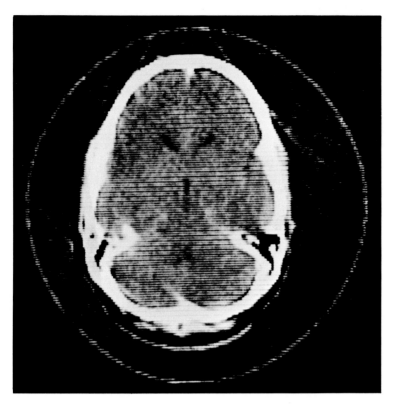
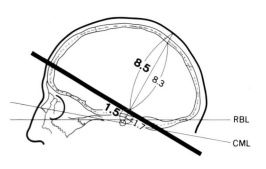

CT scan of 20° section, No. 11.

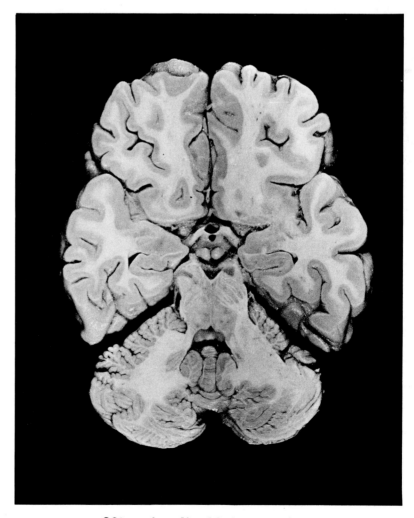

20° section, No. 11, lower surface.

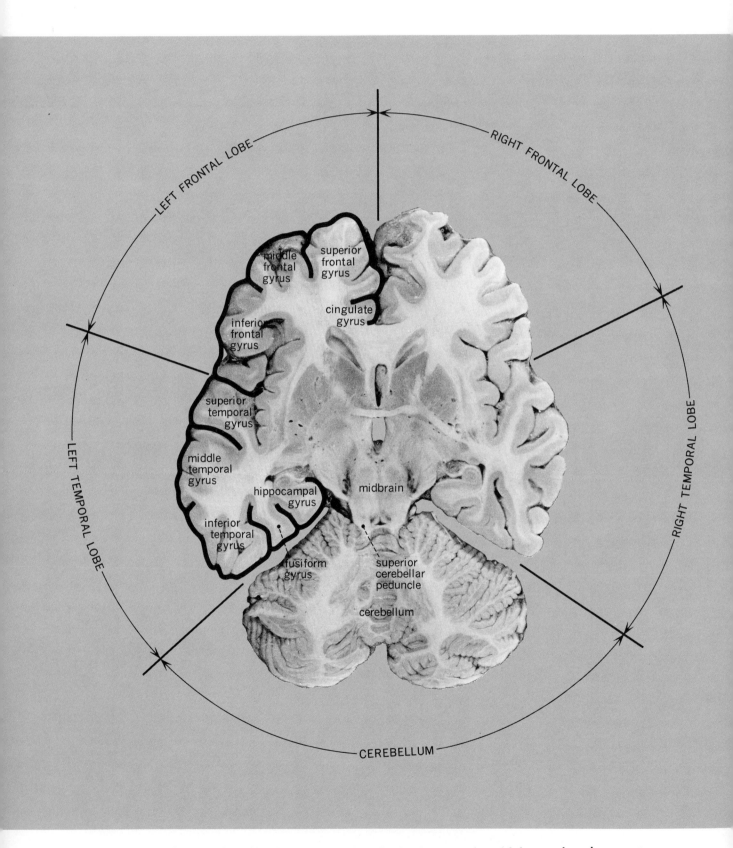

20° section, No. 11, uppersurface indicating prominent lobes and gyri.

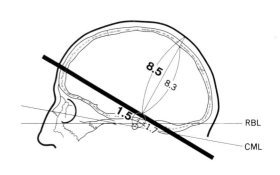

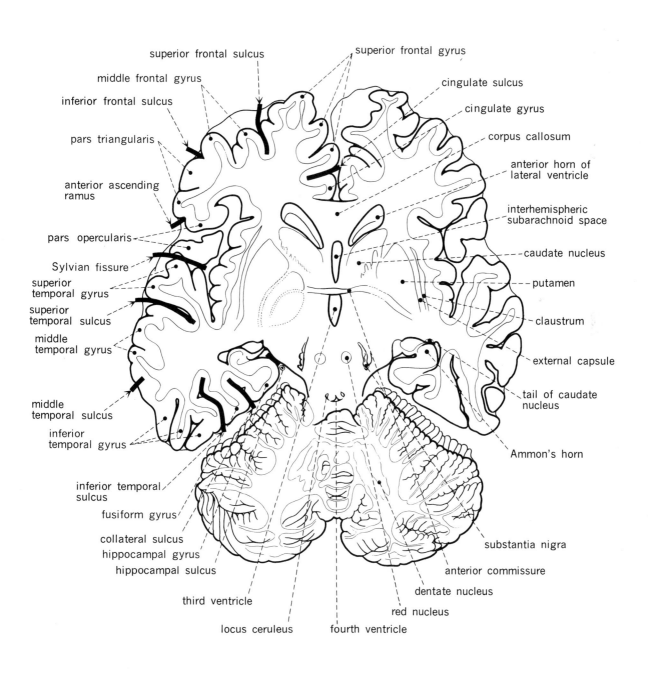

superior frontal sulcus

superior frontal gyrus

middle frontal gyrus

cingulate sulcus

inferior frontal sulcus

cingulate gyrus

corpus callosum

pars triangularis

anterior horn of lateral ventricle

anterior ascending ramus

interhemispheric subarachnoid space

pars opercularis

caudate nucleus

Sylvian fissure

putamen

superior temporal gyrus

superior temporal sulcus

claustrum

middle temporal gyrus

external capsule

tail of caudate nucleus

middle temporal sulcus

Ammon's horn

inferior temporal gyrus

inferior temporal sulcus

fusiform gyrus

collateral sulcus

hippocampal gyrus

substantia nigra

hippocampal sulcus

anterior commissure

third ventricle

dentate nucleus

red nucleus

locus ceruleus   fourth ventricle

20° section, No. 11, uppersurface indicating prominent structures.

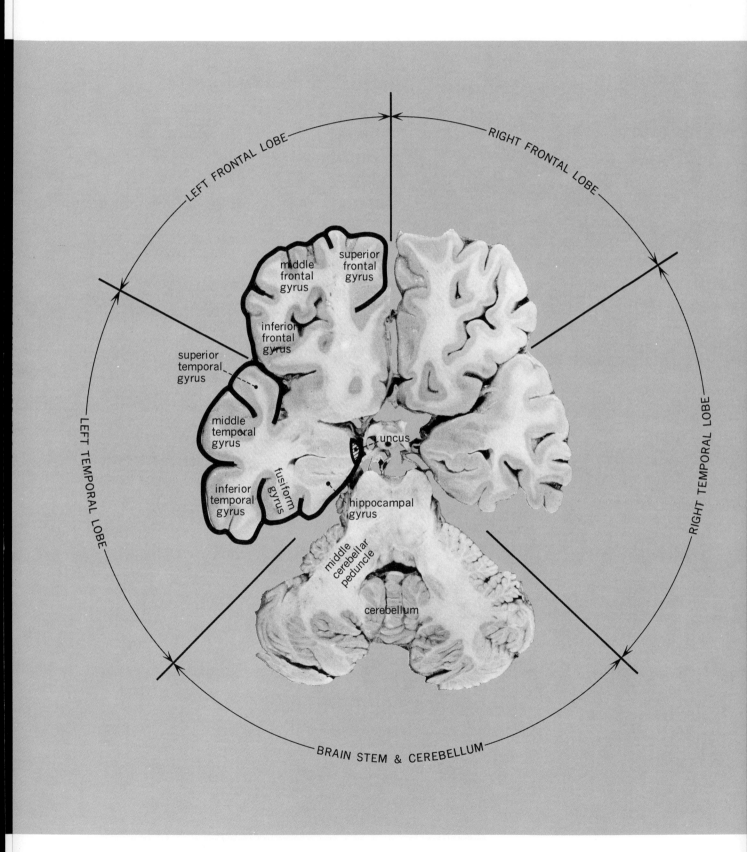

20° section, No. 12, uppersurface indicating prominent lobes and gyri.

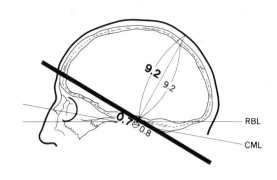

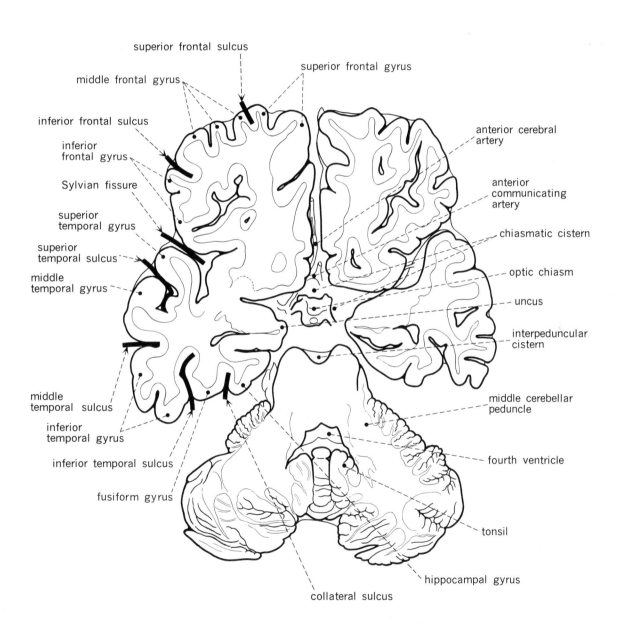

superior frontal sulcus

superior frontal gyrus

middle frontal gyrus

inferior frontal sulcus

inferior frontal gyrus

Sylvian fissure

superior temporal gyrus

superior temporal sulcus

middle temporal gyrus

anterior cerebral artery

anterior communicating artery

chiasmatic cistern

optic chiasm

uncus

interpeduncular cistern

middle cerebellar peduncle

fourth ventricle

middle temporal sulcus

inferior temporal gyrus

inferior temporal sulcus

fusiform gyrus

tonsil

hippocampal gyrus

collateral sulcus

20° section, No. 12, uppersurface indicating prominent structures.

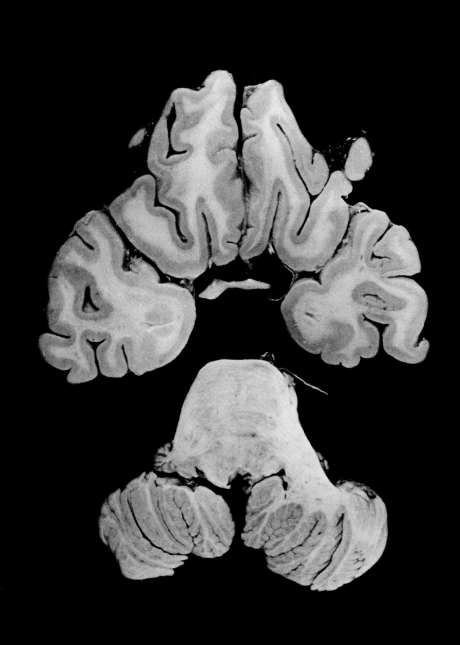

20° section, No. 13, uppersurface.

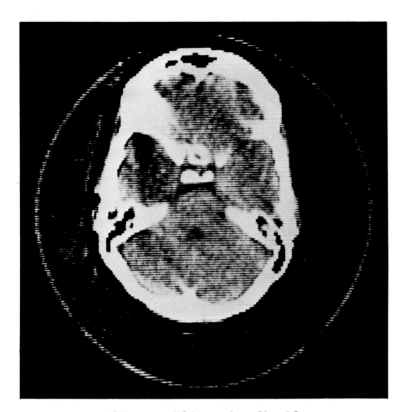

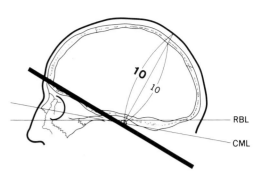

CT scan of 20° section, No. 13.

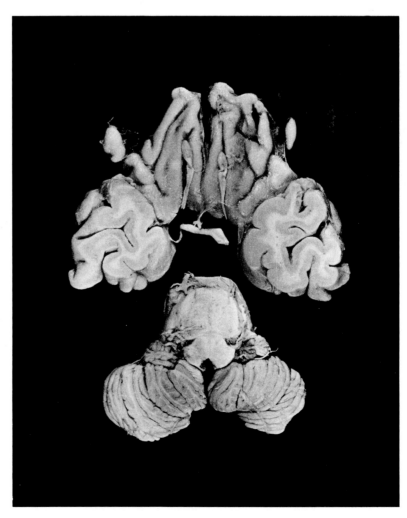

20° section, No. 13, lower surface.

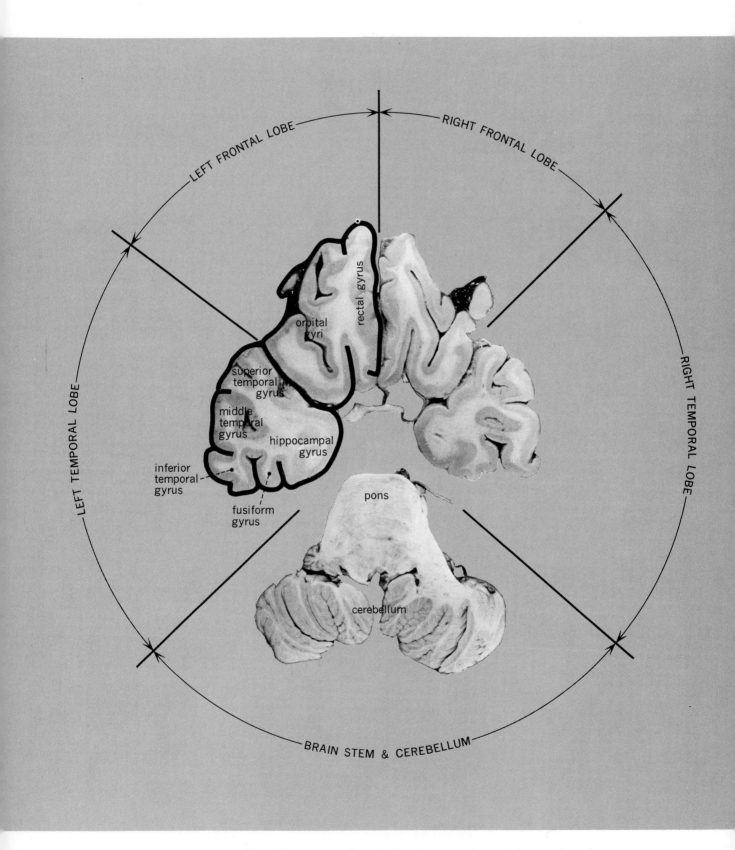

20° section, No. 13, uppersurface indicating prominent lobes and gyri.

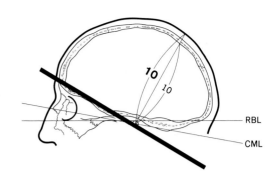

RBL
CML

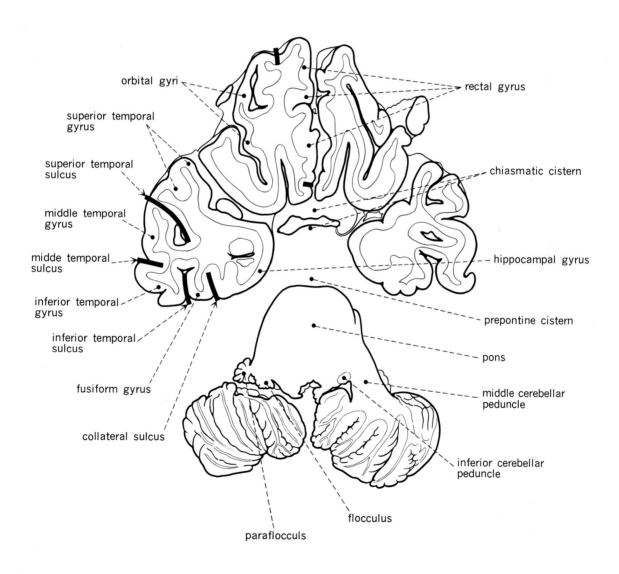

orbital gyri
rectal gyrus

superior temporal
gyrus

superior temporal
sulcus

chiasmatic cistern

middle temporal
gyrus

midde temporal
sulcus

hippocampal gyrus

inferior temporal
gyrus

prepontine cistern

inferior temporal
sulcus

pons

fusiform gyrus

middle cerebellar
peduncle

collateral sulcus

inferior cerebellar
peduncle

paraflocculs

flocculus

20° section, No. 13, uppersurface indicating prominent structures.

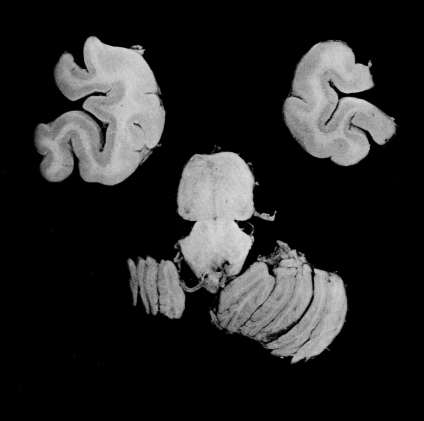

20° section, No. 14, uppersurface.

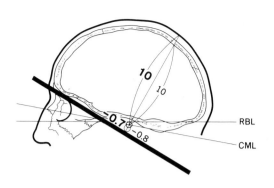

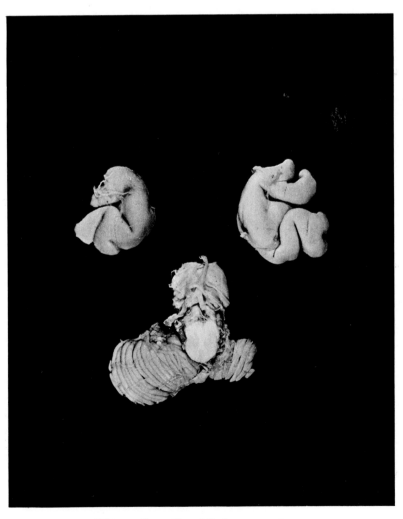

20° section, No. 14, lower surface.

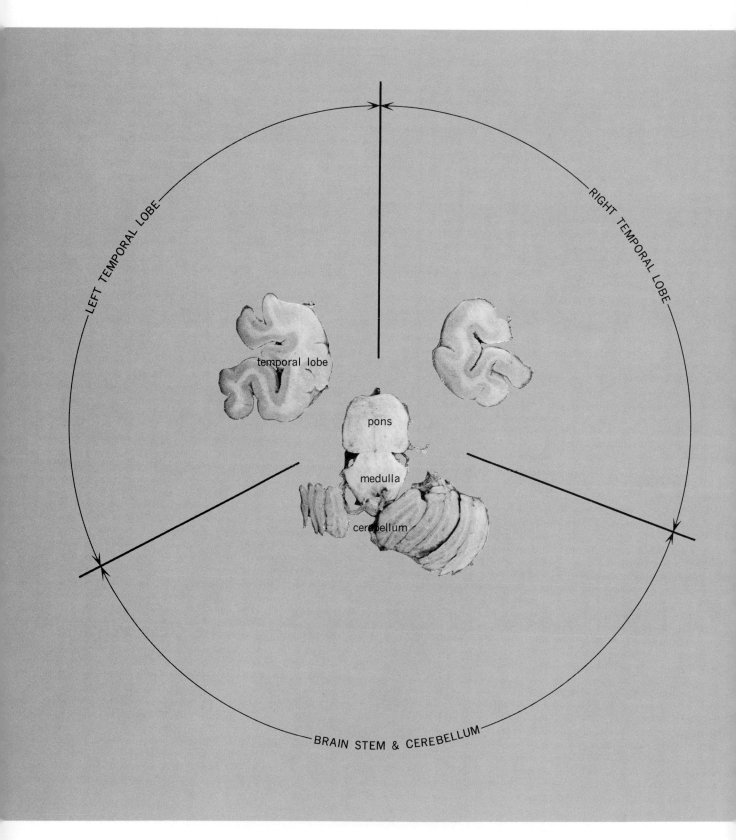

20° section, No. 14, uppersurface indicating prominent lobes and gyri.

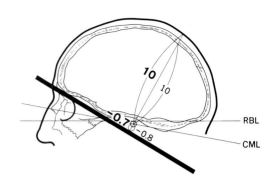

RBL

CML

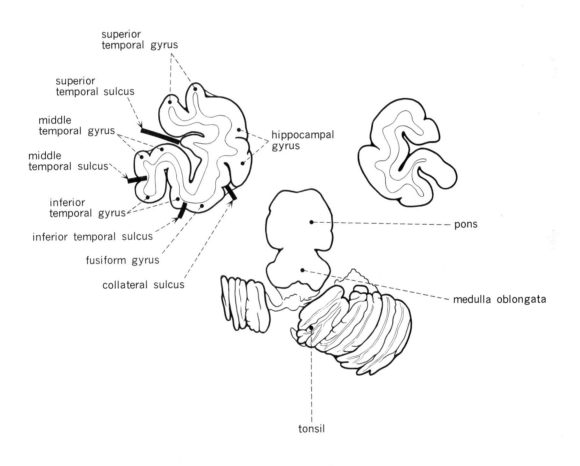

superior
temporal gyrus

superior
temporal sulcus

middle
temporal gyrus

middle
temporal sulcus

inferior
temporal gyrus

inferior temporal sulcus

fusiform gyrus

collateral sulcus

hippocampal
gyrus

pons

medulla oblongata

tonsil

20° section, No. 14, uppersurface indicating prominent structures.

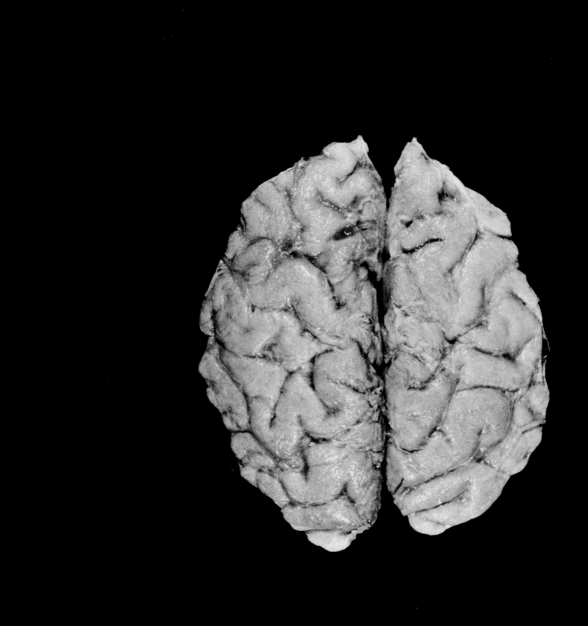

0° section, No. 1, uppersurface.

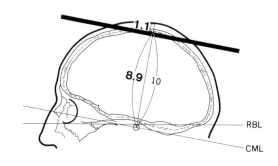

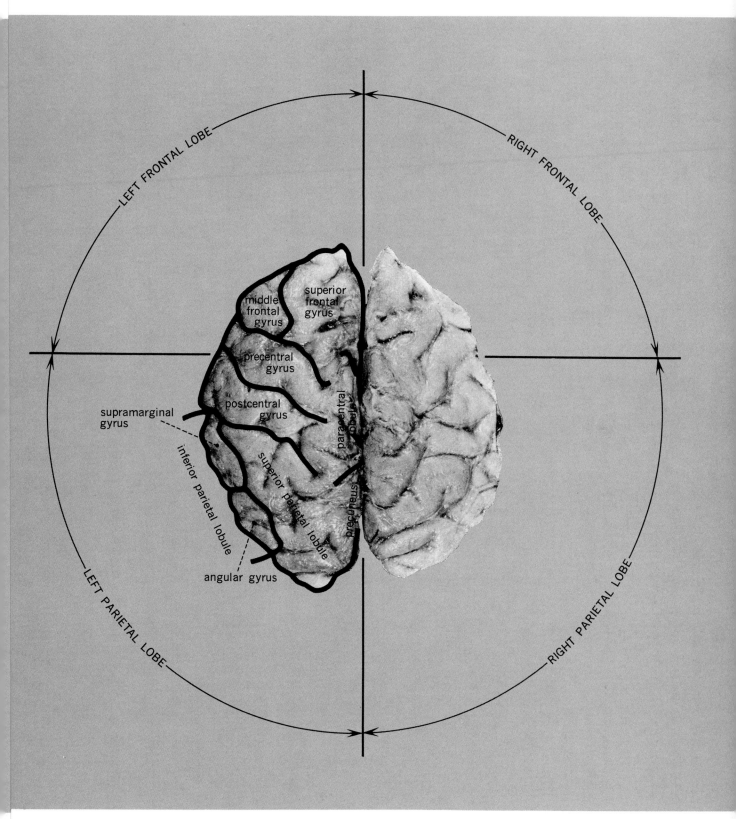

0° section, No. 1, uppersurface indicating prominent lobes and gyri.

LEFT FRONTAL LOBE

RIGHT FRONTAL LOBE

middle frontal gyrus

superior frontal gyrus

precentral gyrus

postcentral gyrus

supramarginal gyrus

inferior parietal lobule

superior parietal lobule

paracentral lobule

precuneus

angular gyrus

LEFT PARIETAL LOBE

RIGHT PARIETAL LOBE

0°-3

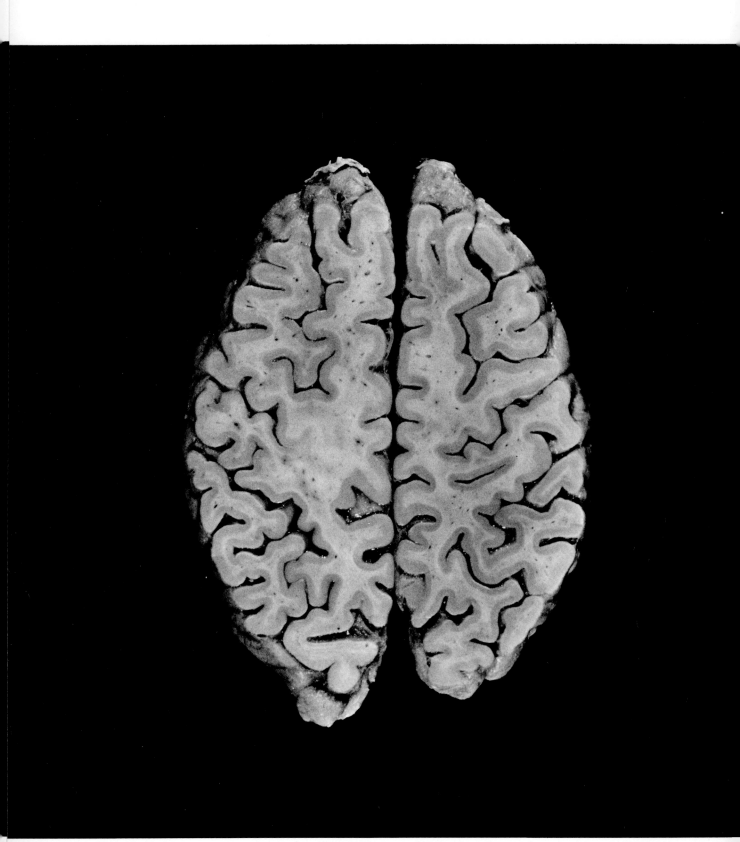

0° section, No. 3, uppersurface.

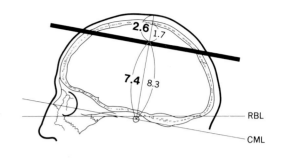

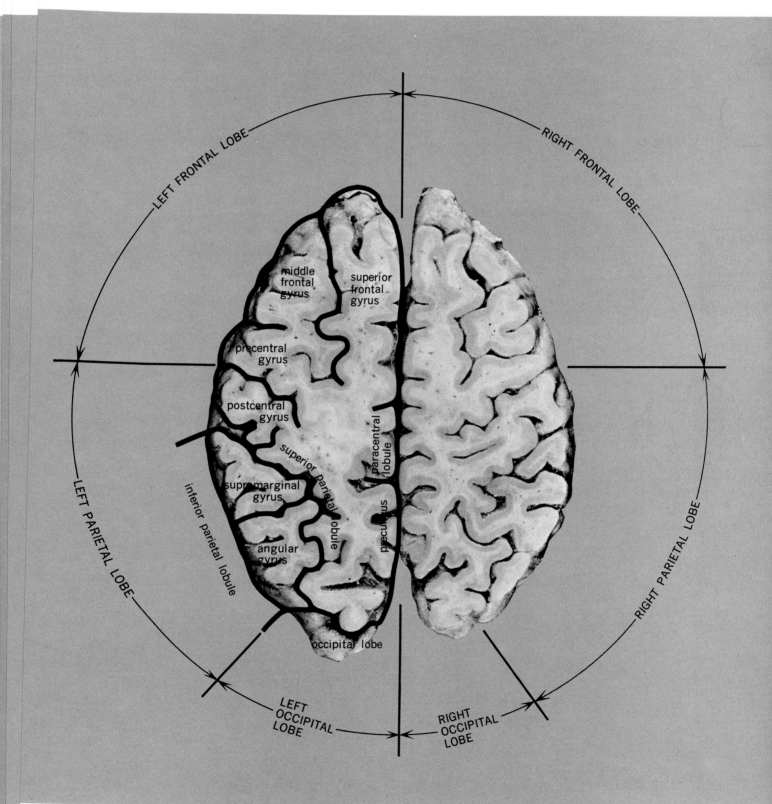

0° section, No. 3, uppersurface indicating prominent lobes and gyri.

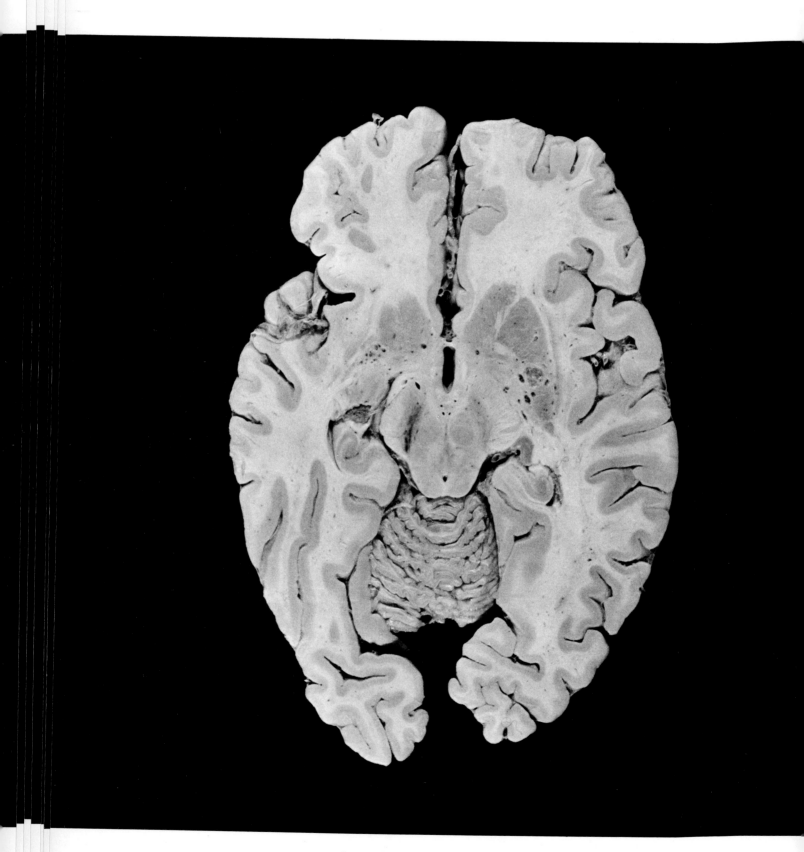

0° section, No. 10, uppersurface.

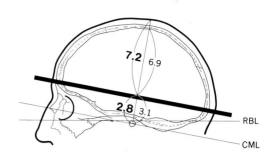

7.2 6.9

2.8 3.1

RBL

CML

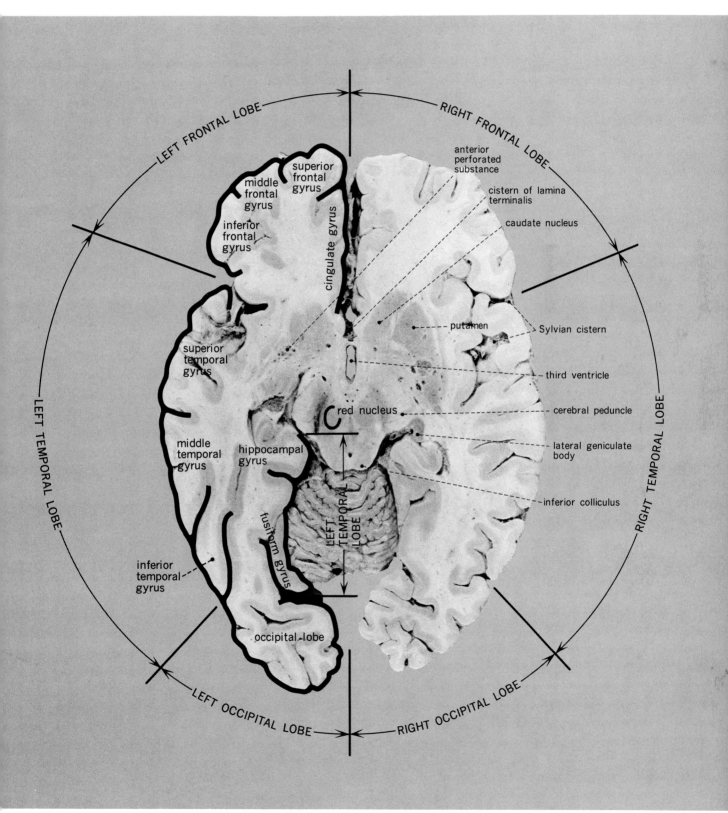

LEFT FRONTAL LOBE

RIGHT FRONTAL LOBE

anterior
perforated
substance

cistern of lamina
terminalis

caudate nucleus

superior
frontal
gyrus

middle
frontal
gyrus

inferior
frontal
gyrus

cingulate gyrus

superior
temporal
gyrus

putamen

Sylvian cistern

third ventricle

red nucleus

cerebral peduncle

lateral geniculate
body

middle
temporal
gyrus

hippocampal
gyrus

inferior colliculus

LEFT TEMPORAL LOBE

RIGHT TEMPORAL LOBE

LEFT TEMPORAL LOBE

fusiform gyrus

inferior
temporal
gyrus

occipital lobe

LEFT OCCIPITAL LOBE

RIGHT OCCIPITAL LOBE

0° section, No. 10, uppersurface indicating prominent structures, lobes and gyri.

157

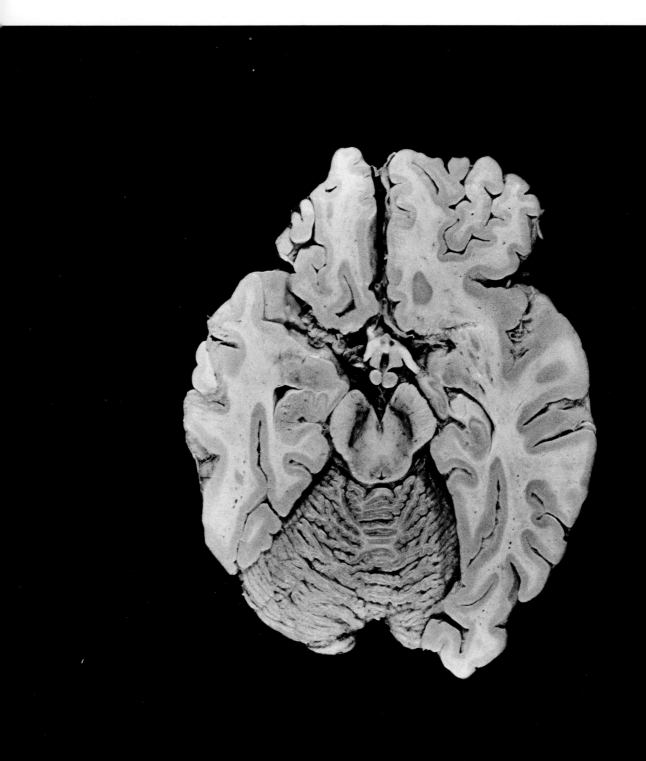

0° section, No. 11, uppersurface.

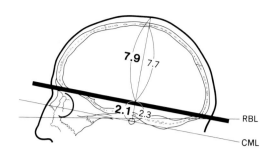

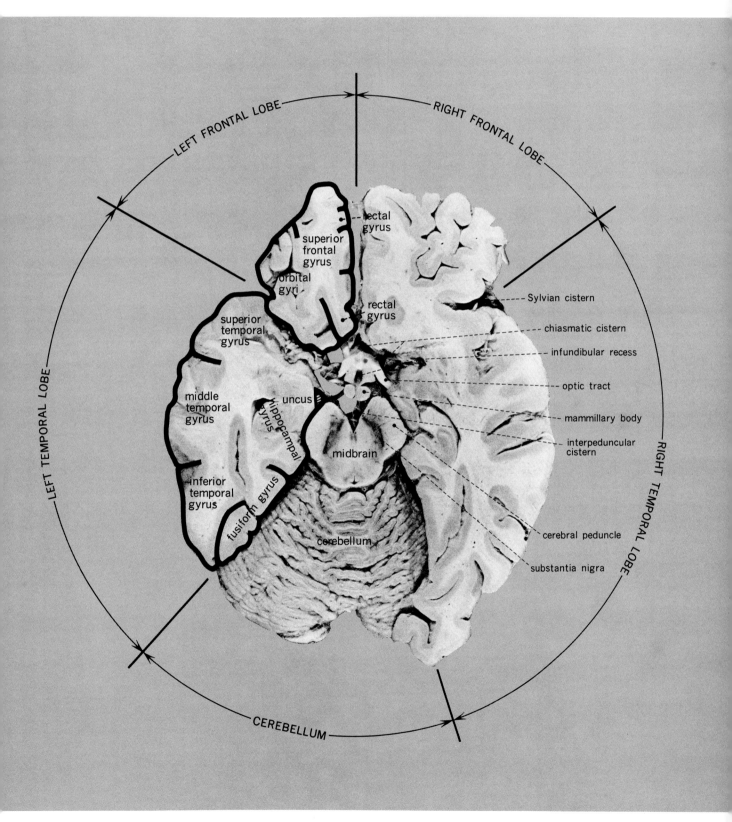

0° section, No. 11, uppersurface indicating prominent structures, lobes and gyri.

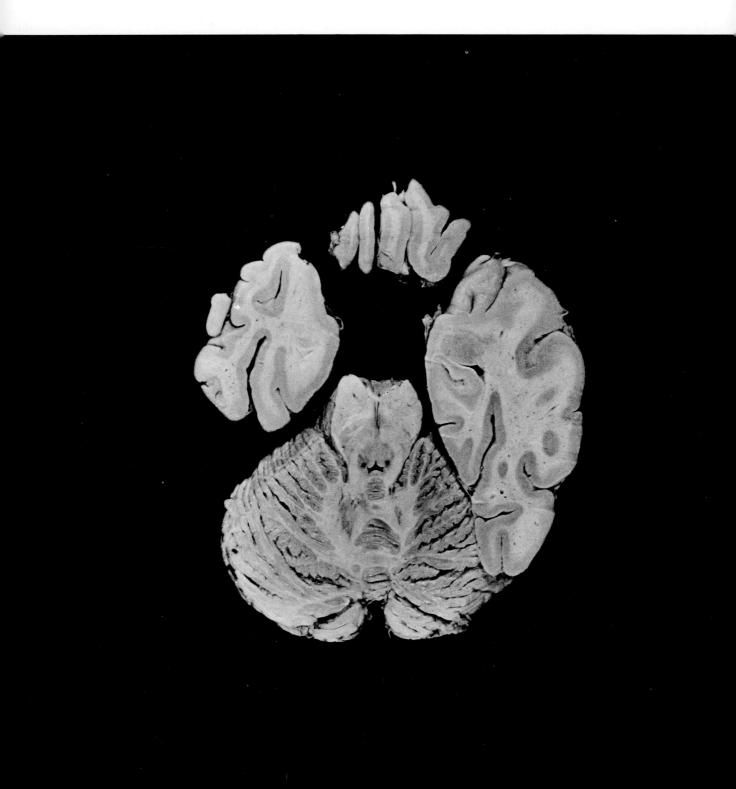

0° section, No. 12, uppersurface.

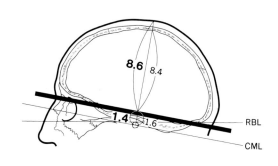

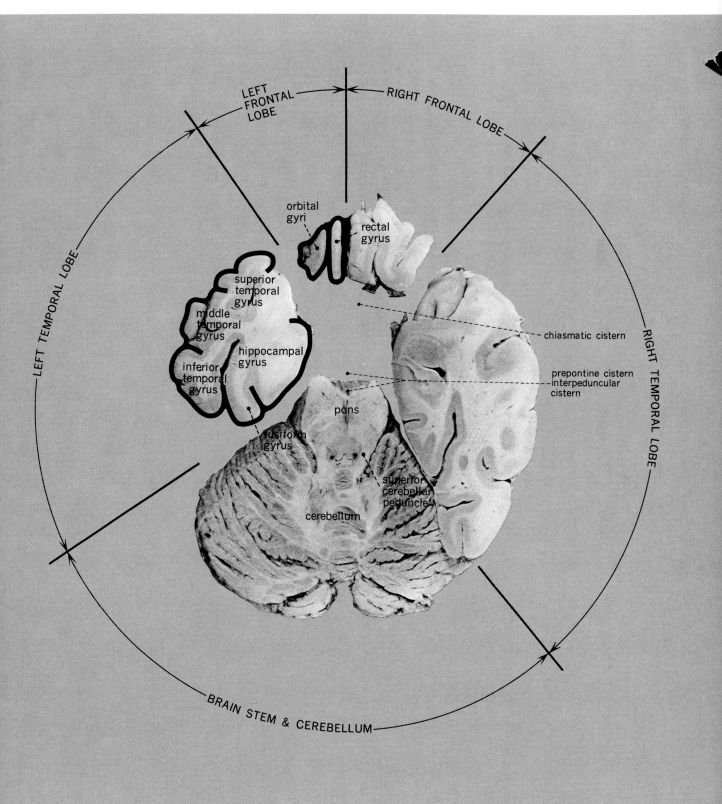

0° section, No. 12, uppersurface indicating prominent structures, lobes and gyri.

161

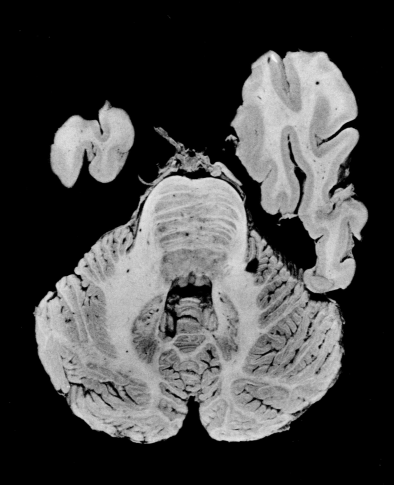

0° section, No. 13, uppersurface.

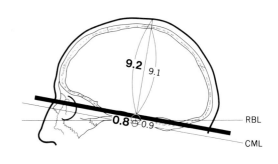

9.2 9.1

0.8 0.9

RBL

CML

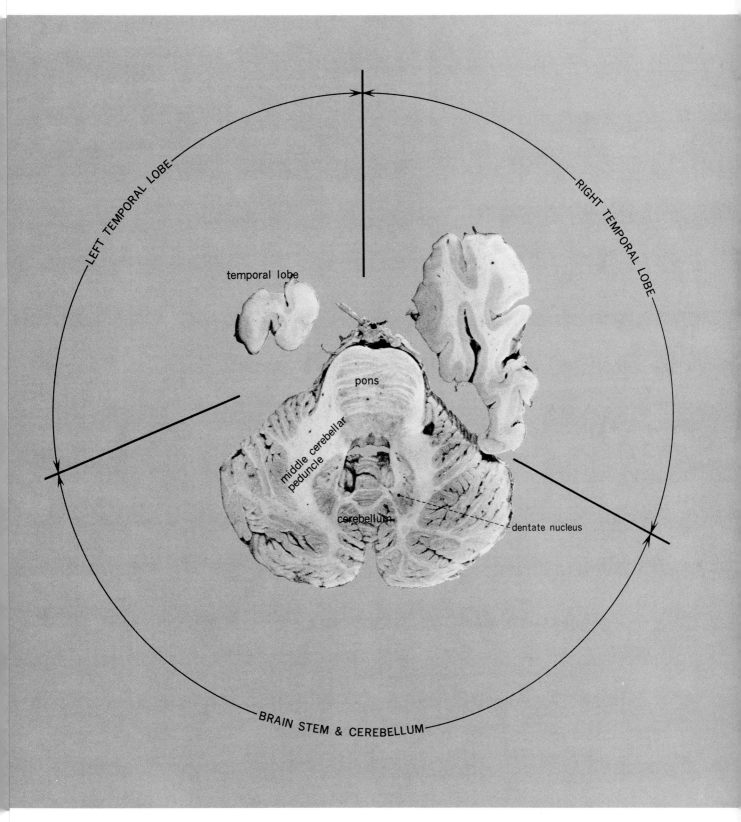

LEFT TEMPORAL LOBE

RIGHT TEMPORAL LOBE

temporal lobe

pons

middle cerebellar peduncle

cerebellum

dentate nucleus

BRAIN STEM & CEREBELLUM

0° section, No. 13, uppersurface indicating prominent structures, lobes and gyri.

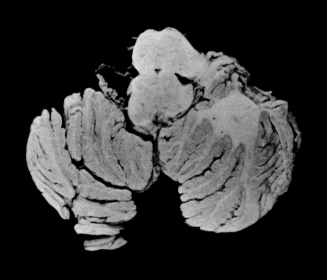

0° section, No. 15, uppersurface.

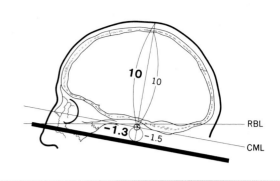

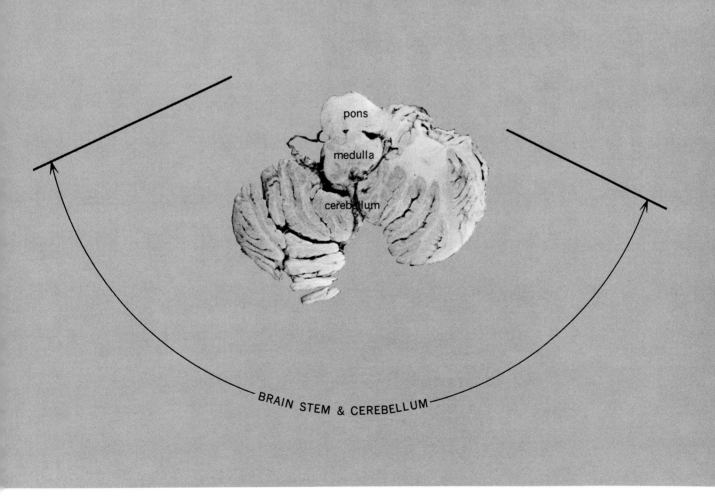

0° section, No. 15, uppersurface indicating prominent lobes and gyri.

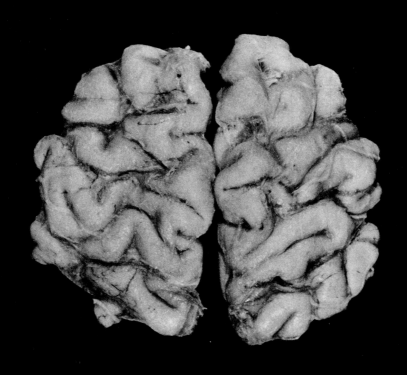

10° section, No. 1, uppersurface.

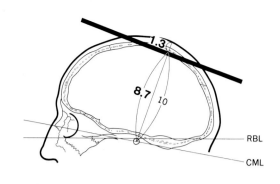

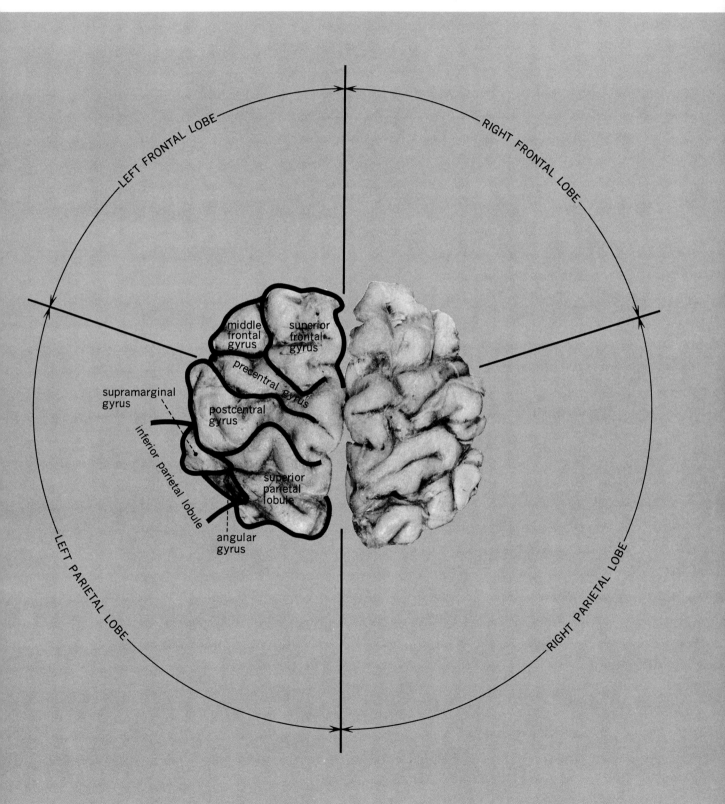

10° section, No. 1, uppersurface indicating prominent lobes and gyri.

169

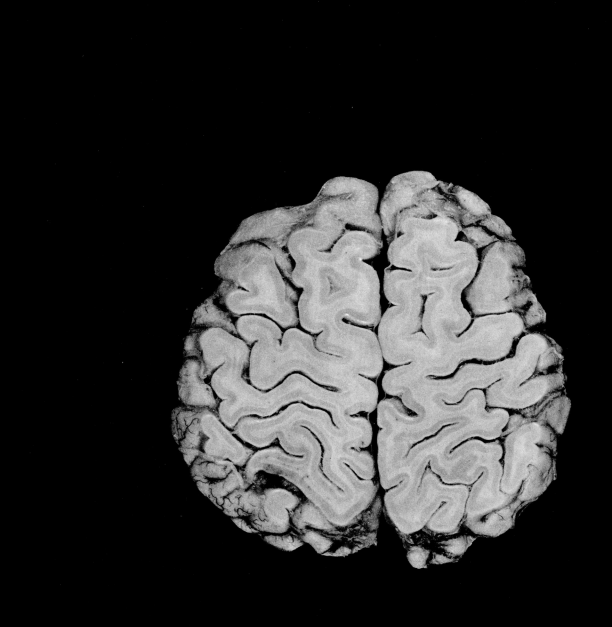

10° section, No. 2, uppersurface.

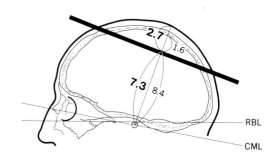

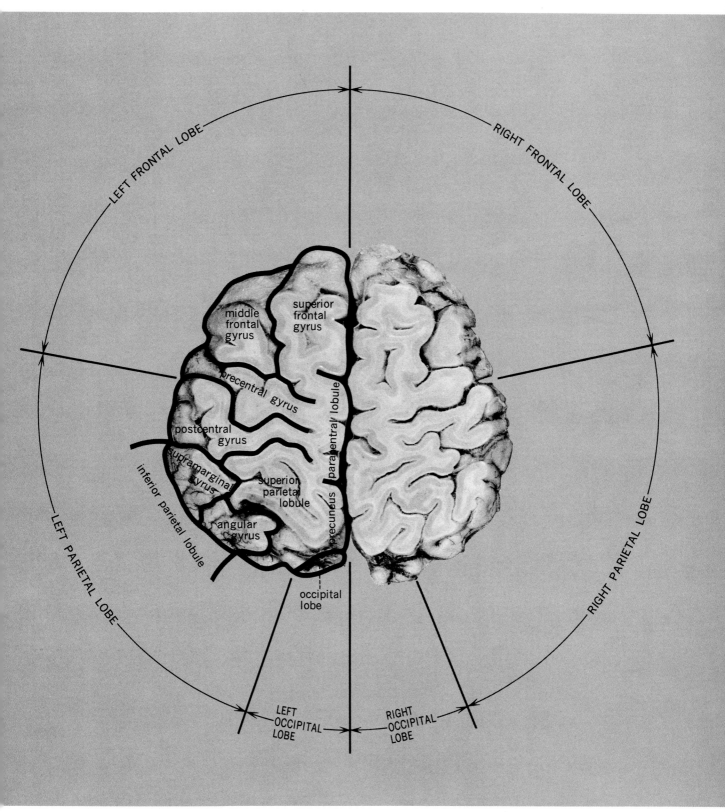

10° section, No. 2, uppersurface indicating prominent lobes and gyri.

171

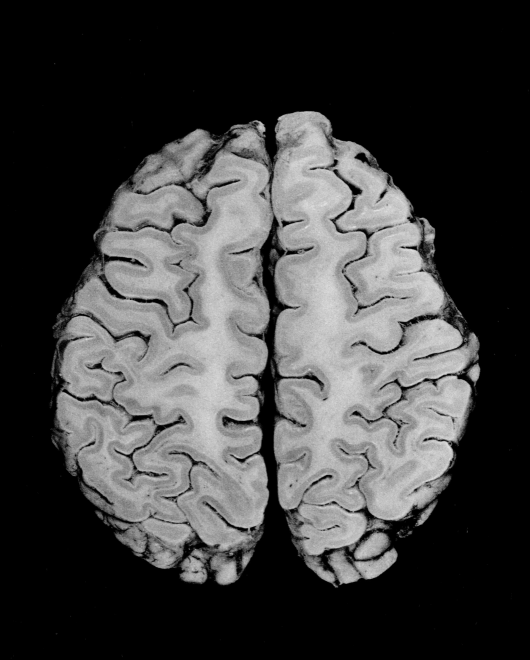

10° section, No. 3, uppersurface.

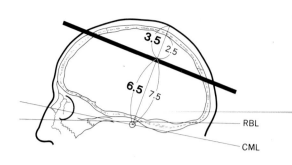

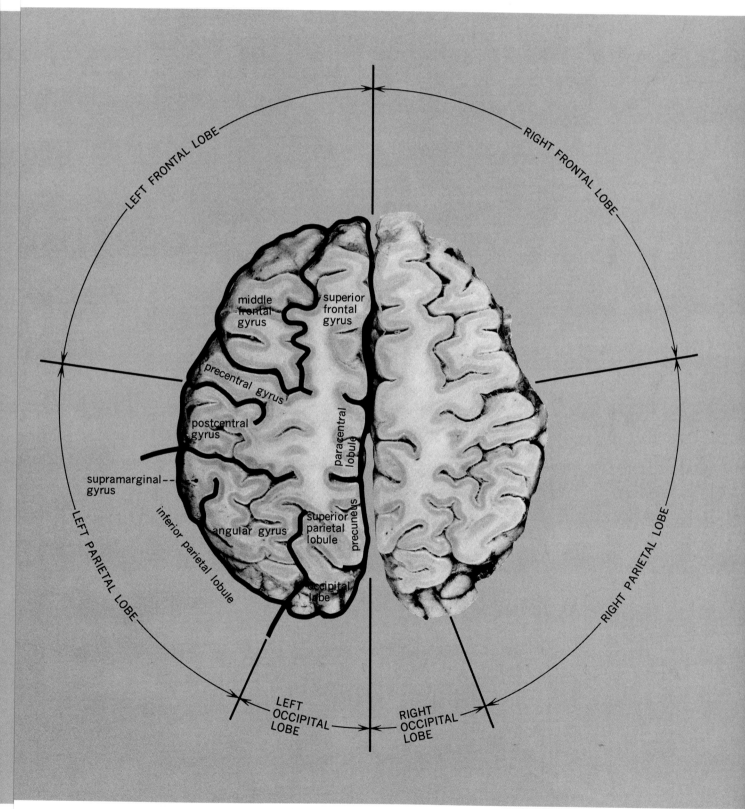

middle frontal gyrus

superior frontal gyrus

precentral gyrus

postcentral gyrus

paracentral lobule

supramarginal gyrus

inferior parietal lobule

angular gyrus

superior parietal lobule

precuneus

occipital lobe

LEFT FRONTAL LOBE

RIGHT FRONTAL LOBE

LEFT PARIETAL LOBE

RIGHT PARIETAL LOBE

LEFT OCCIPITAL LOBE

RIGHT OCCIPITAL LOBE

RBL

CML

10° section, No. 3, uppersurface indicating prominent lobes and gyri.

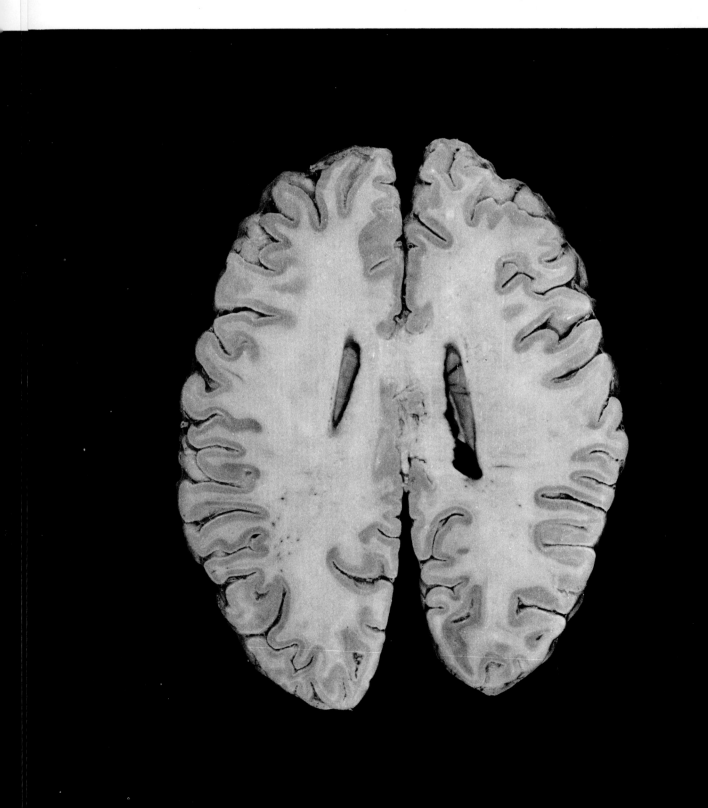

10° section, No. 6, uppersurface.

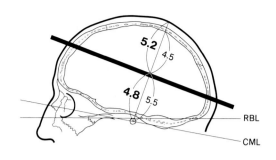

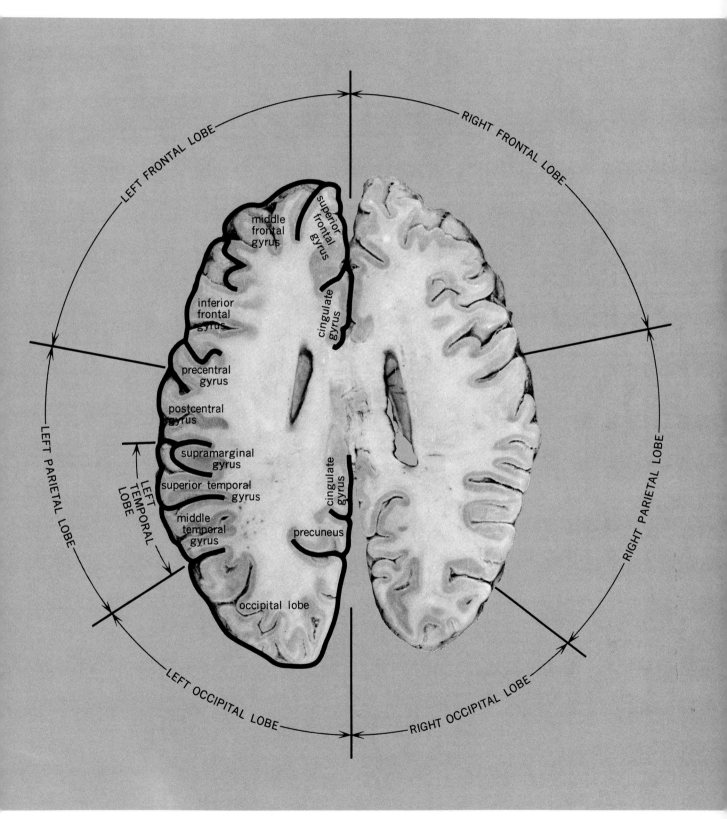

LEFT FRONTAL LOBE

RIGHT FRONTAL LOBE

middle
frontal
gyrus

superior
frontal
gyrus

cingulate
gyrus

inferior
frontal
gyrus

precentral
gyrus

postcentral
gyrus

supramarginal
gyrus

**LEFT
TEMPORAL
LOBE**

superior temporal
gyrus

cingulate
gyrus

middle
temporal
gyrus

precuneus

occipital lobe

LEFT PARIETAL LOBE

RIGHT PARIETAL LOBE

LEFT OCCIPITAL LOBE

RIGHT OCCIPITAL LOBE

10° section, No. 6, uppersurface indicating prominent lobes and gyri.

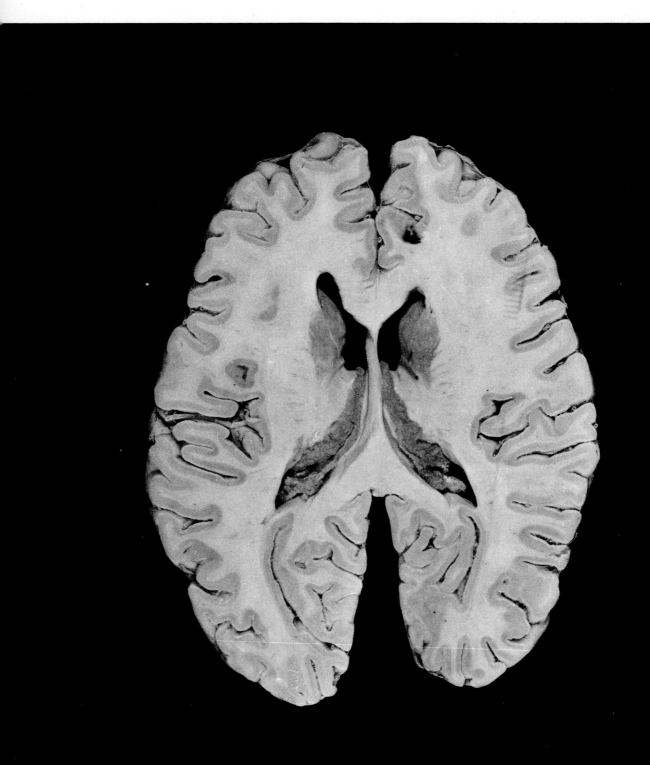

10° section, No. 7, uppersurface.

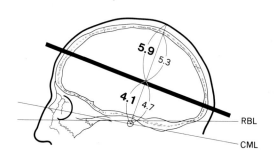

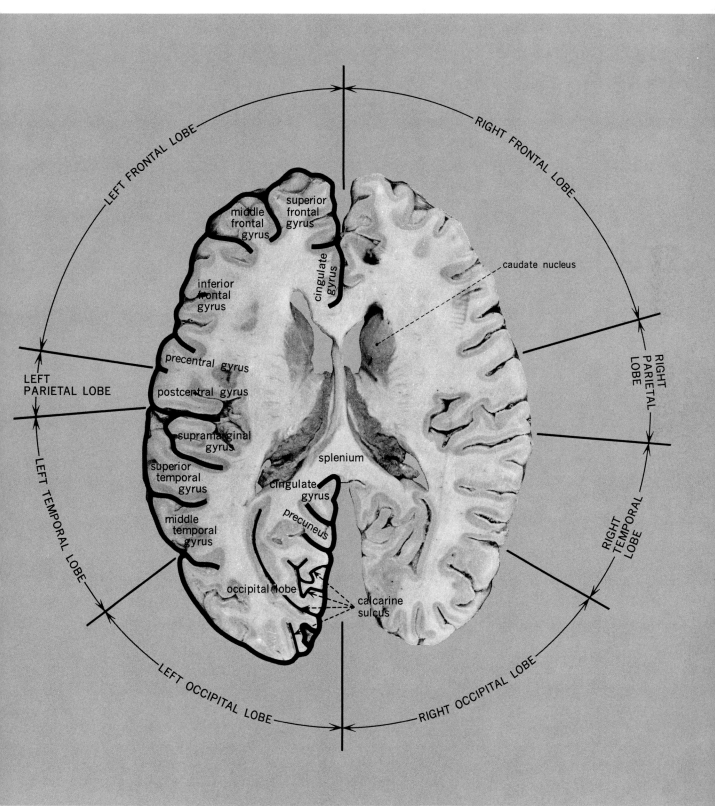

10° section, No. 7, uppersurface indicating prominent structures, lobes and gyri.

181

10°-8

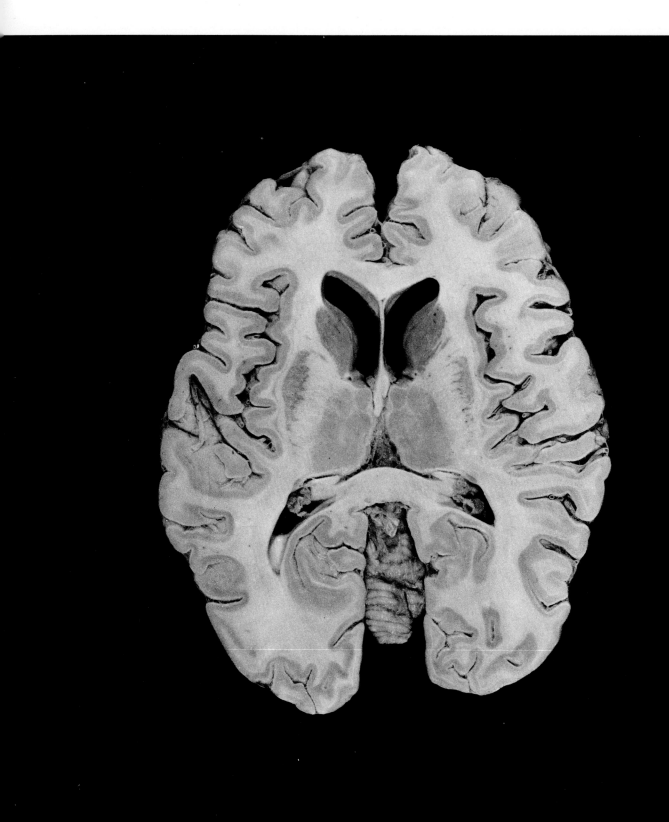

10° section, No. 8, uppersurface.

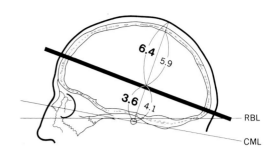

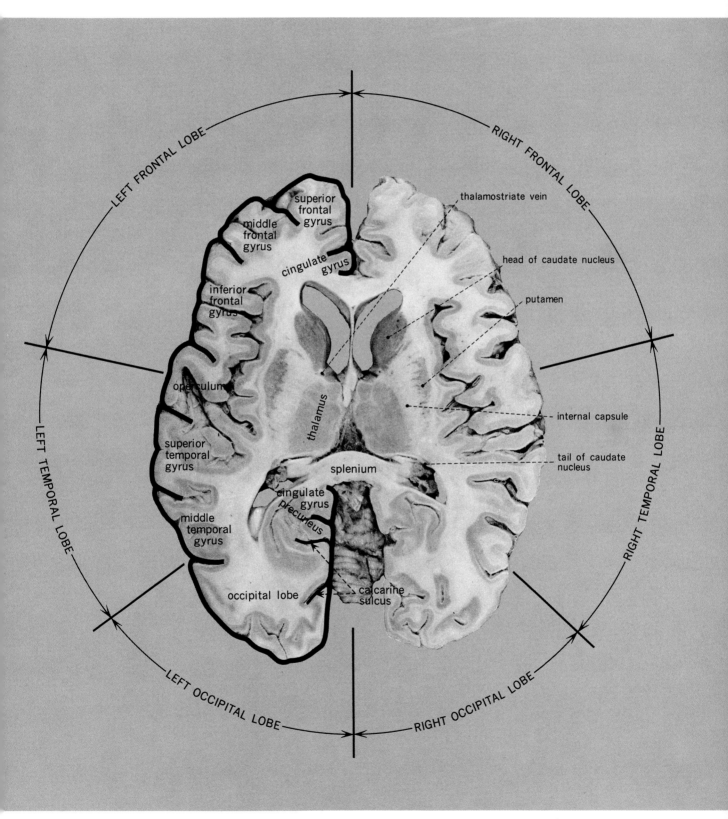

10° section, No. 8, uppersurface indicating prominent structures, lobes and gyri.

10°-9

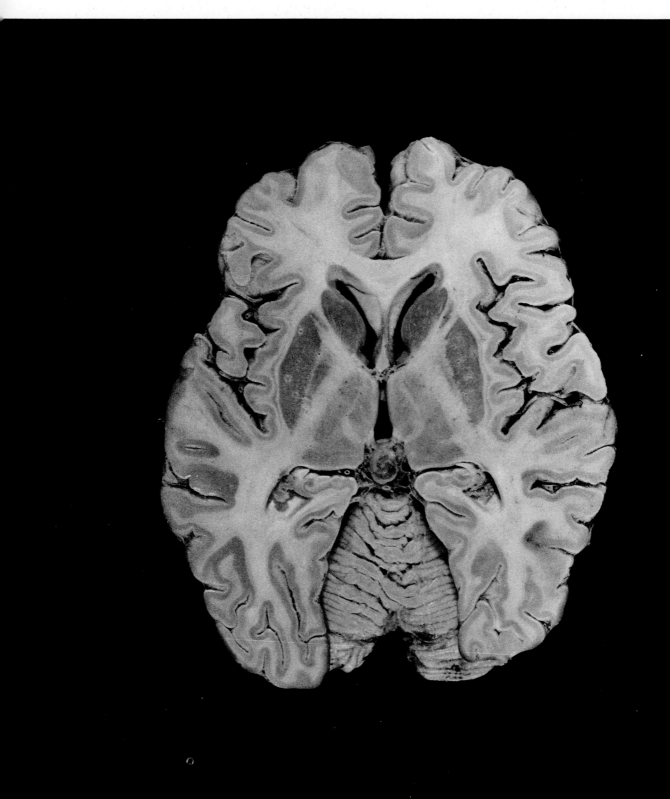

10° section, No. 9, uppersurface.

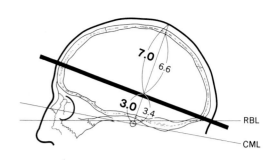

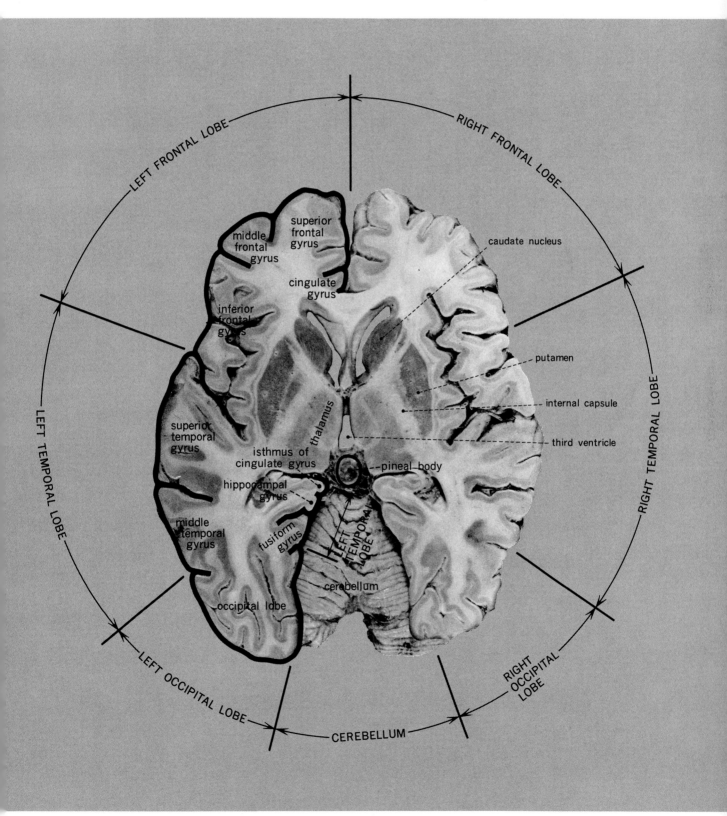

10° section, No. 9, uppersurface indicating prominent structures, lobes and gyri.

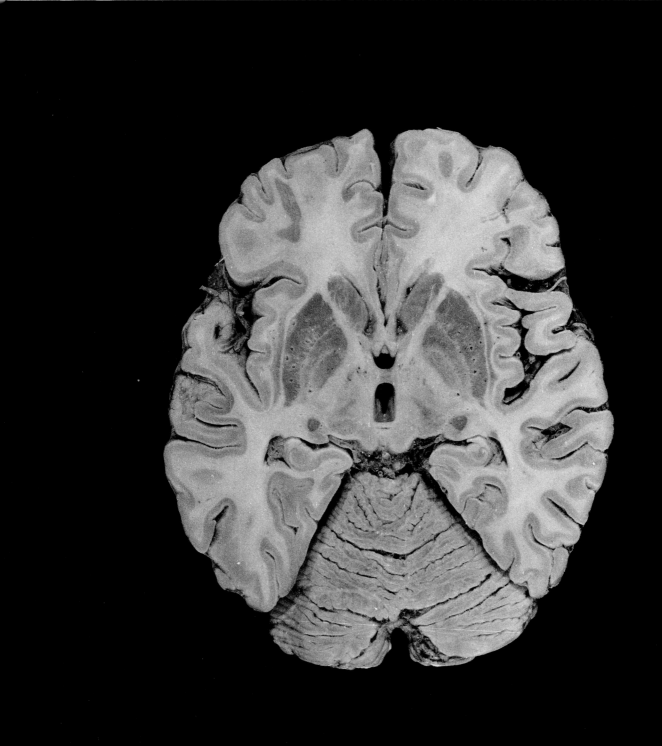

10° section, No. 10, uppersurface.

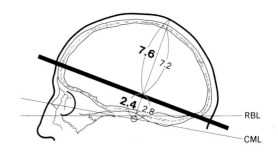

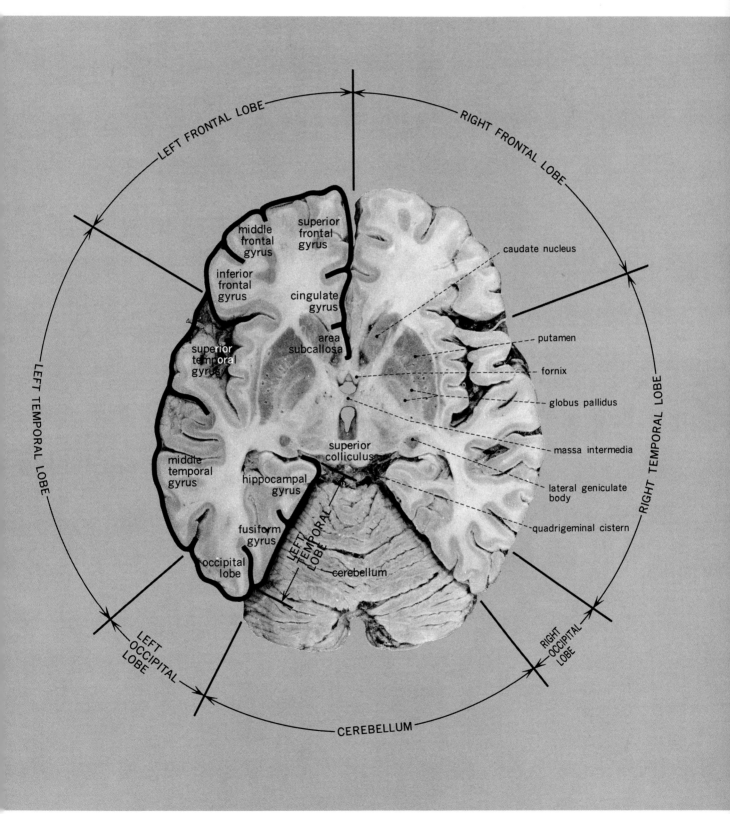

10° section, No. 10, uppersurface indicating prominent structures, lobes and gyri.

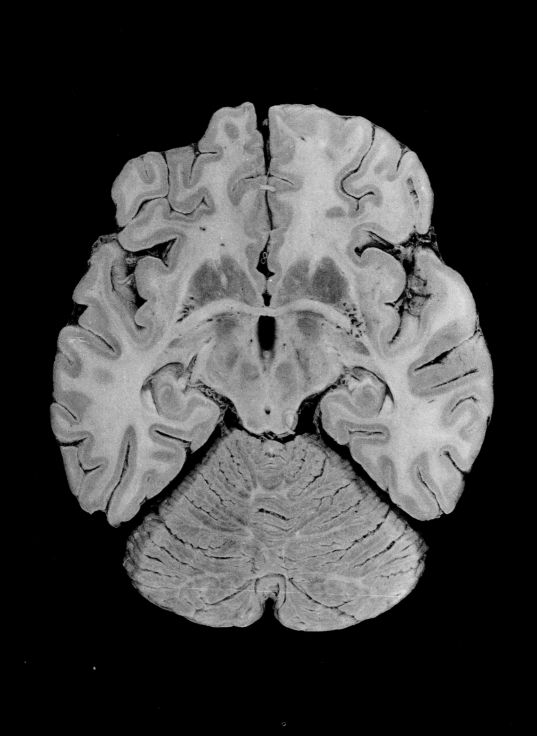

10° section, No. 11, uppersurface.

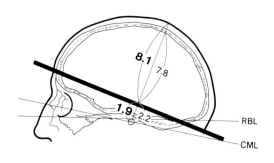

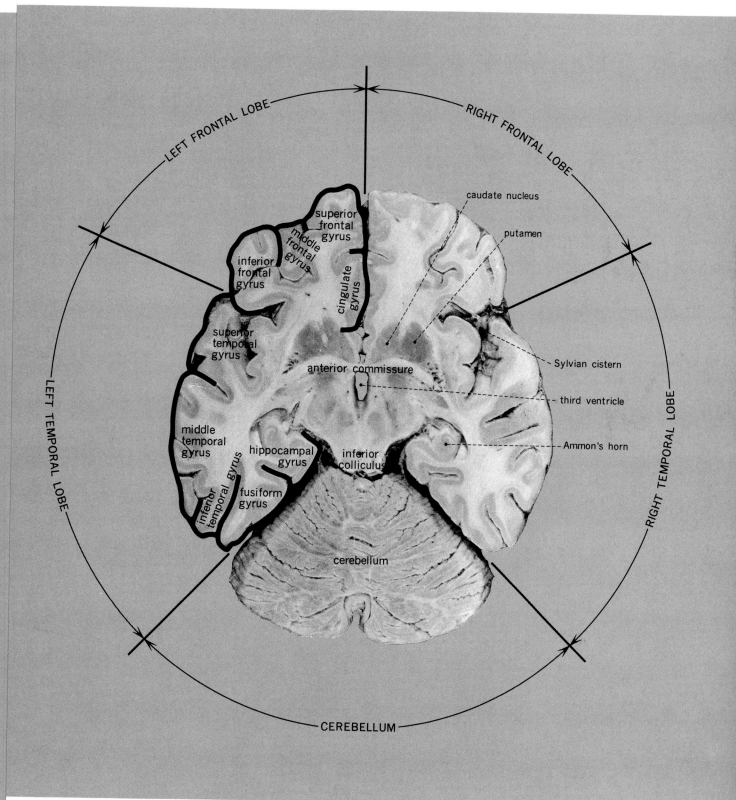

LEFT FRONTAL LOBE

RIGHT FRONTAL LOBE

LEFT TEMPORAL LOBE

RIGHT TEMPORAL LOBE

CEREBELLUM

superior frontal gyrus

middle frontal gyrus

inferior frontal gyrus

cingulate gyrus

superior temporal gyrus

middle temporal gyrus

inferior temporal gyrus

hippocampal gyrus

fusiform gyrus

inferior colliculus

cerebellum

anterior commissure

caudate nucleus

putamen

Sylvian cistern

third ventricle

Ammon's horn

10° section, No. 11, uppersurface indicating prominent structures, lobes and gyri.

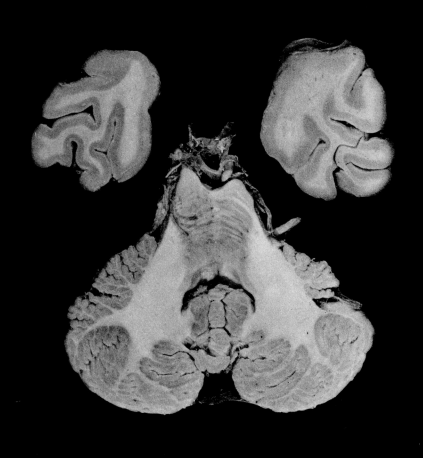

10° section, No. 14, uppersurface.

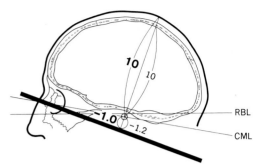

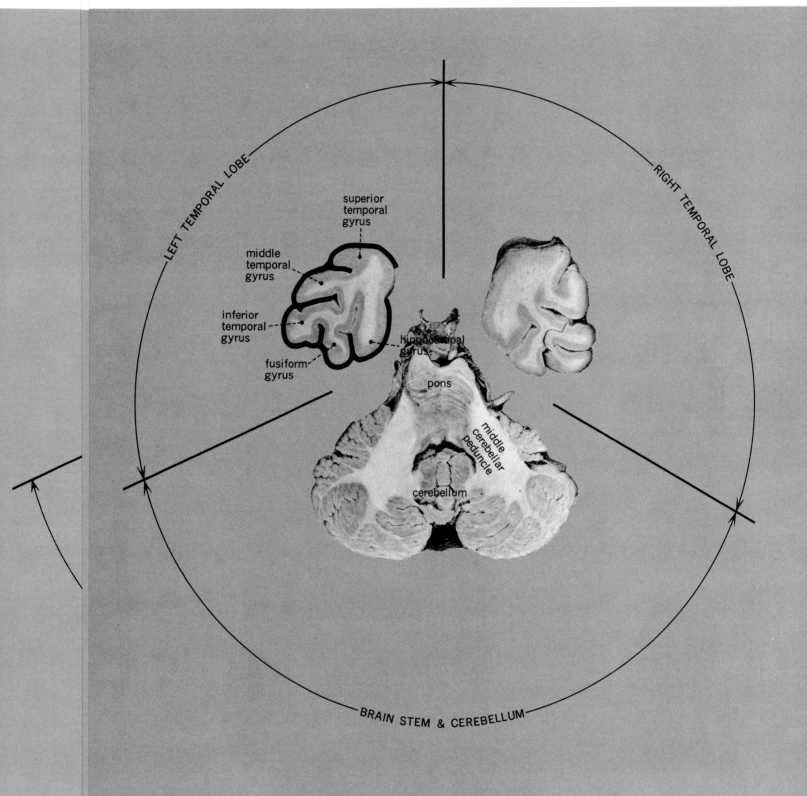

10° section, No. 14, uppersurface indicating prominent lobes and gyri.

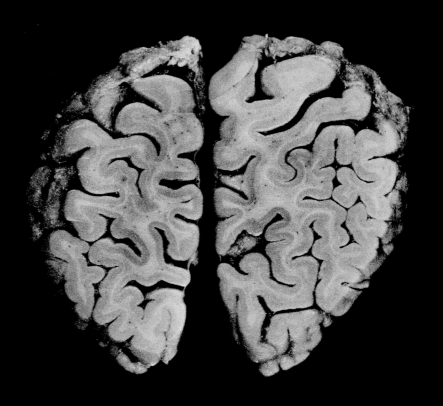

25° section, No. 3, uppersurface.

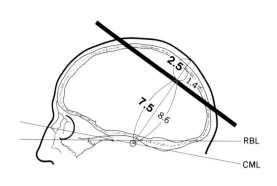

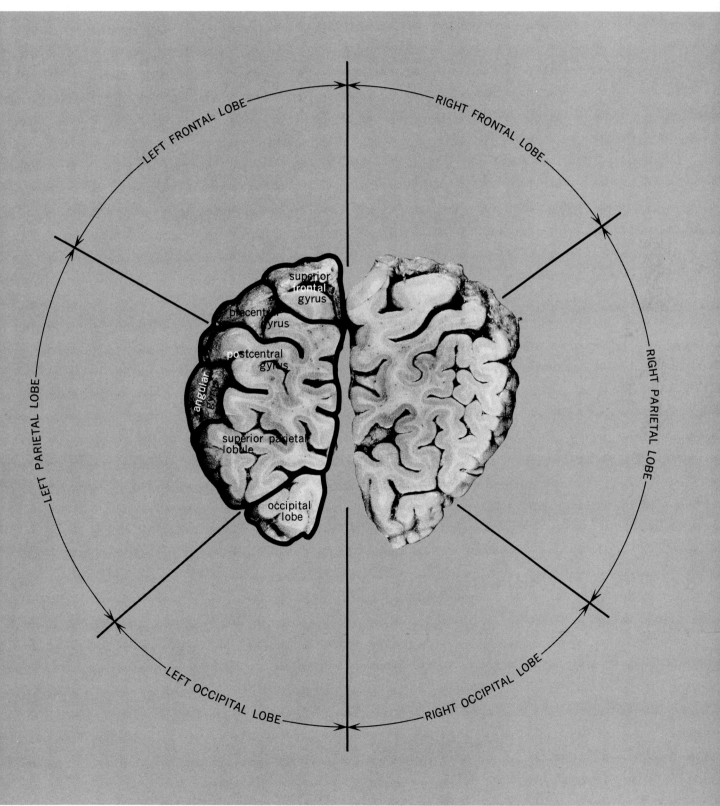

25° section, No. 3, uppersurface indicating prominent lobes and gyri.

LEFT FRONTAL LOBE

RIGHT FRONTAL LOBE

LEFT PARIETAL LOBE

RIGHT PARIETAL LOBE

LEFT OCCIPITAL LOBE

RIGHT OCCIPITAL LOBE

superior frontal gyrus

precentral gyrus

postcentral gyrus

angular

superior parietal lobule

occipital lobe

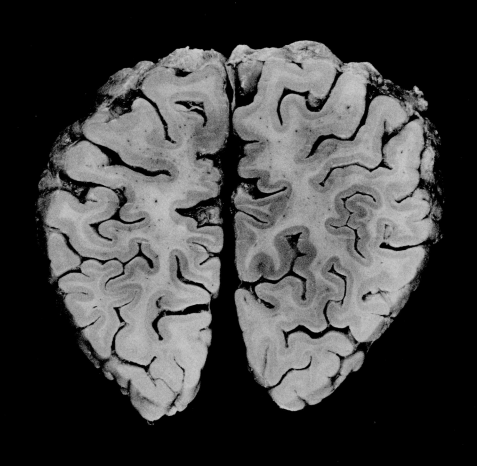

25° section, No. 4, uppersurface.

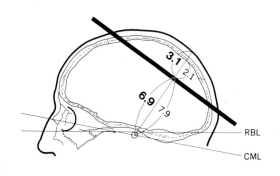

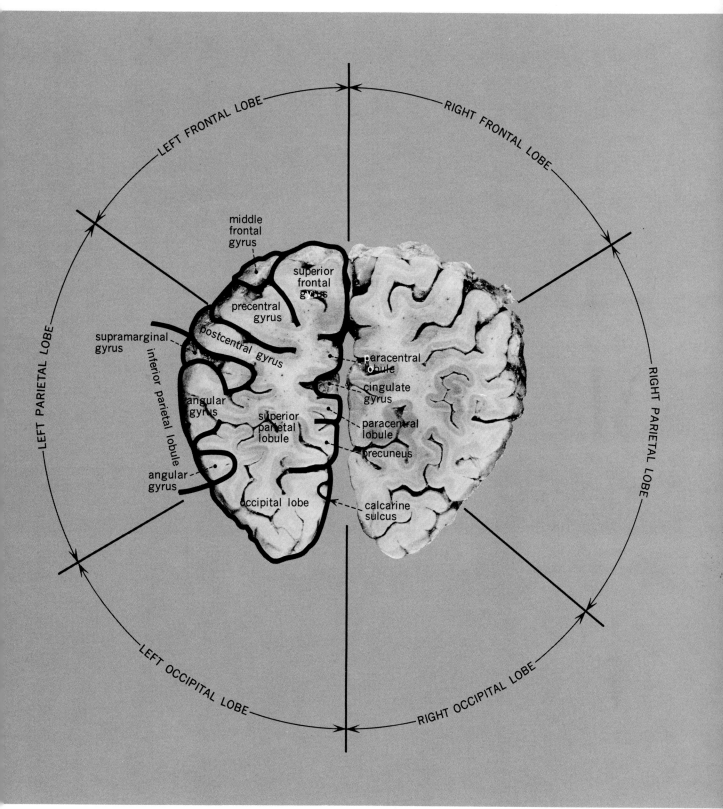

25° section, No. 4, uppersurface indicating prominent lobes and gyri.

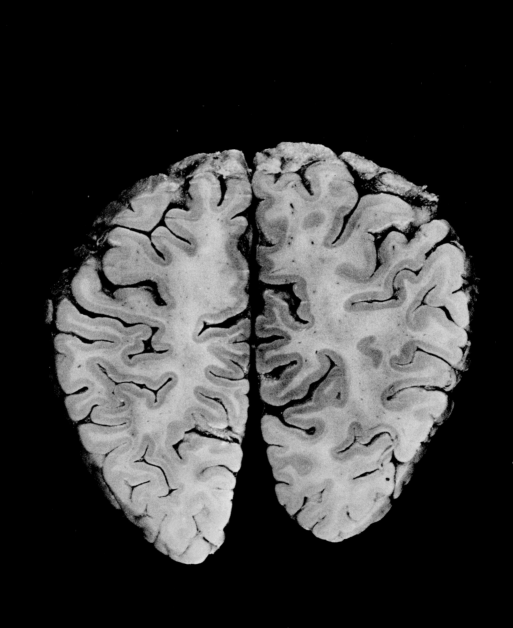

25° section, No. 5, uppersurface.

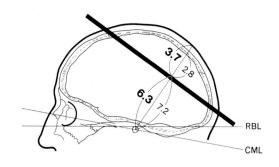

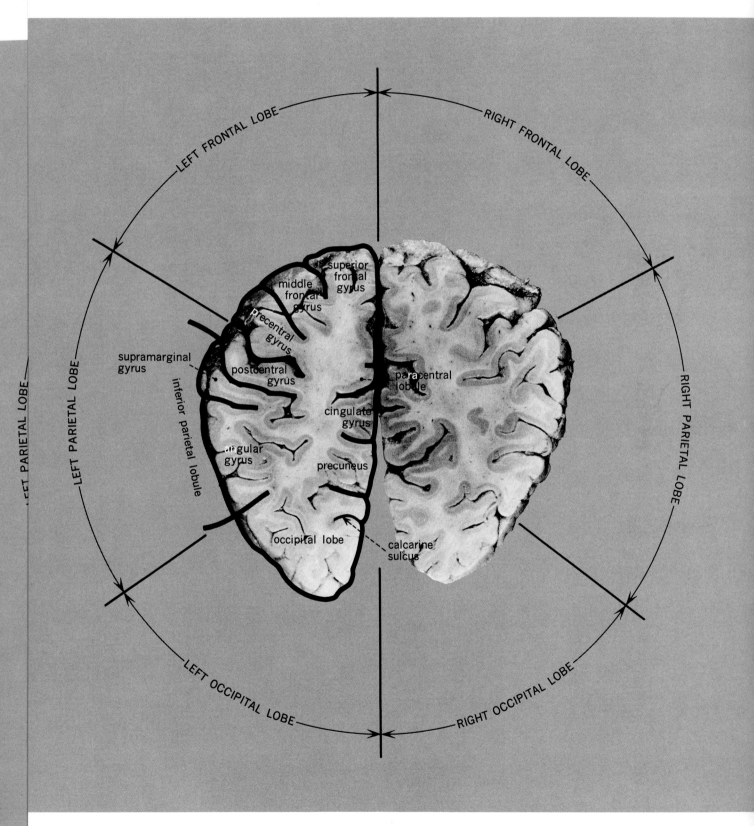

25° section, No. 5, uppersurface indicating prominent lobes and gyri.

25°-7

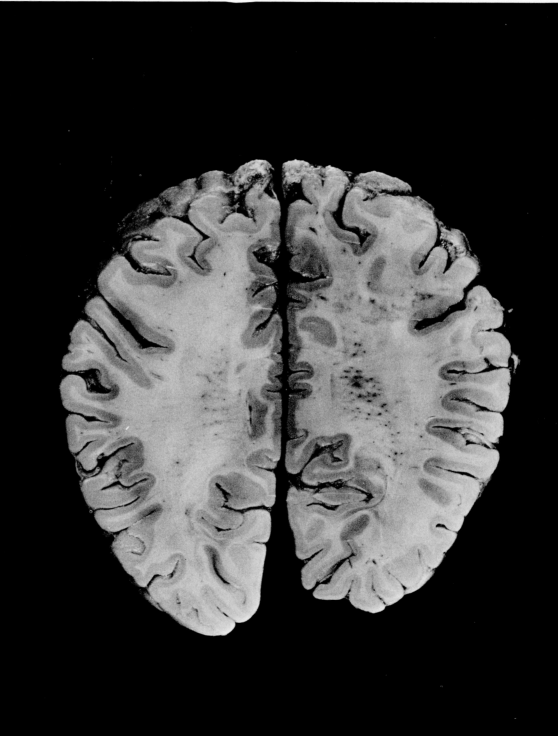

25° section, No. 7, uppersurface.

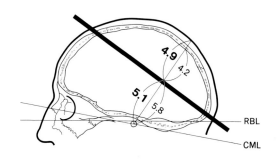

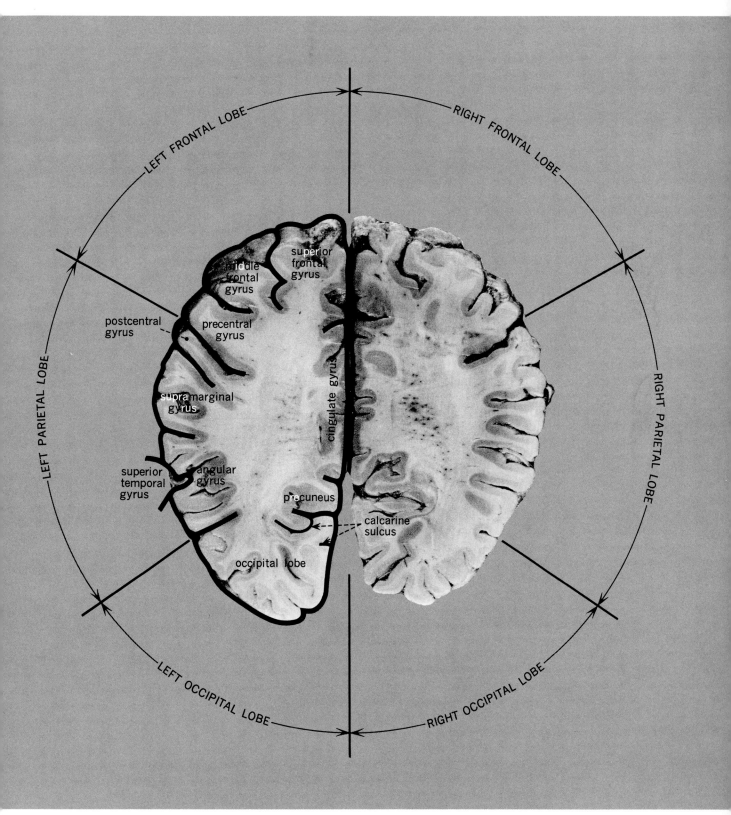

25° section, No. 7, uppersurface indicating prominent lobes and gyri.

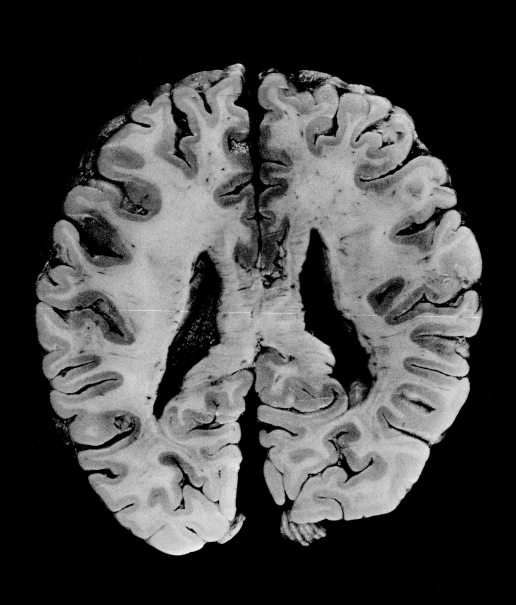

25° section, No. 8, uppersurface.

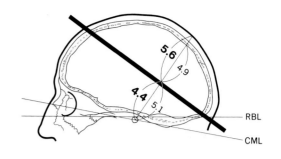

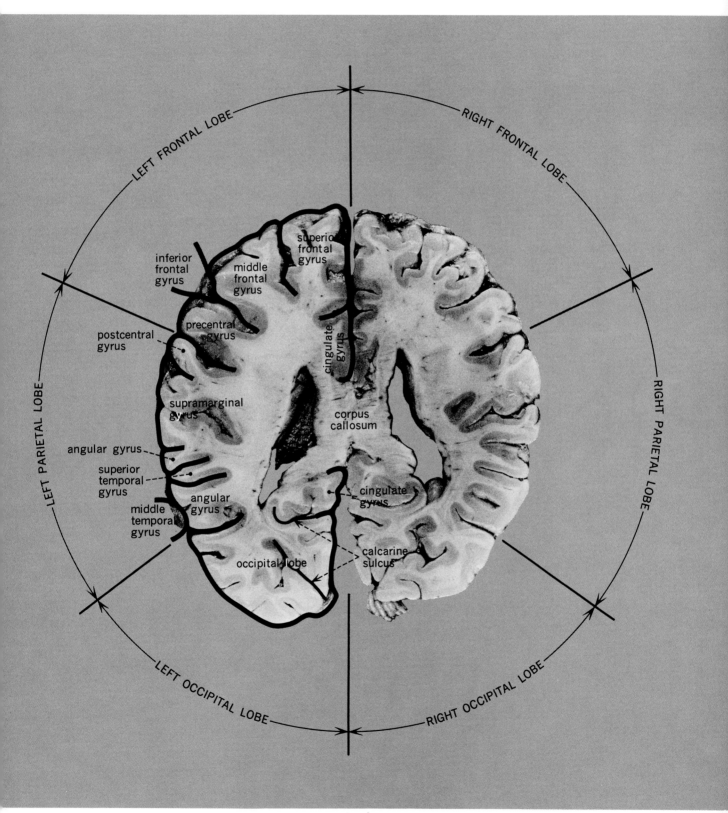

25° section, No. 8, uppersurface indicating prominent lobes and gyri.

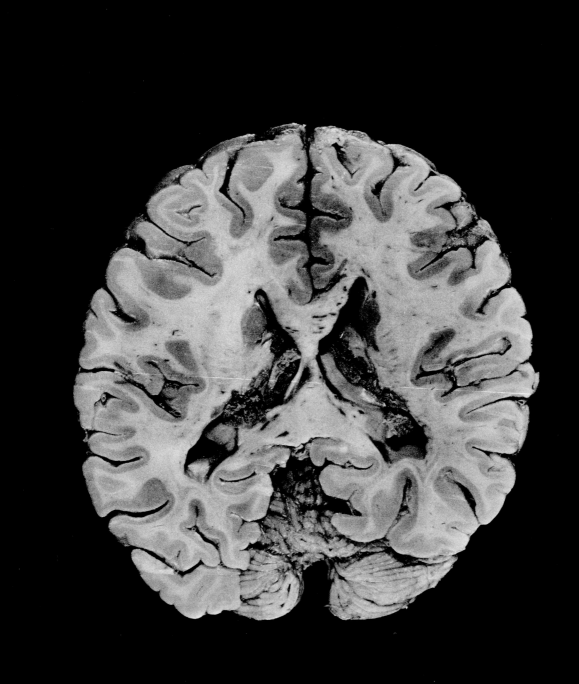

25° section, No. 9, uppersurface.

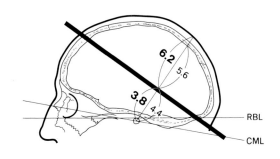

RBL
CML

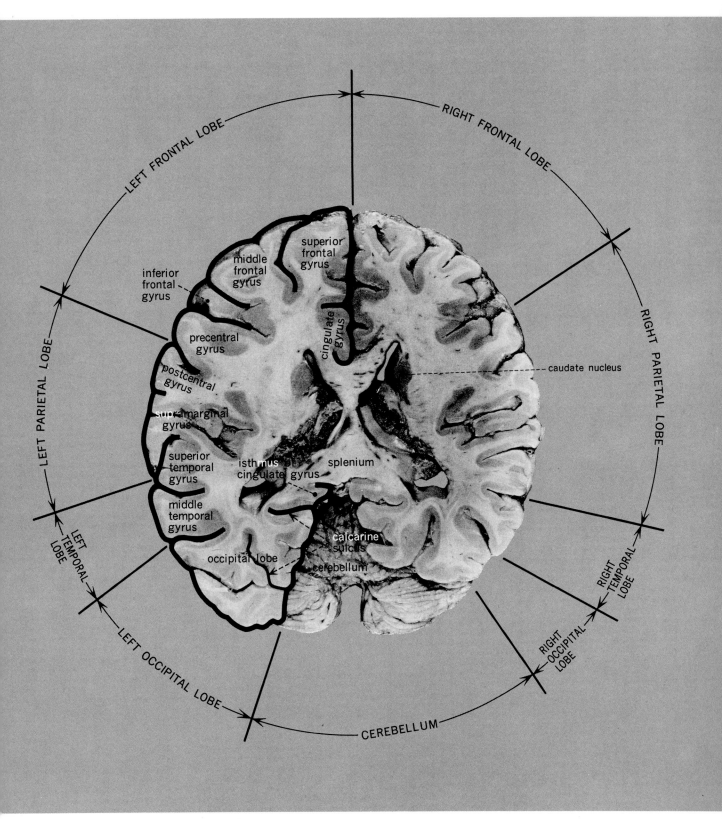

LEFT FRONTAL LOBE

RIGHT FRONTAL LOBE

superior
frontal
gyrus

middle
frontal
gyrus

inferior
frontal
gyrus

cingulate
gyrus

caudate nucleus

precentral
gyrus

postcentral
gyrus

supramarginal
gyrus

LEFT PARIETAL LOBE

RIGHT PARIETAL LOBE

superior
temporal
gyrus

isthmus of
cingulate gyrus

splenium

middle
temporal
gyrus

LEFT TEMPORAL LOBE

RIGHT TEMPORAL LOBE

calcarine
sulcus

occipital lobe

cerebellum

RIGHT OCCIPITAL LOBE

LEFT OCCIPITAL LOBE

CEREBELLUM

25° section, No. 9, uppersurface indicating prominent structures, lobes and gyri.

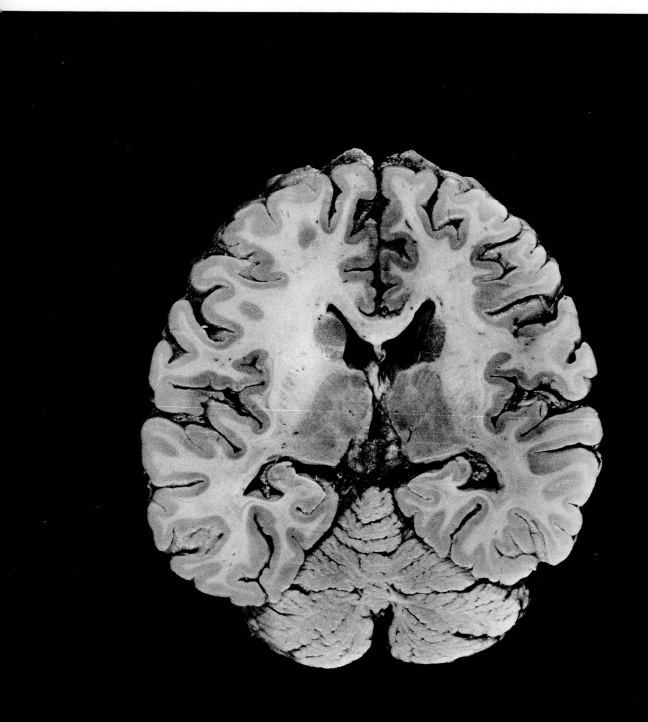

25° section, No. 10, uppersurface.

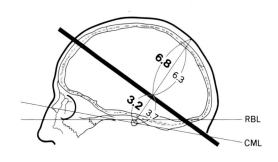

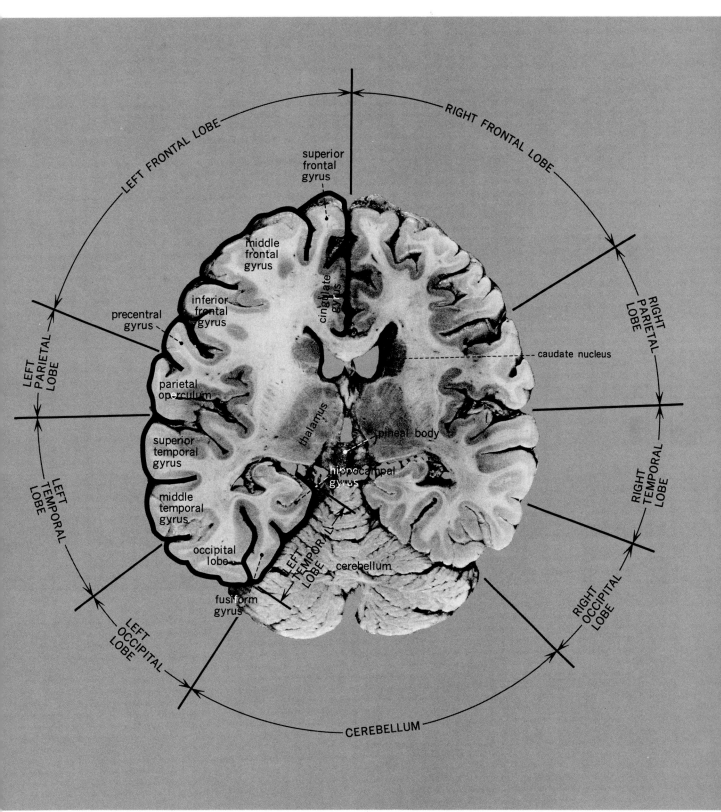

25° section, No. 10, uppersurface indicating prominent structures, lobes and gyri.

219

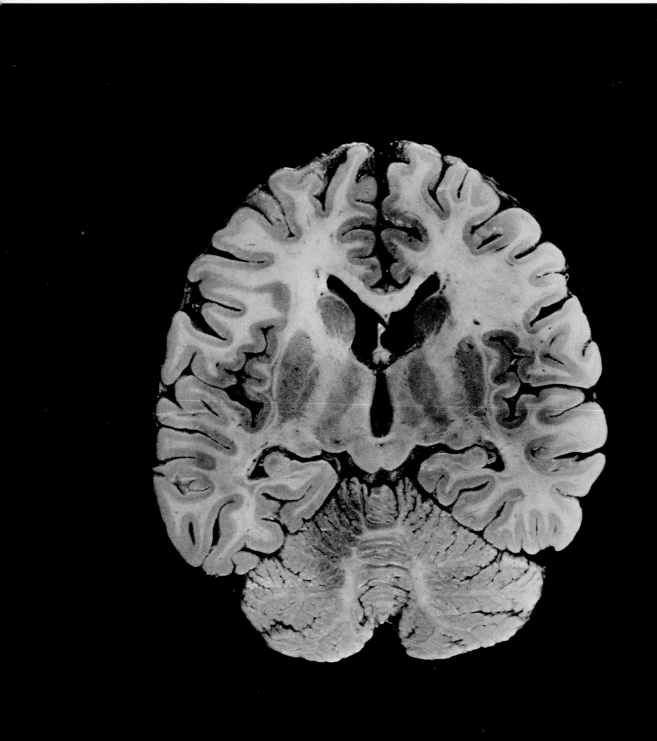

25° section, No. 11, uppersurface.

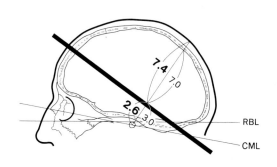

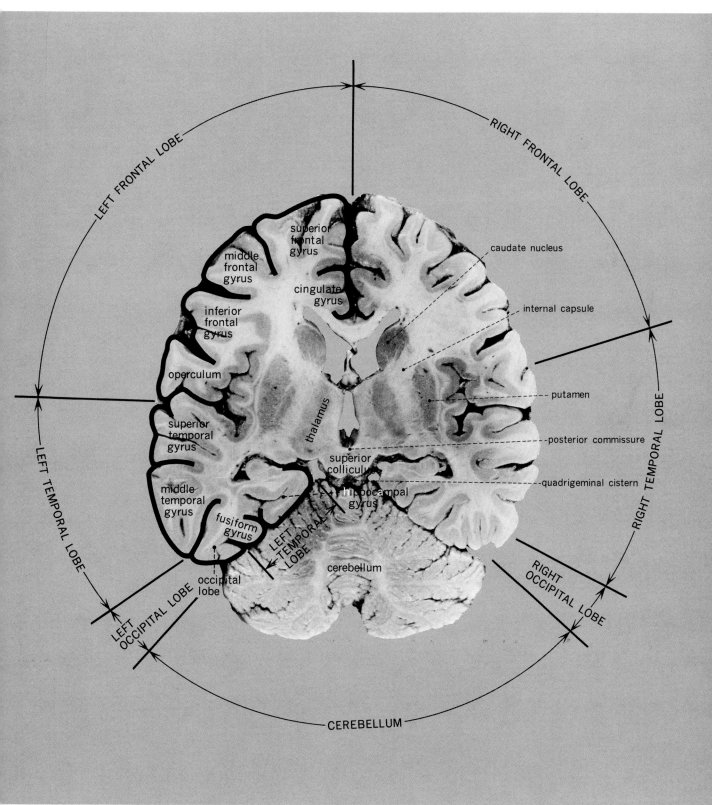

25° section, No. 11, uppersurface indicating prominent structures, lobes and gyri.

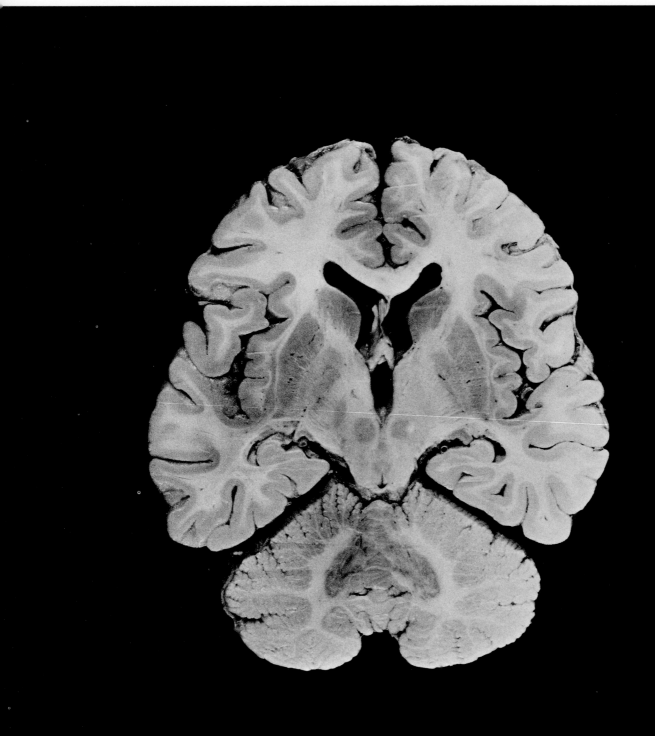

25° section, No. 12, uppersurface.

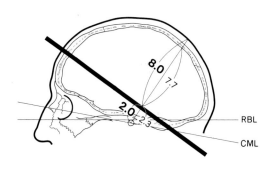

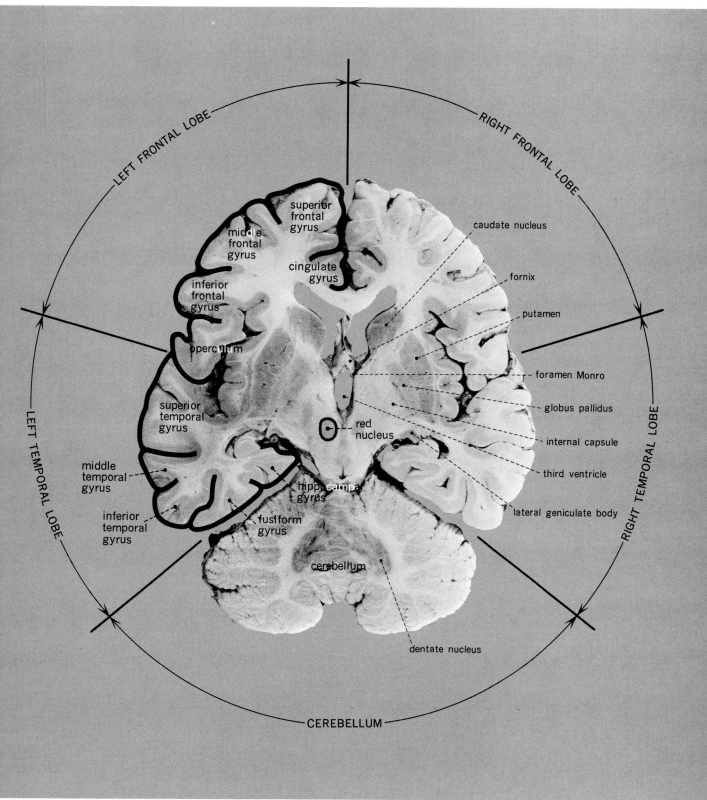

25° section, No. 12, uppersurface indicating prominent structures, lobes and gyri.

223

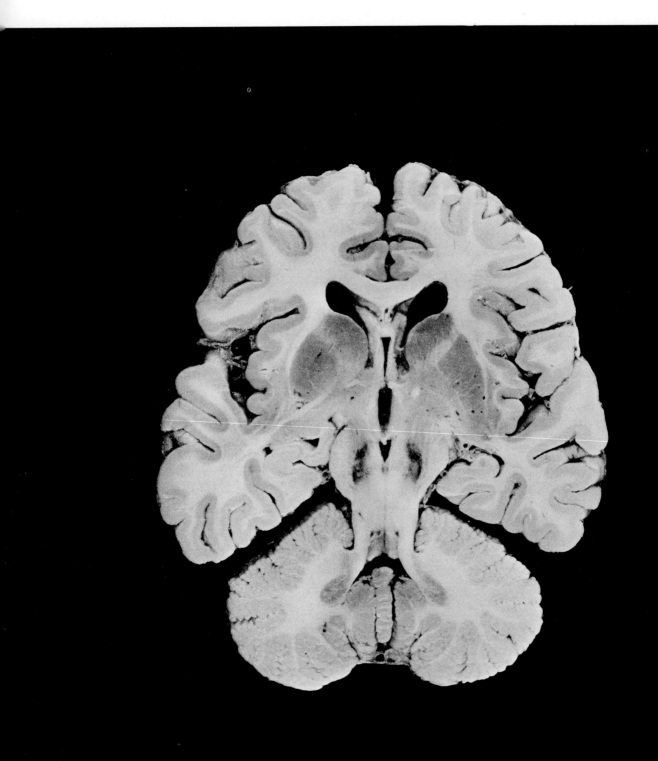

25° section, No. 13, uppersurface.

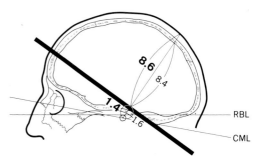

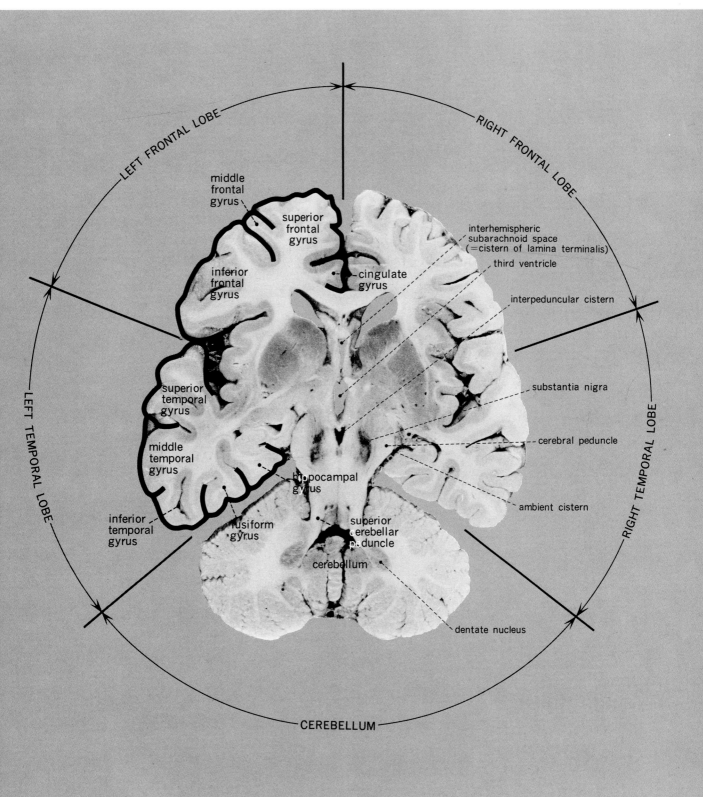

25° section, No. 13, uppersurface indicating prominent structures, lobes and gyri.

25°- 14

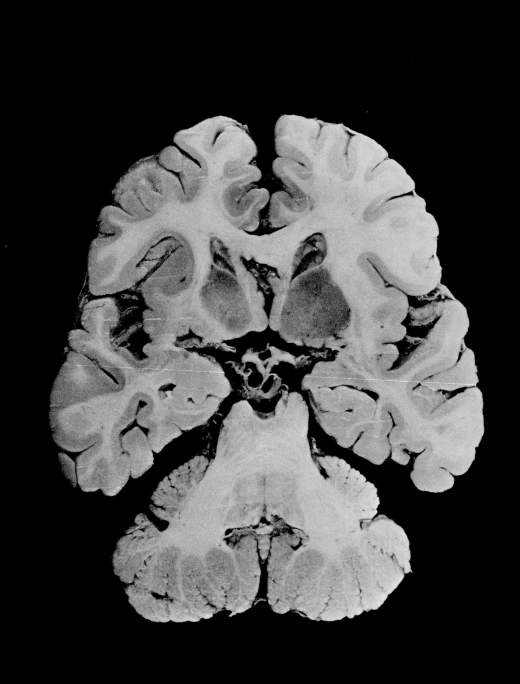

25° section, No. 14, uppersurface.

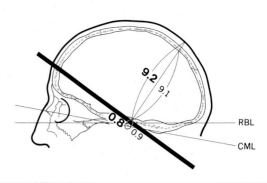

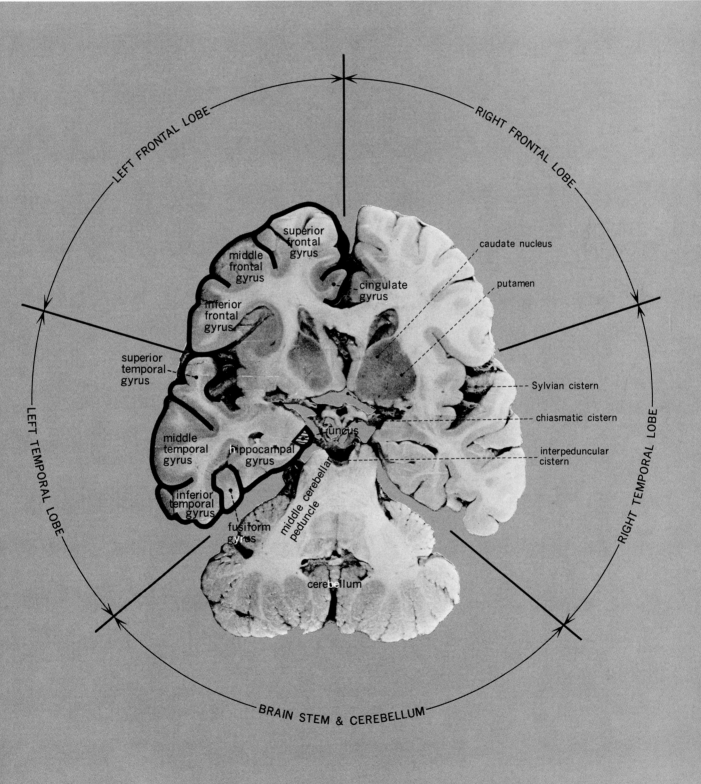

25° section, No. 14, uppersurface indicating prominent structures, lobes and gyri.

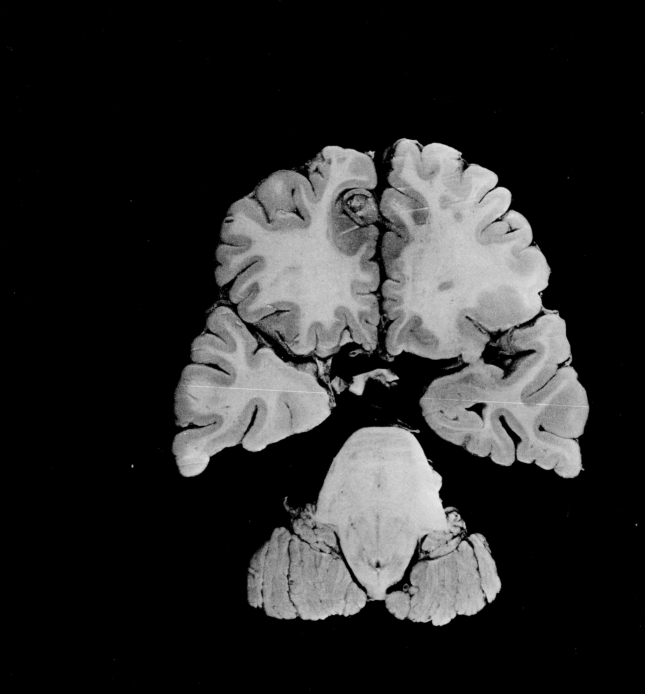

25° section, No. 15, uppersurface.

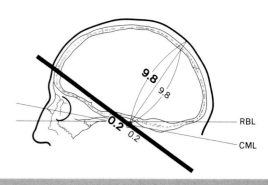

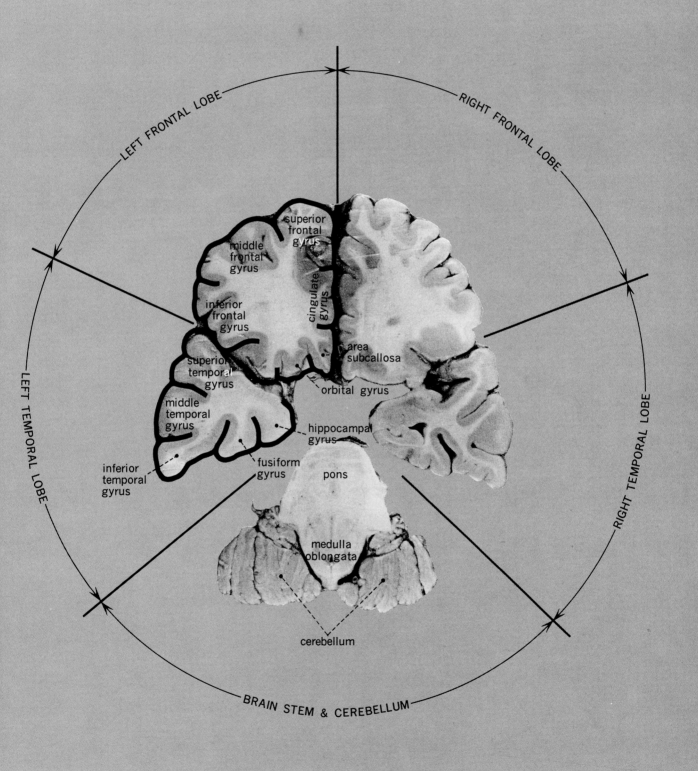

25° section, No. 15, uppersurface indicating prominent lobes and gyri.

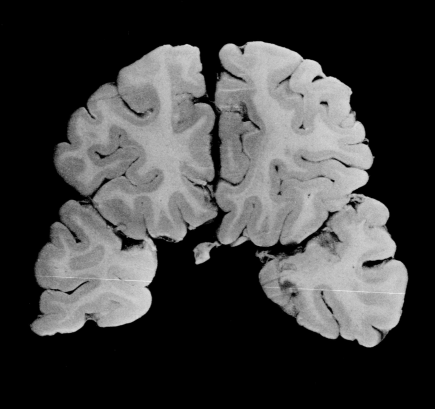

25° section, No. 16, uppersurface.

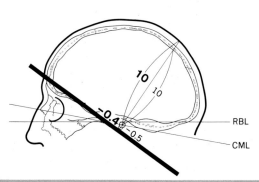

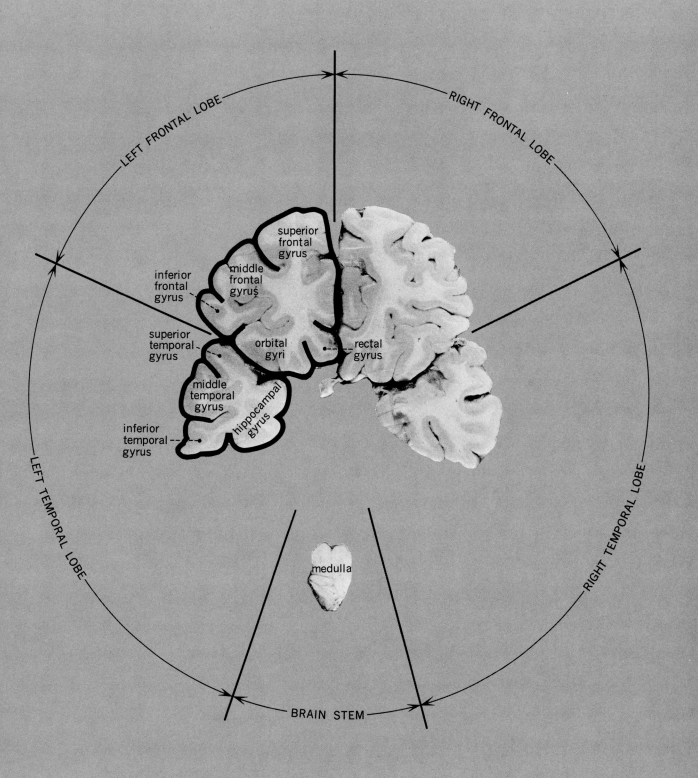

25° section, No. 16, uppersurface indicating prominent lobes and gyri.

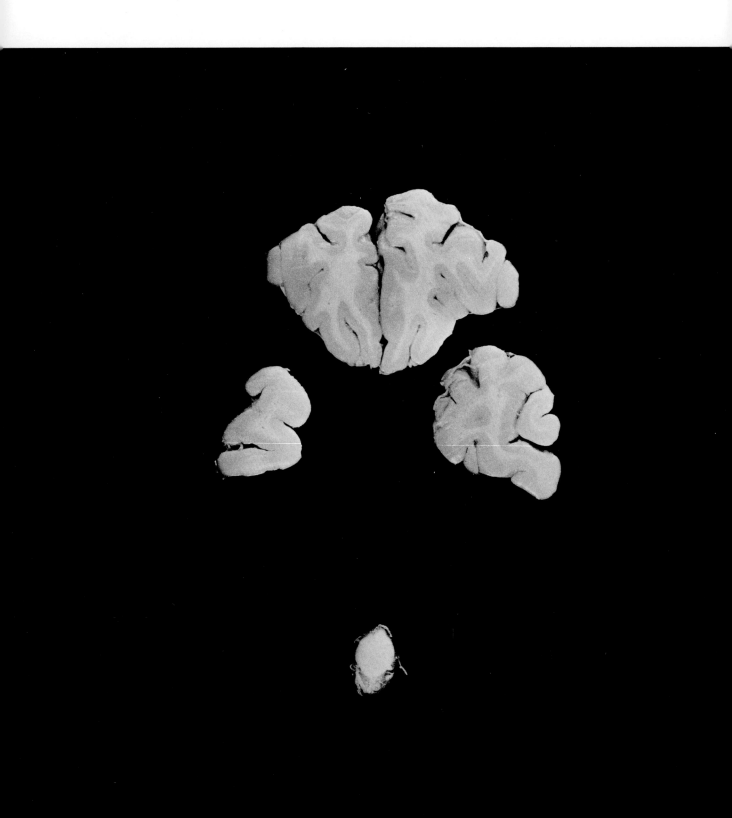

25° section, No. 17, uppersurface.

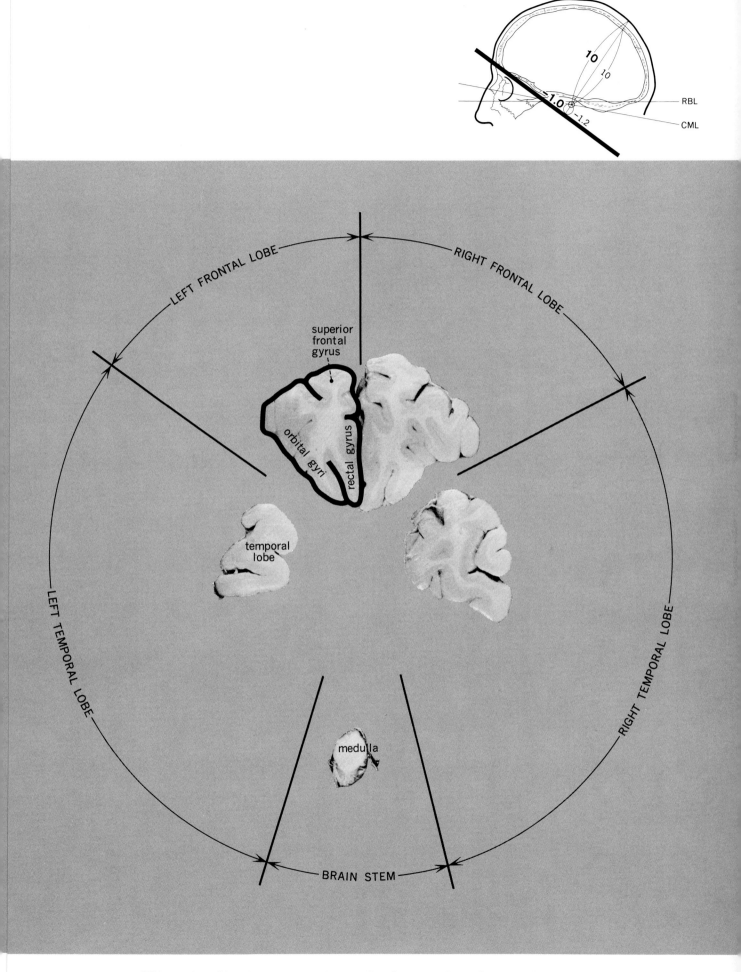

25° section, No. 17, uppersurface indicating prominent lobes and gyri.

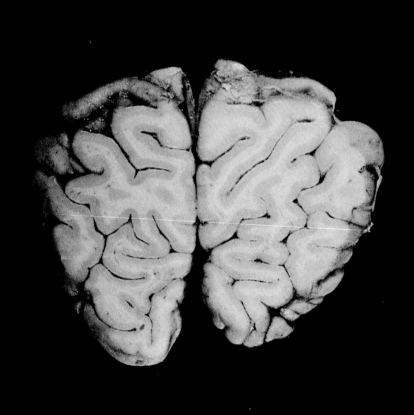

30° section, No. 2, uppersurface.

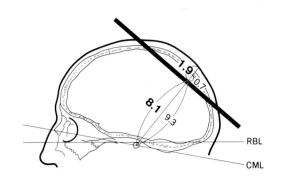

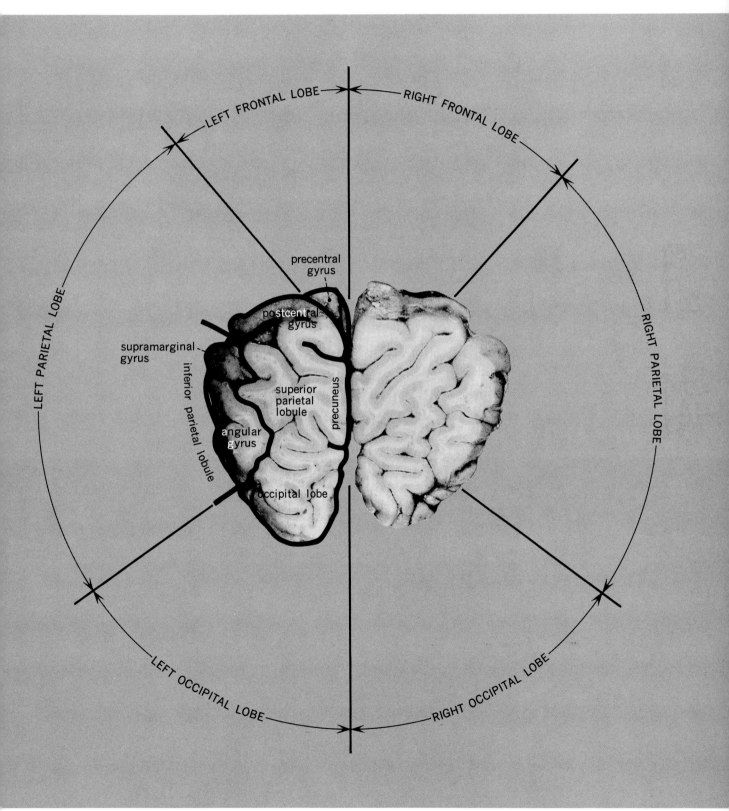

RBL

CML

precentral gyrus

postcentral gyrus

supramarginal gyrus

inferior parietal lobule

superior parietal lobule

precuneus

angular gyrus

occipital lobe

LEFT FRONTAL LOBE

RIGHT FRONTAL LOBE

LEFT PARIETAL LOBE

RIGHT PARIETAL LOBE

LEFT OCCIPITAL LOBE

RIGHT OCCIPITAL LOBE

30° section, No. 2, uppersurface indicating prominent lobes and gyri.

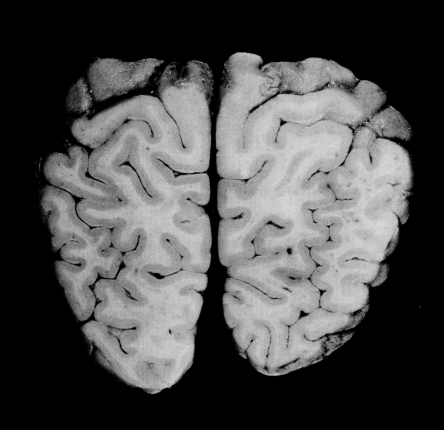

30° section, No. 3, uppersurface.

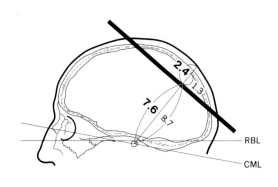

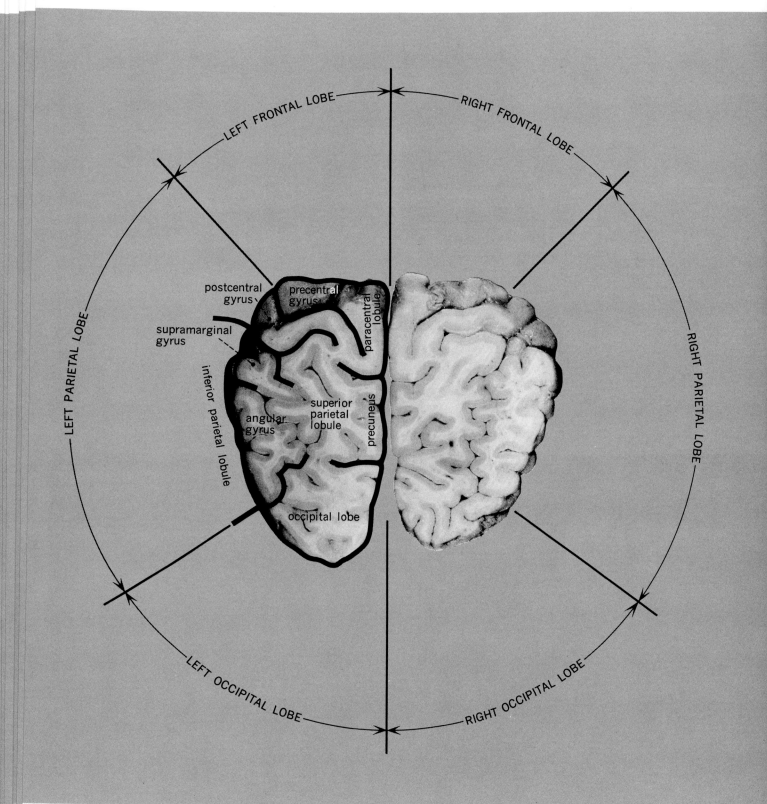

postcentral gyrus

precentral gyrus

paracentral lobule

supramarginal gyrus

inferior parietal lobule

angular gyrus

superior parietal lobule

precuneus

occipital lobe

LEFT FRONTAL LOBE

RIGHT FRONTAL LOBE

LEFT PARIETAL LOBE

RIGHT PARIETAL LOBE

LEFT OCCIPITAL LOBE

RIGHT OCCIPITAL LOBE

RBL

CML

2.4 1.3

7.6 8.7

30° section, No. 3, uppersurface indicating prominent lobes and gyri.

239

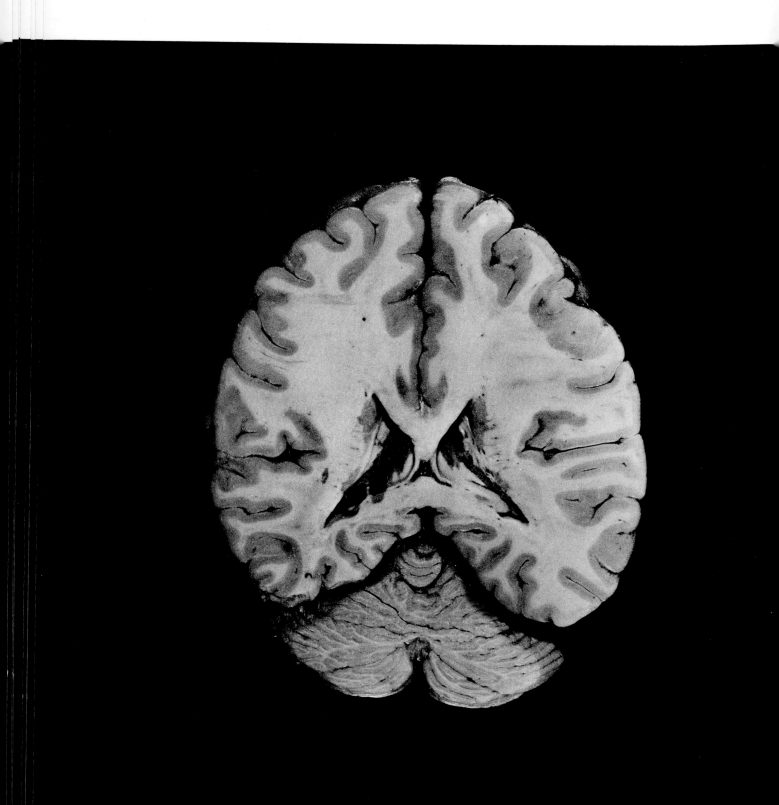

30° section, No. 10, uppersurface.

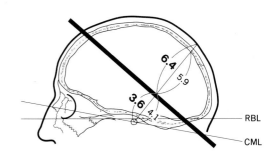

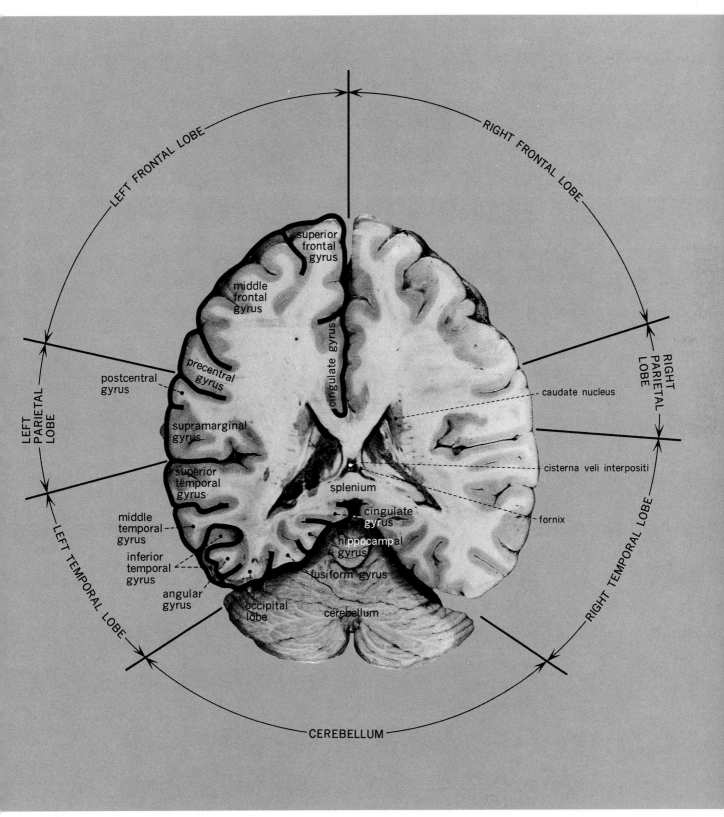

30° section, No. 10, uppersurface indicating prominent structures, lobes and gyri.

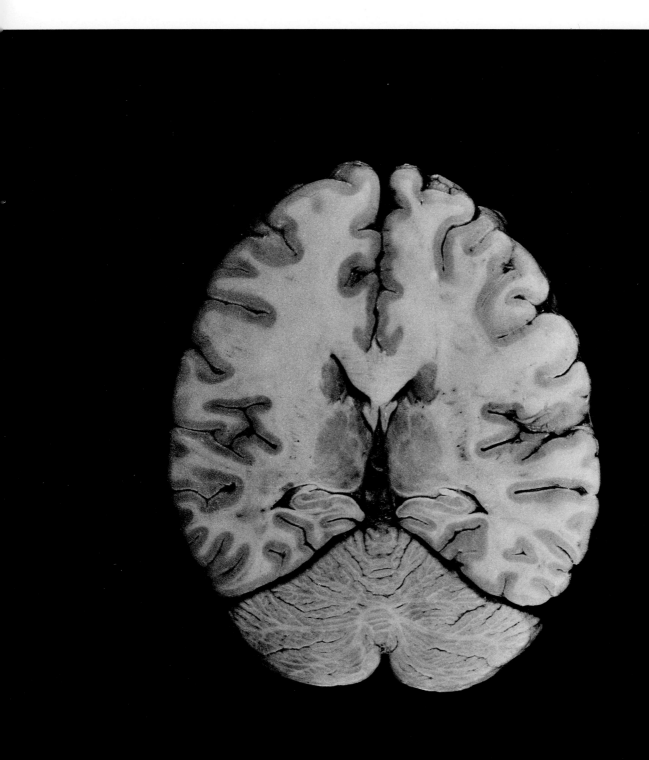

30° section, No. 11, uppersurface.

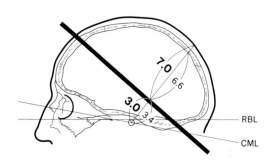

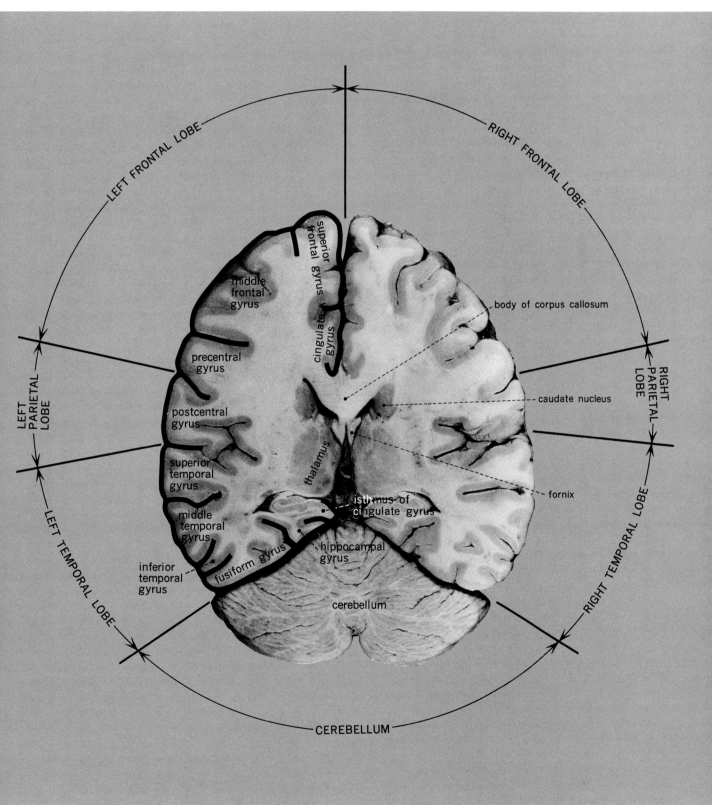

30° section, No. 11, uppersurface indicating prominent structures, lobes and gyri.

255

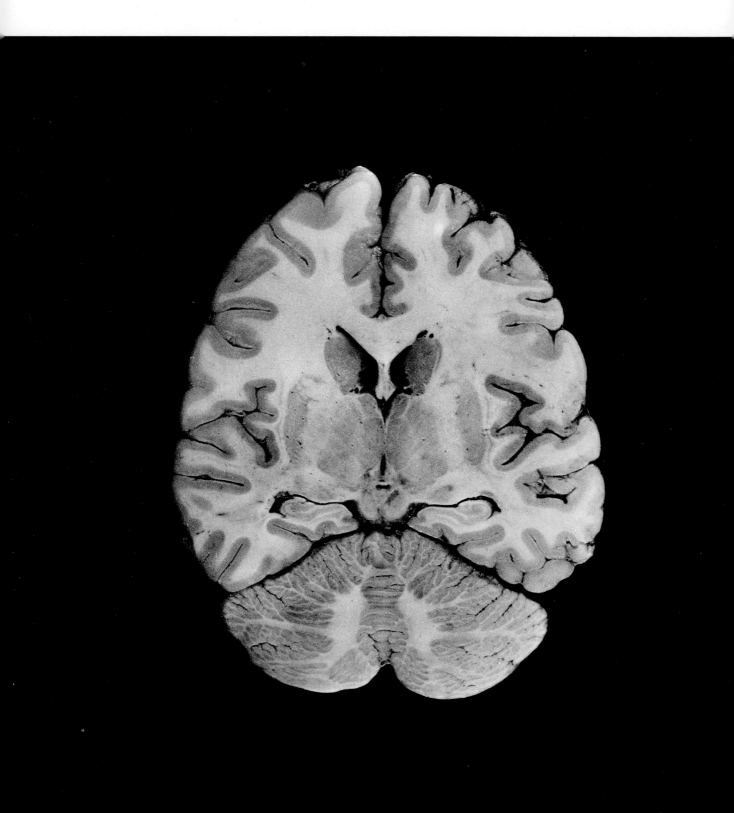

30° section, No. 12, uppersurface.

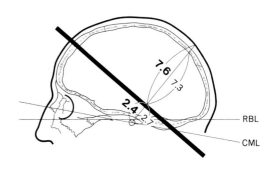

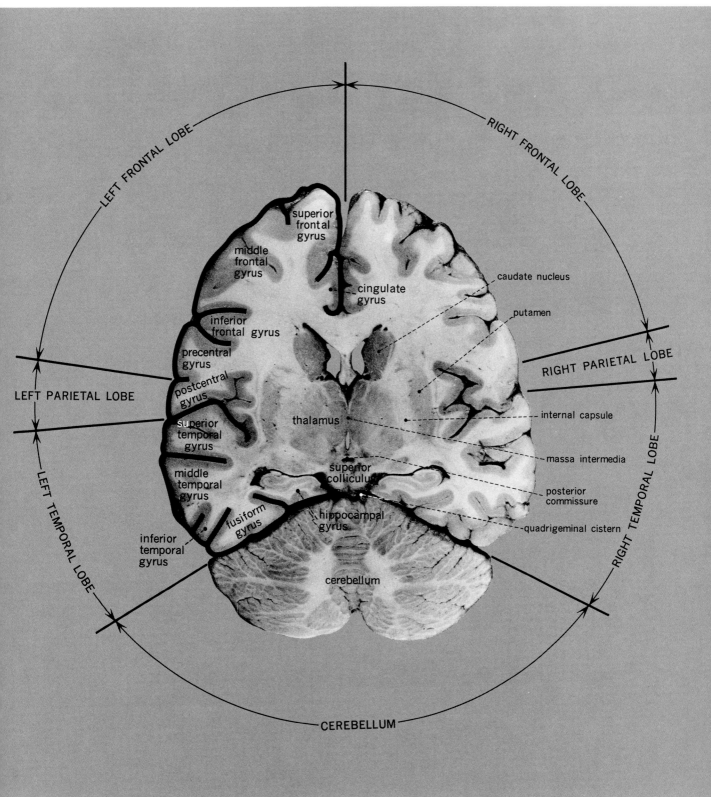

30° section, No. 12, uppersurface indicating prominent structures, lobes and gyri.

30°- 13

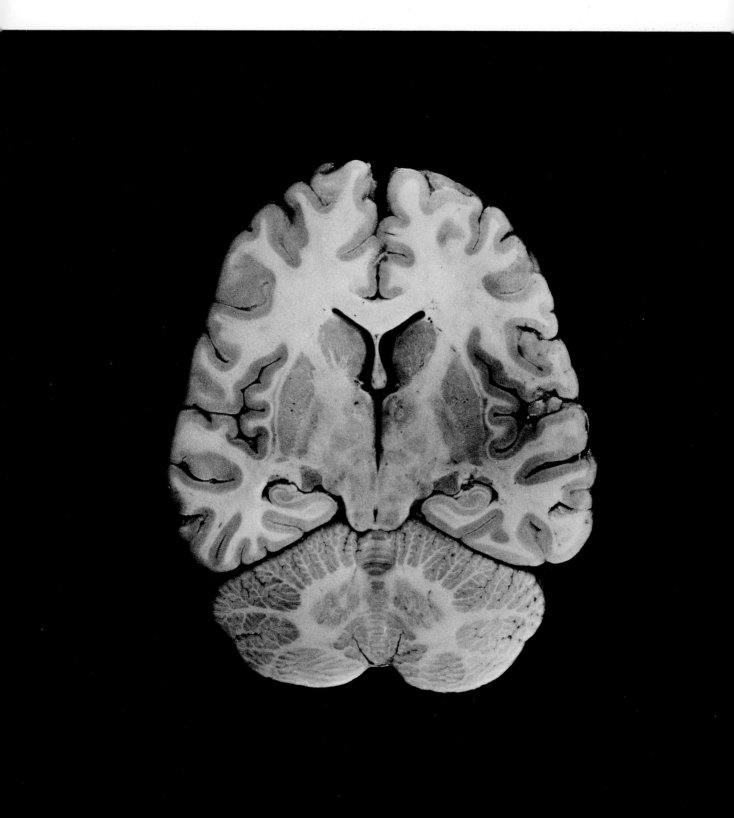

30° section, No. 13, uppersurface.

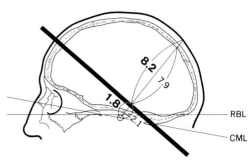

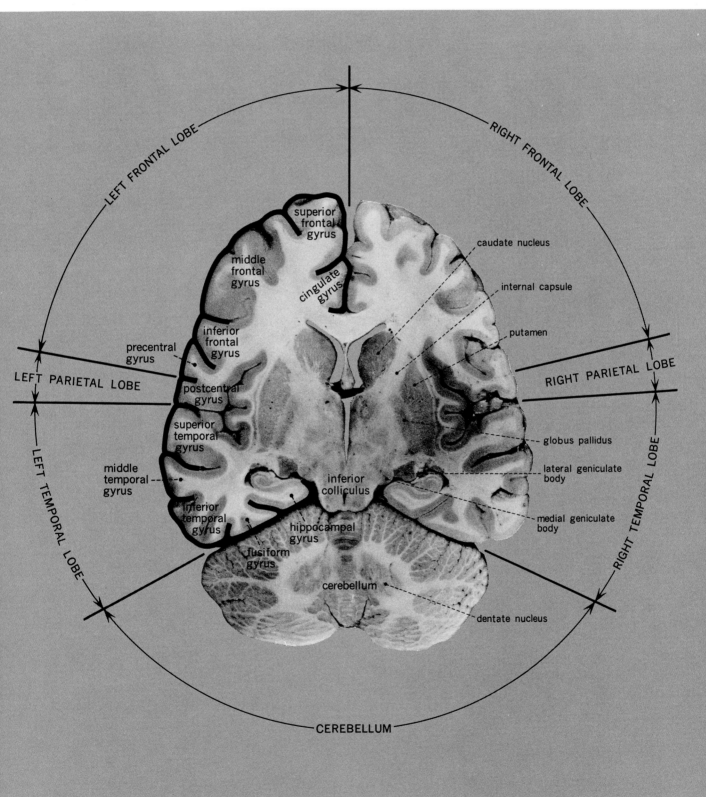

30° section, No. 13, uppersurface indicating prominent structures, lobes and gyri.

259

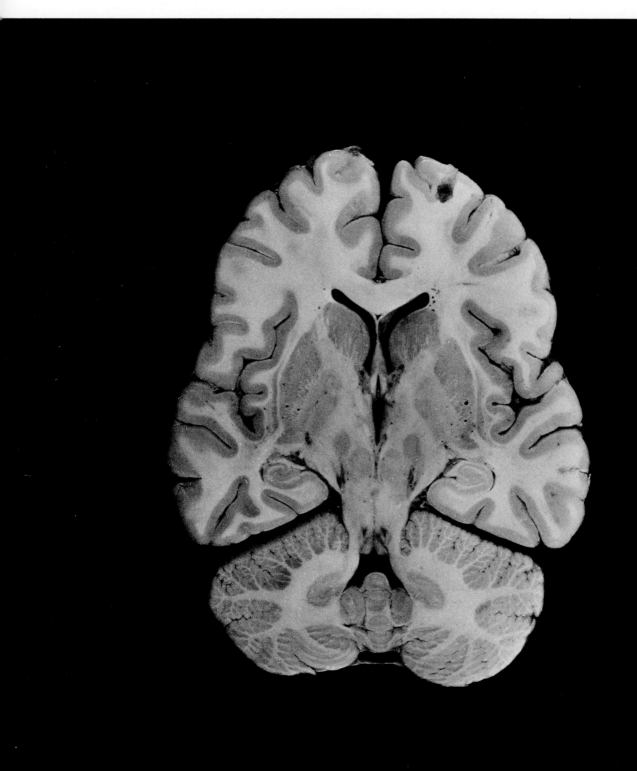

30° section, No. 14, uppersurface.

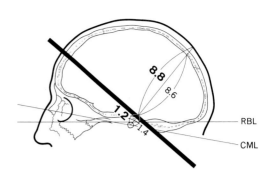

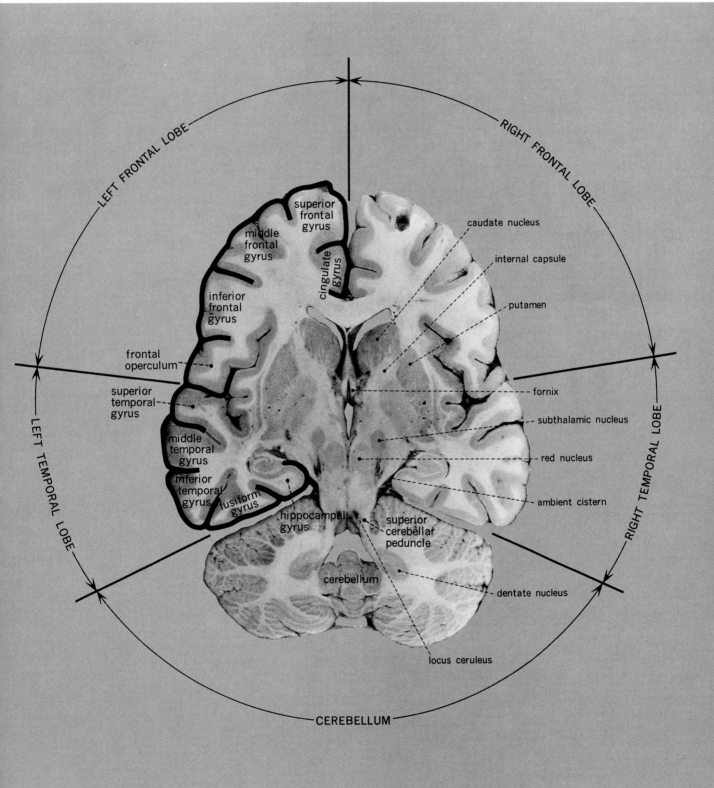

30° section, No. 14, uppersurface indicating prominent structures, lobes and gyri.

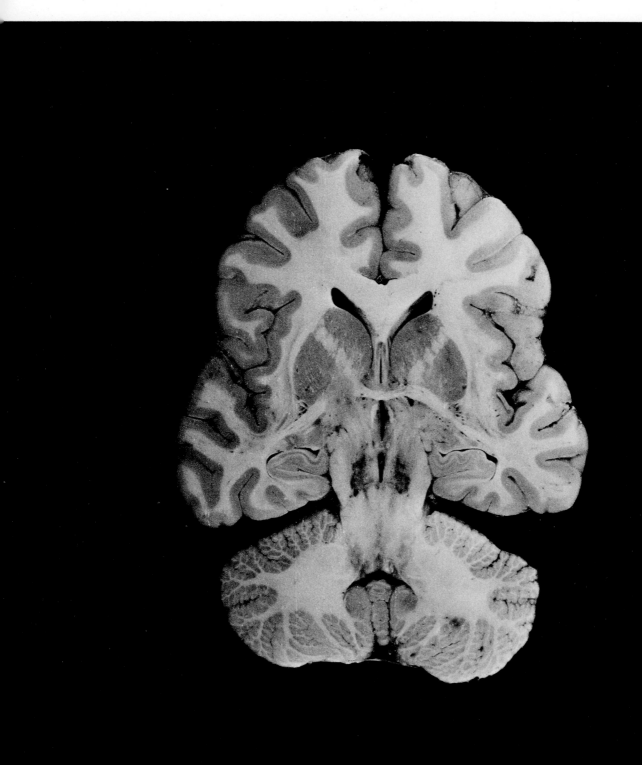

30° section, No. 15, uppersurface.

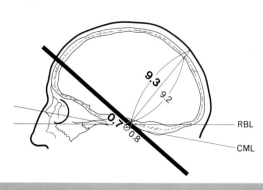

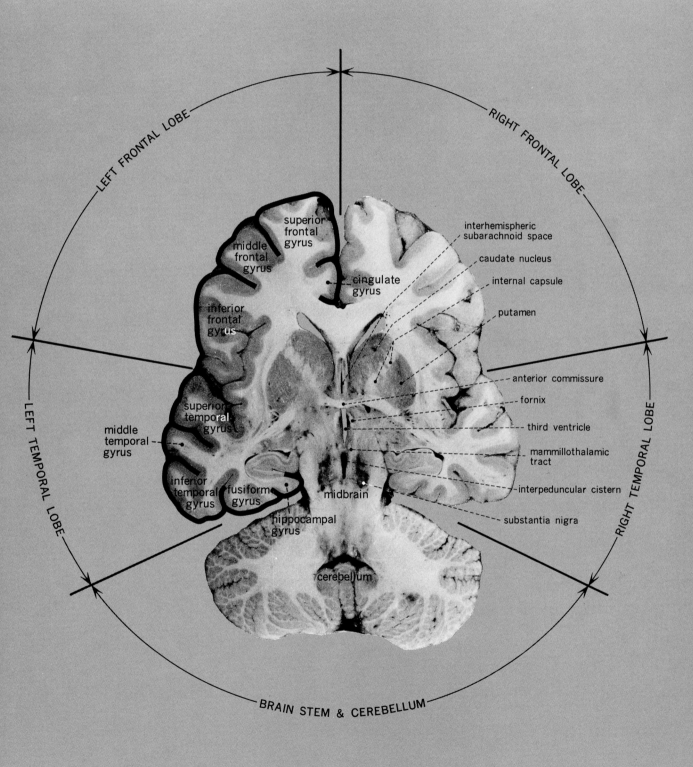

30° section, No. 15, uppersurface indicating prominent structures, lobes and gyri.

263

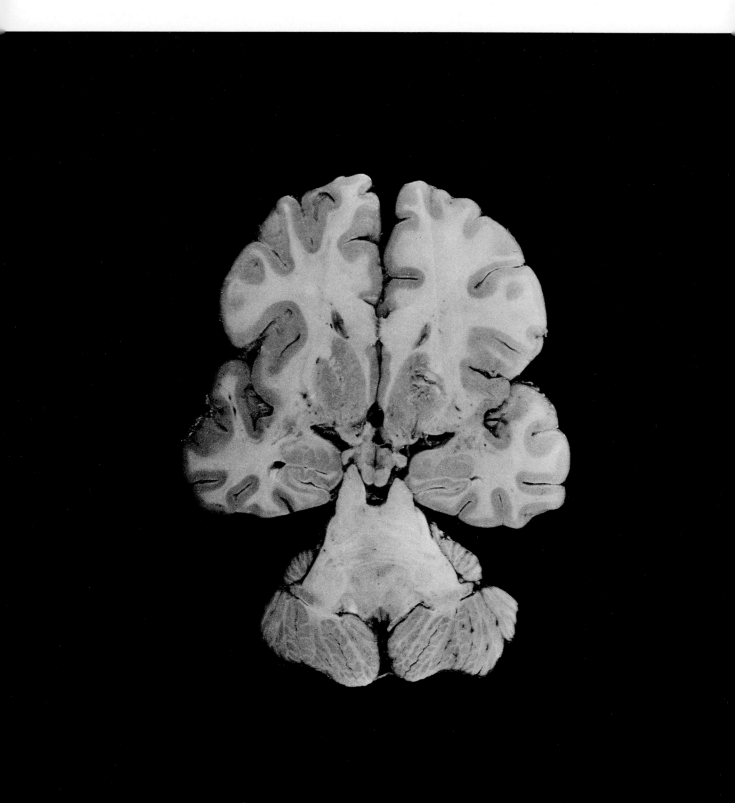

30° section, No. 16, uppersurface.

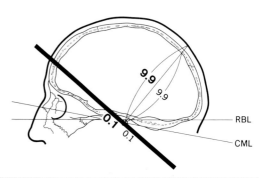

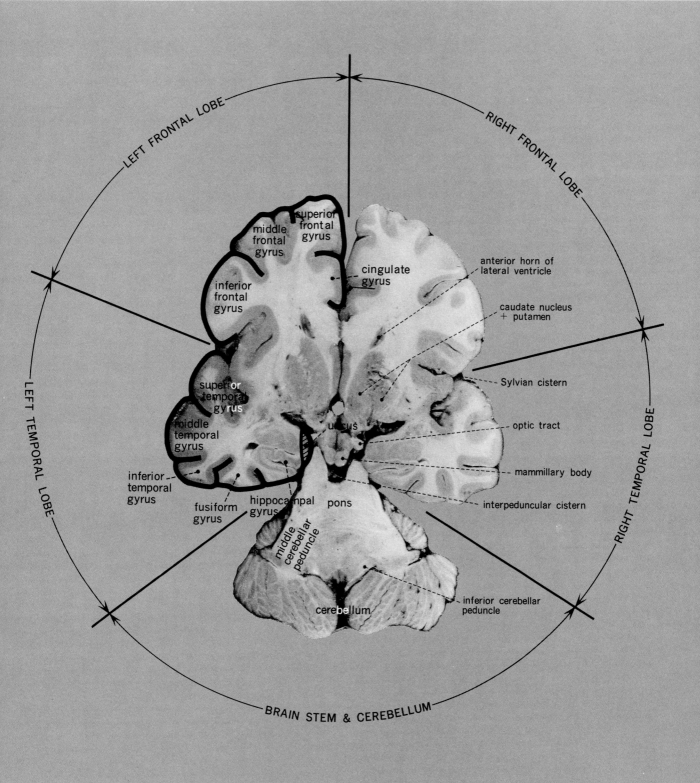

30° section, No. 16, uppersurface indicating prominent structures, lobes and gyri.

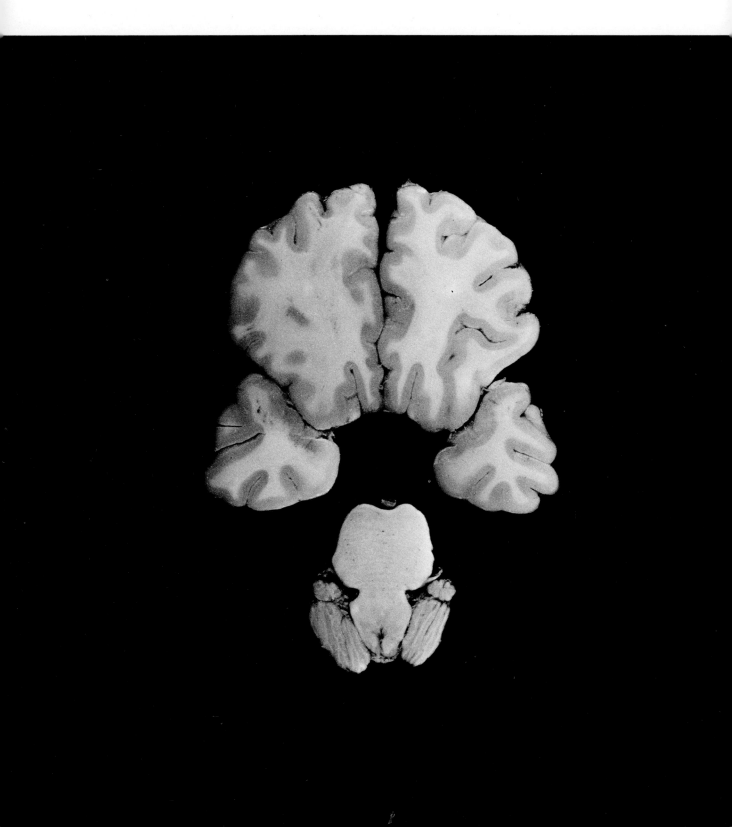

30° section, No. 17, uppersurface.

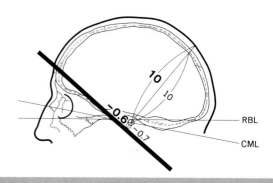

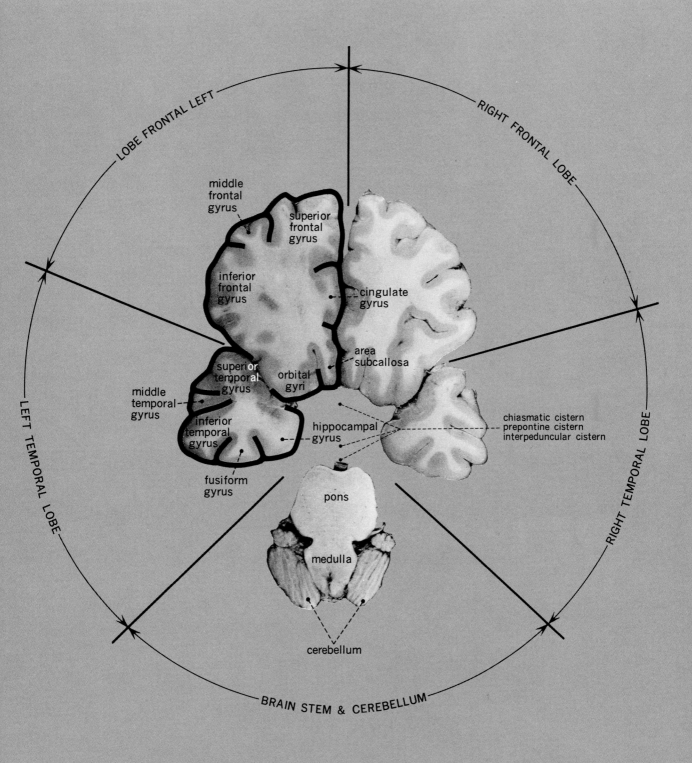

30° section, No. 17, uppersurface indicating prominent structures, lobes and gyri.

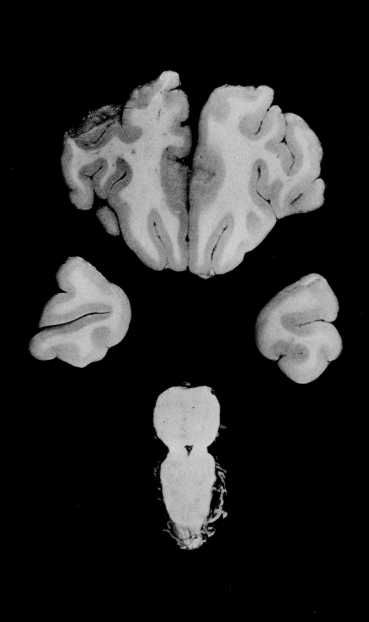

30° section, No. 18, uppersurface.

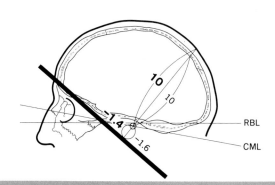

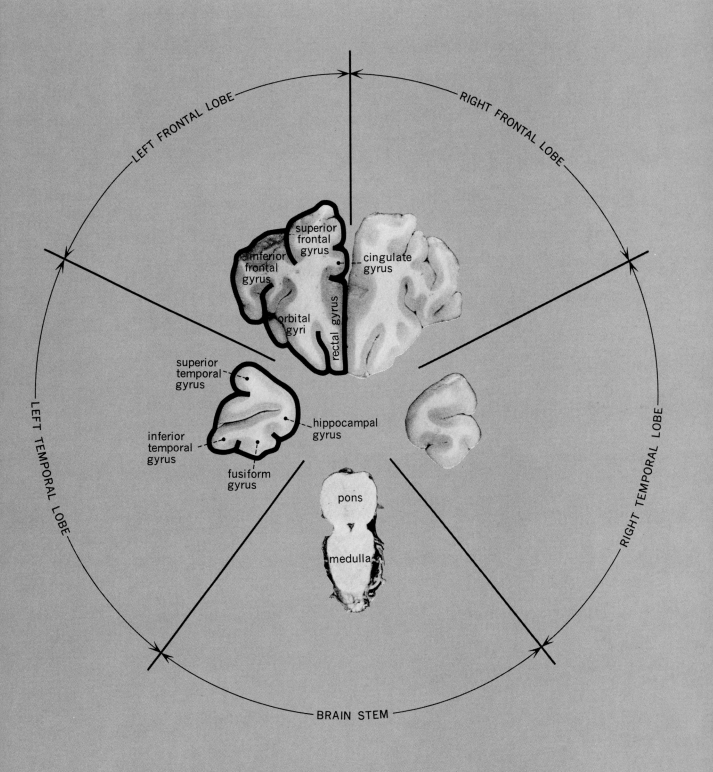

30° section, No. 18, uppersurface indicating prominent lobes and gyri.

40°-1

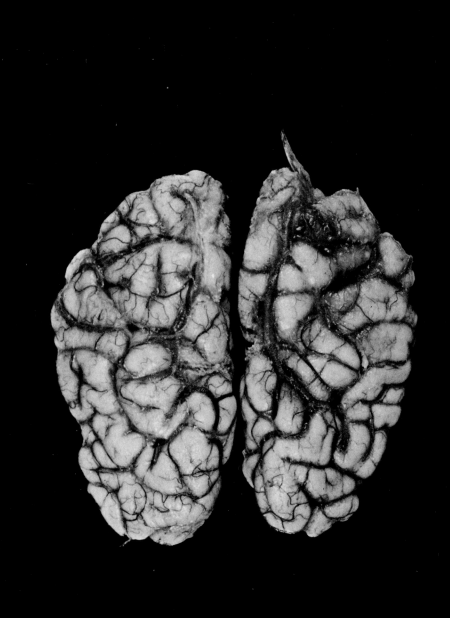

40° section, No. 1, uppersurface.

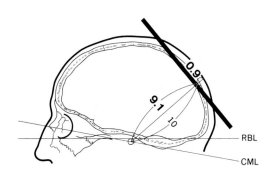

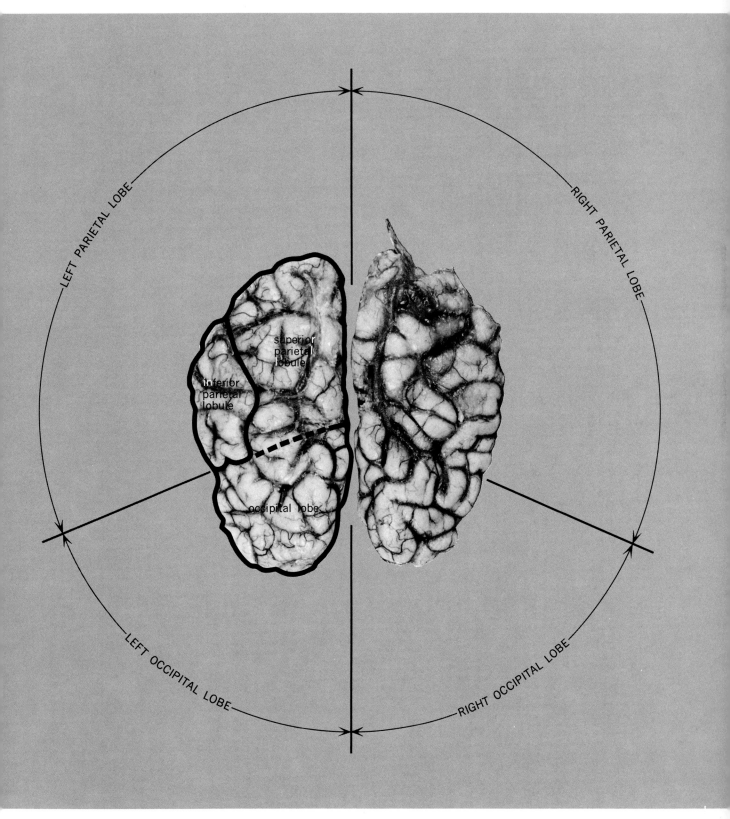

40° section, No. 1, uppersurface indicating prominent lobes and gyri.

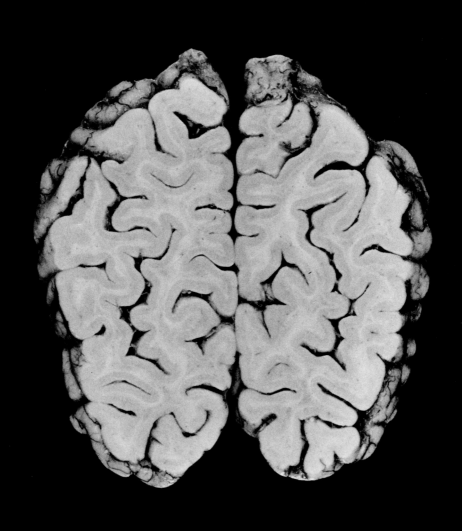

40° section, No. 2, uppersurface.

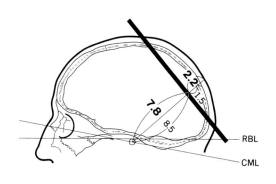

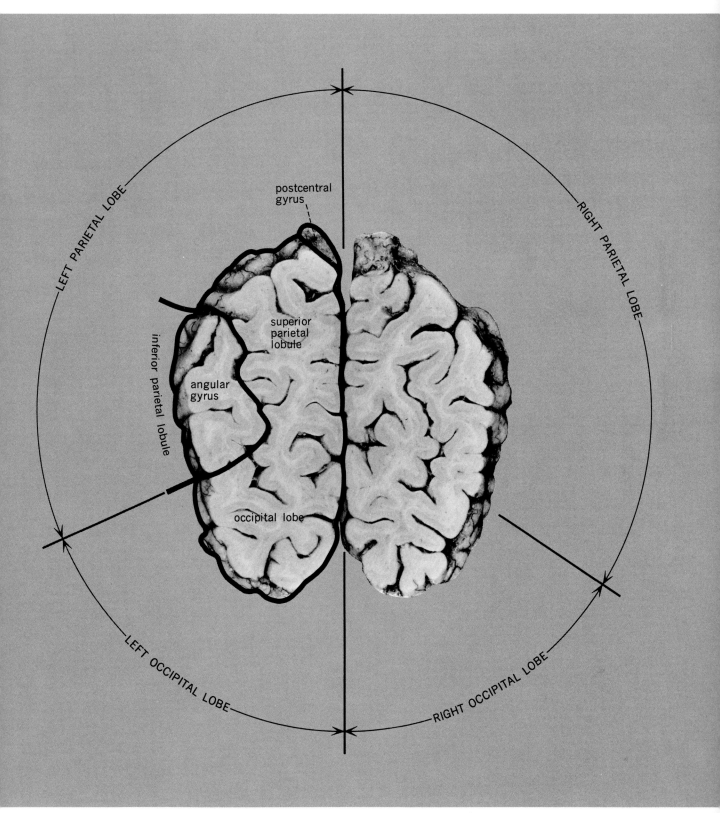

40° section, No. 2, uppersurface indicating prominent lobes and gyri.

275

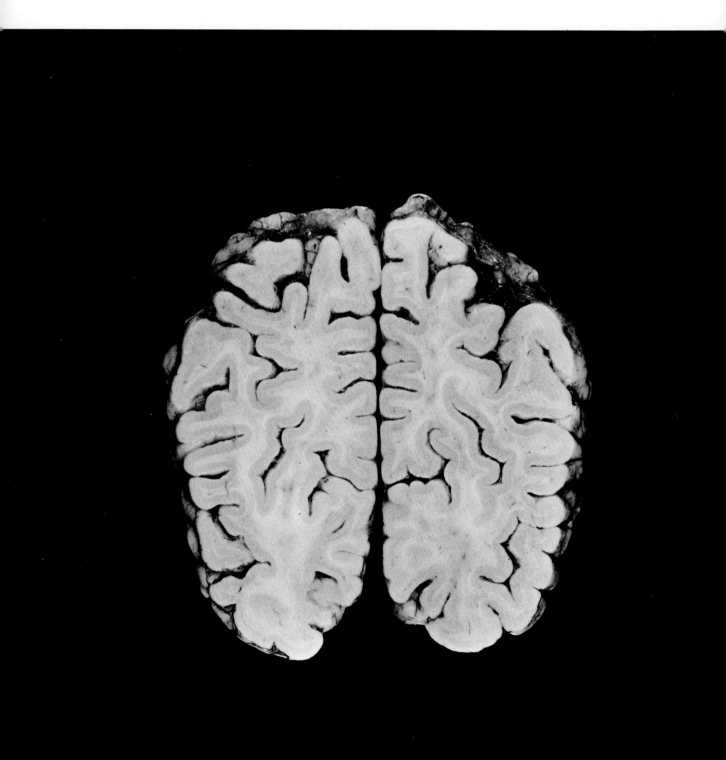

40° section, No. 3, uppersurface.

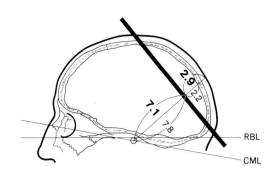

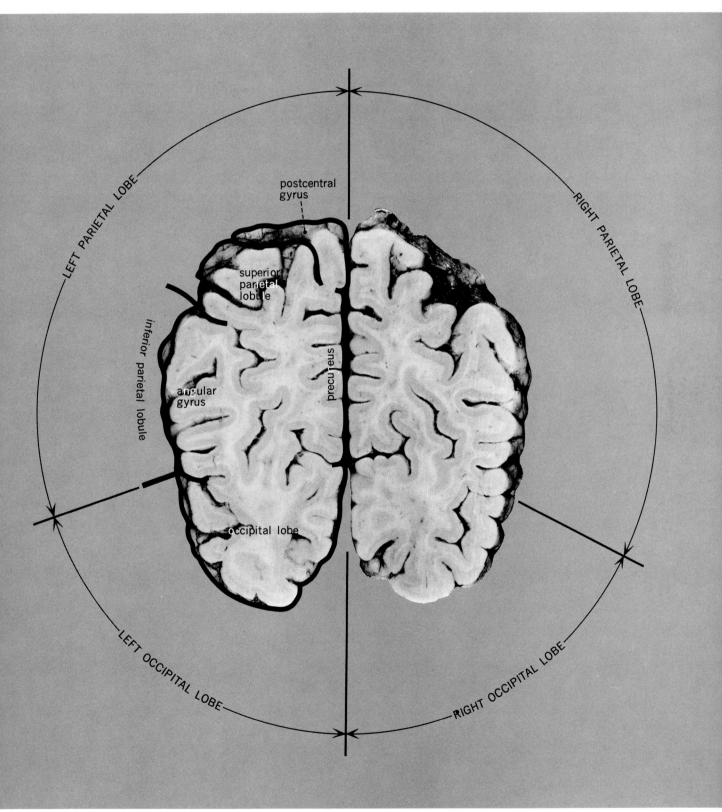

40° section, No. 3, uppersurface indicating prominent lobes and gyri.

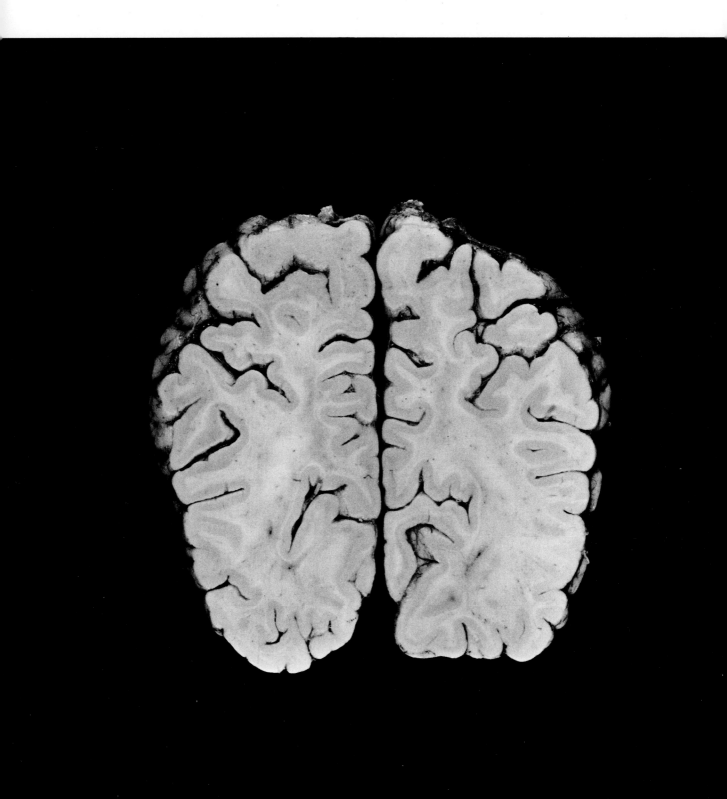

40° section, No. 4, uppersurface.

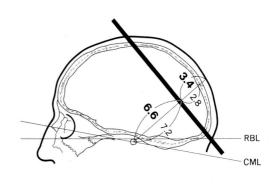

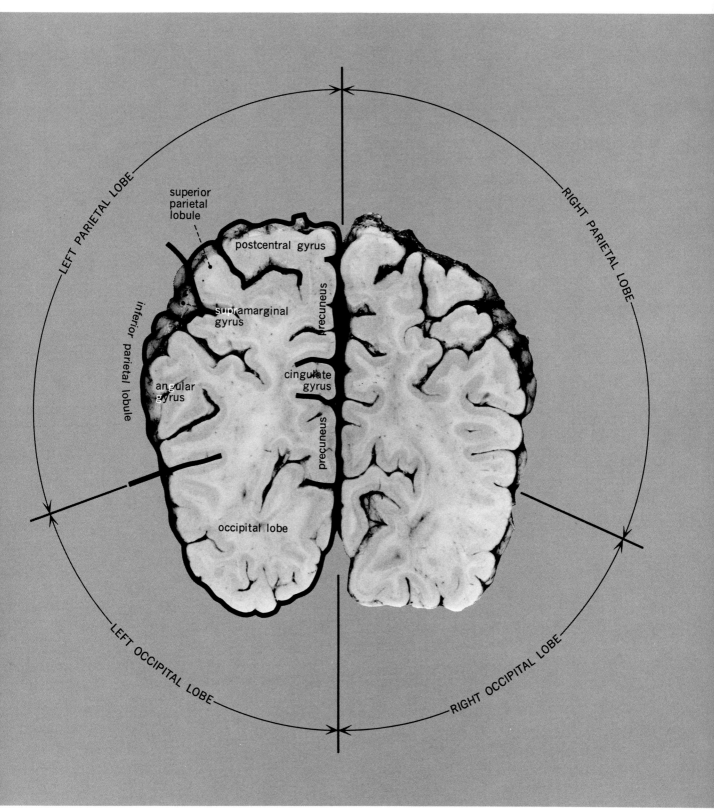

40° section, No. 4, uppersurface indicating prominent lobes and gyri.

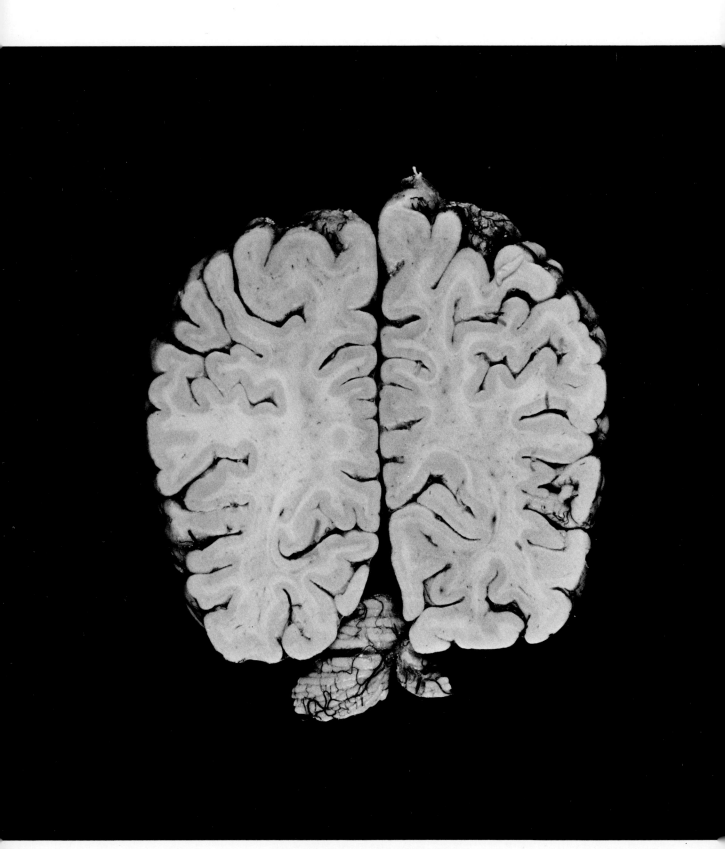

40° section, No. 5, uppersurface.

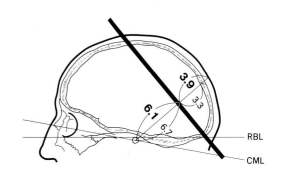

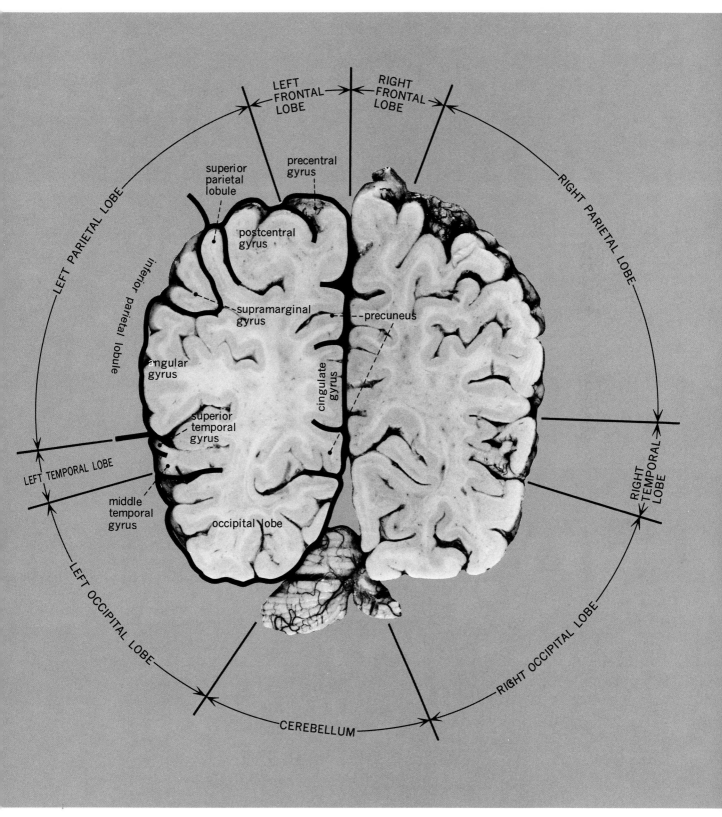

40° section, No. 5, uppersurface indicating prominent lobes and gyri.

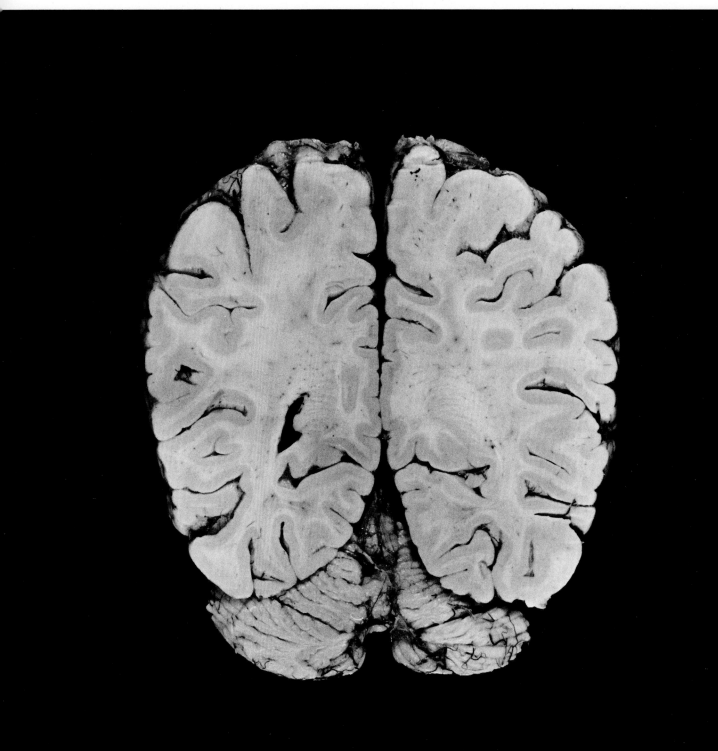

40° section, No. 6, uppersurface.

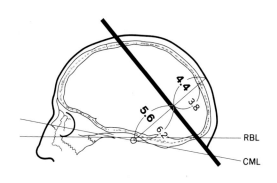

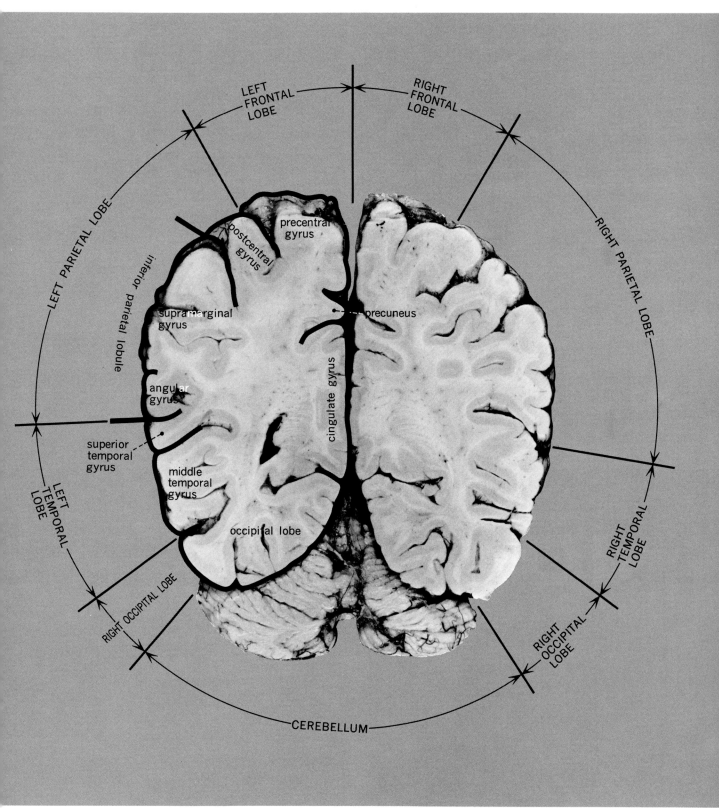

40° section, No. 6, uppersurface indicating prominent lobes and gyri.

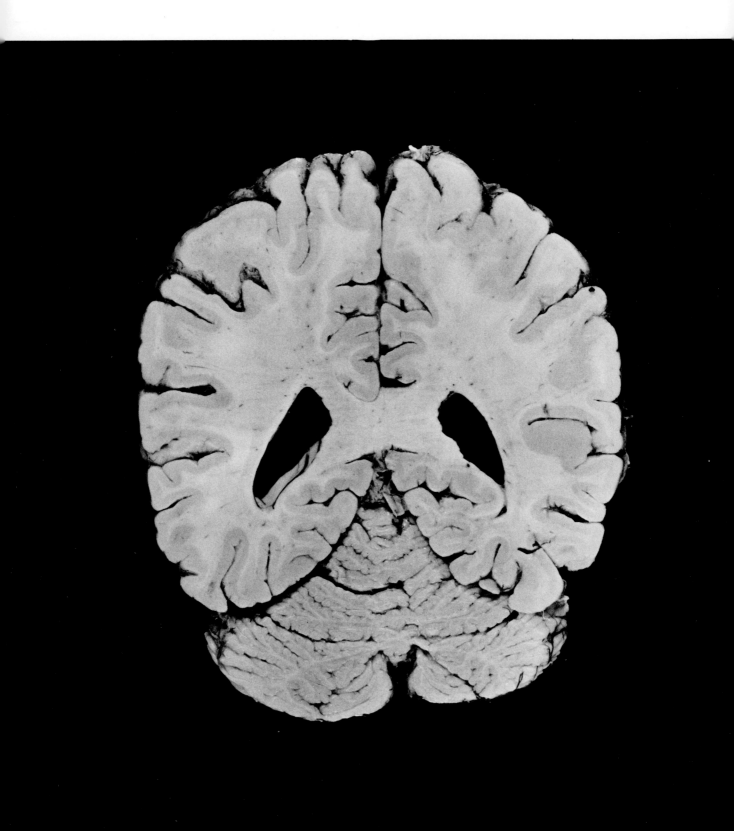

40° section, No. 7, uppersurface.

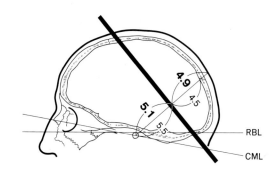

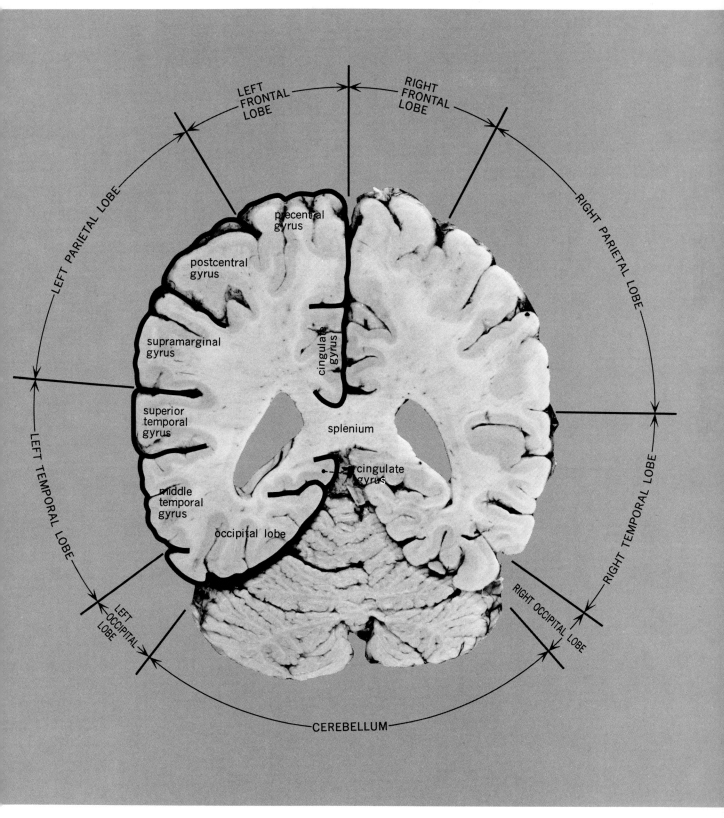

40° section, No. 7, uppersurface indicating prominent lobes and gyri.

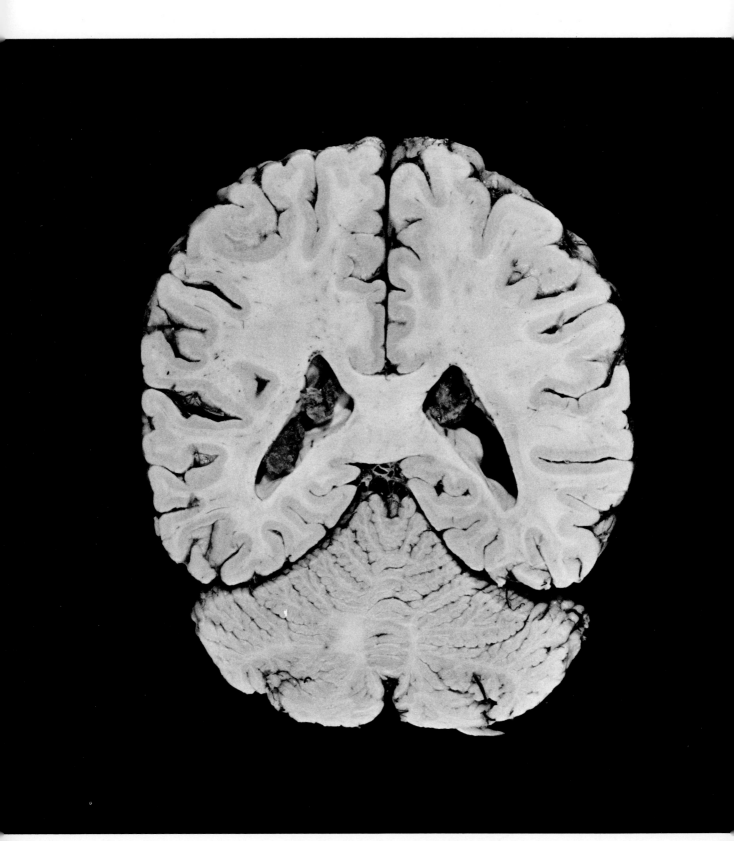

40° section, No. 8, uppersurface.

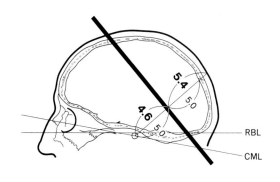

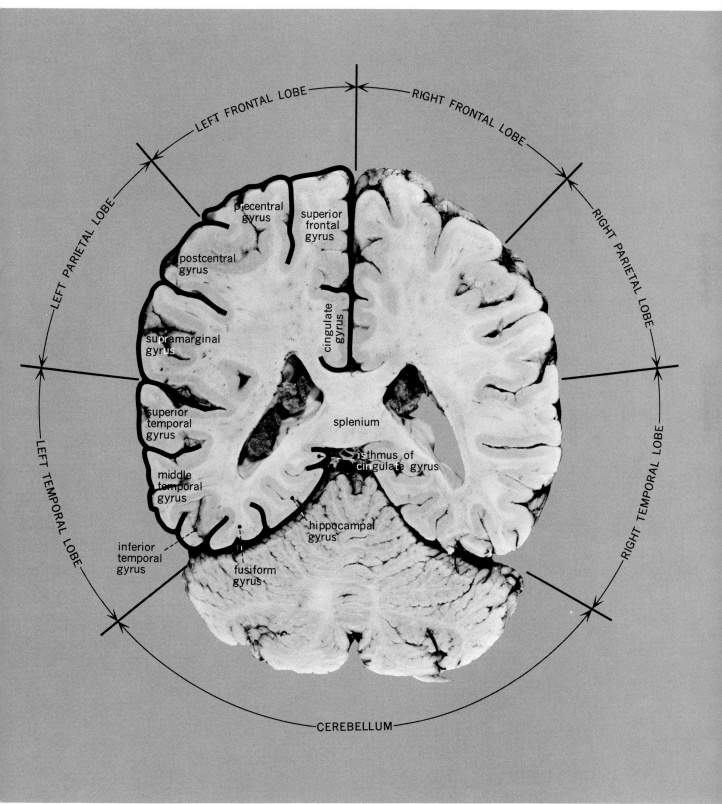

40° section, No. 8, uppersurface indicating prominent lobes and gyri.

40°-9

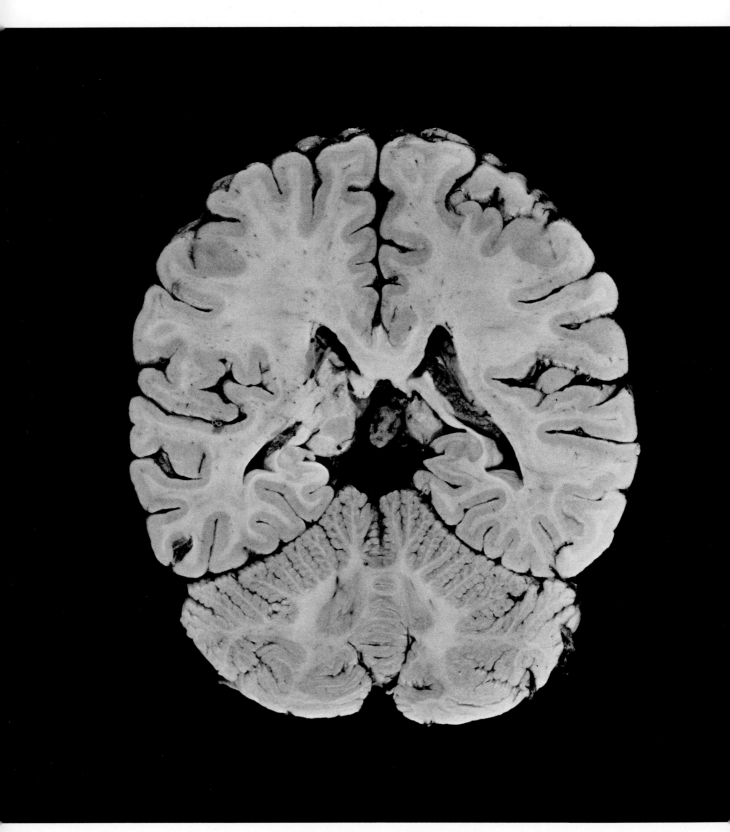

40° section, No. 9, uppersurface.

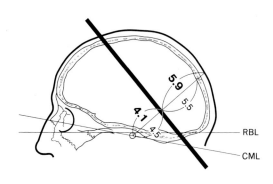

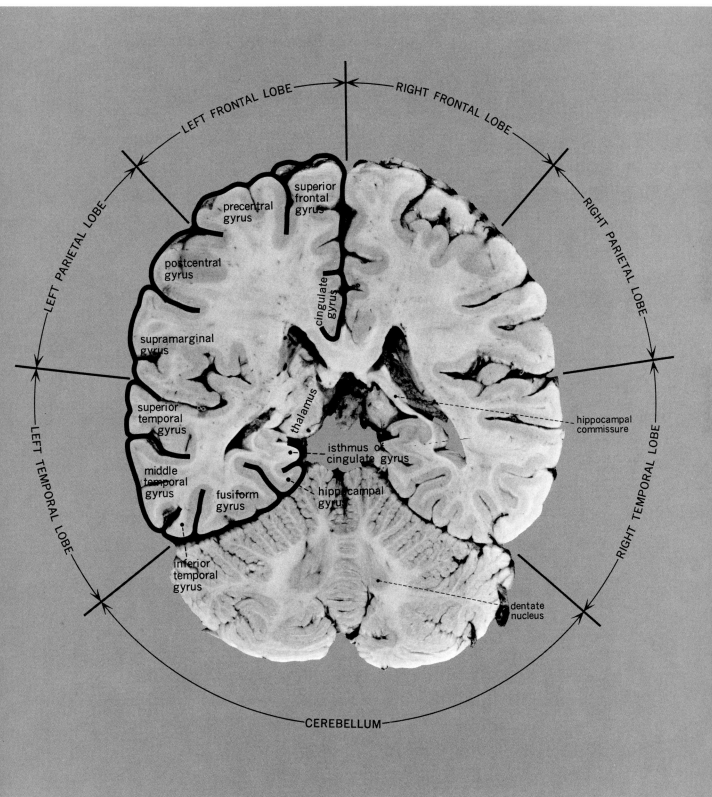

40° section, No. 9, uppersurface indicating prominent structures, lobes and gyri.

289

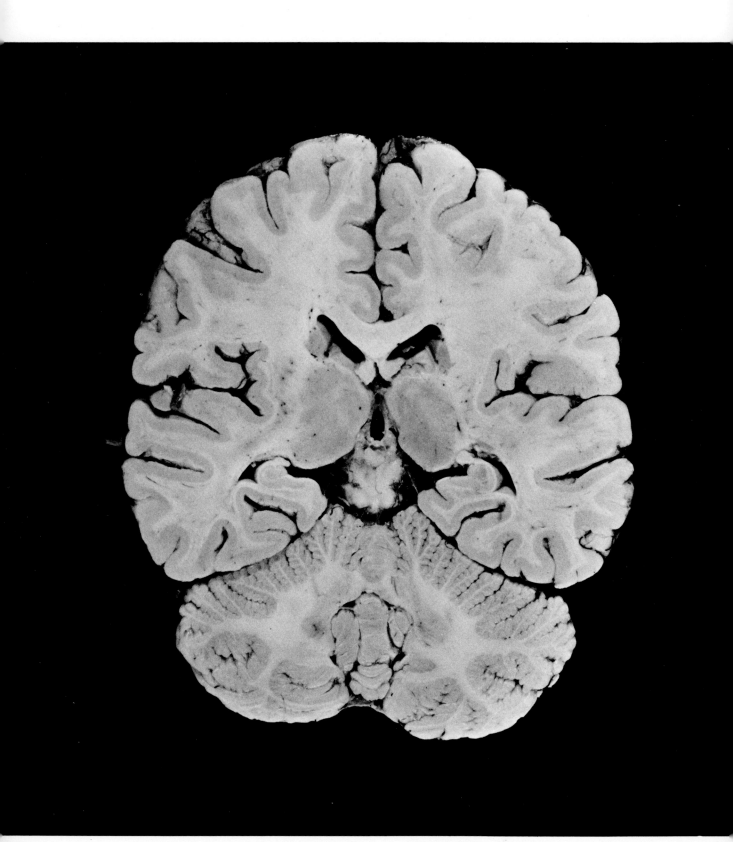

40° section, No. 10, uppersurface.

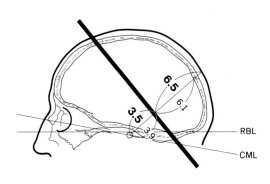

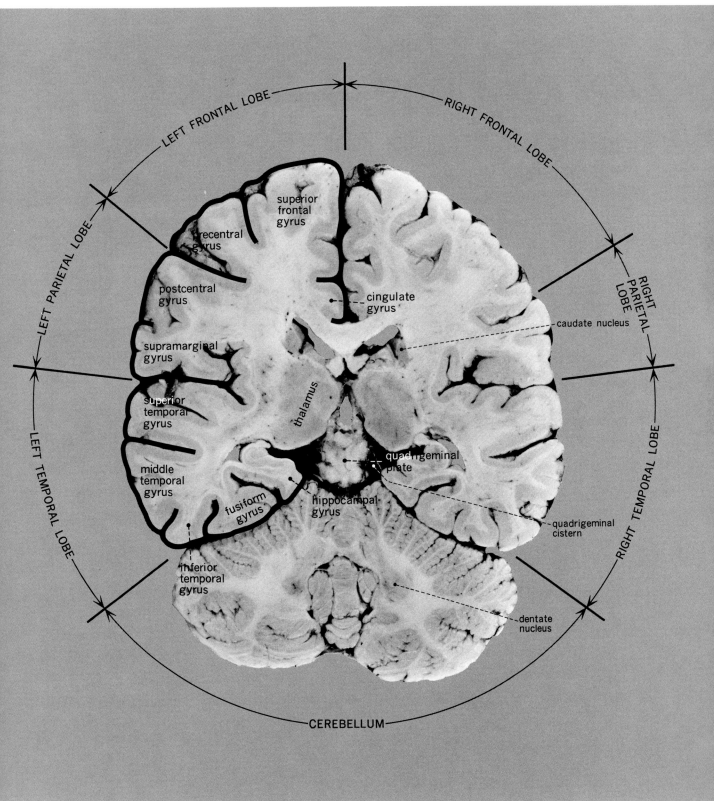

40° section, No. 10, uppersurface indicating prominent structures, lobes and gyri.

291

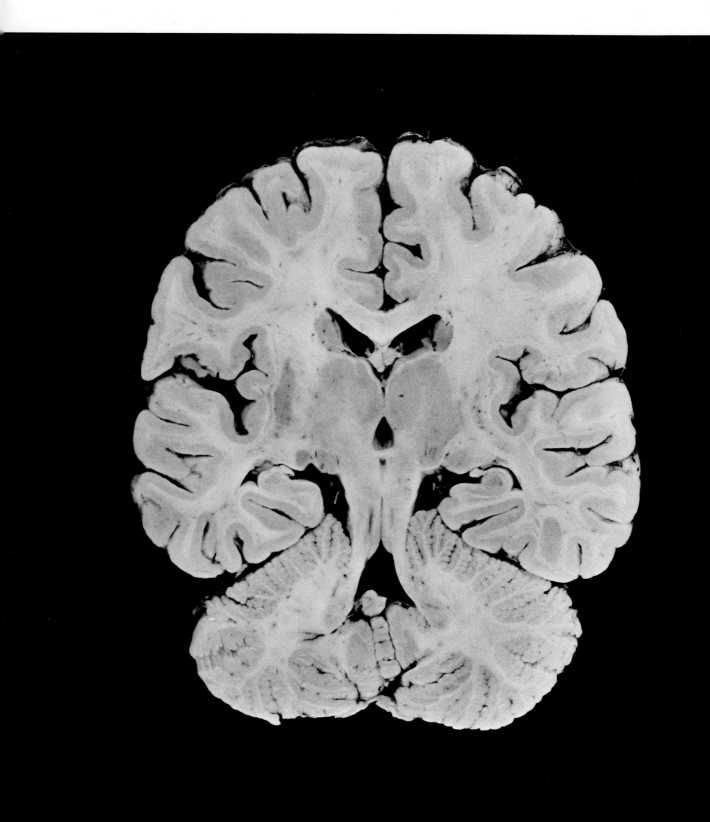

40° section, No. 11, uppersurface.

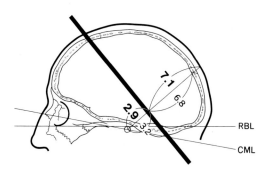

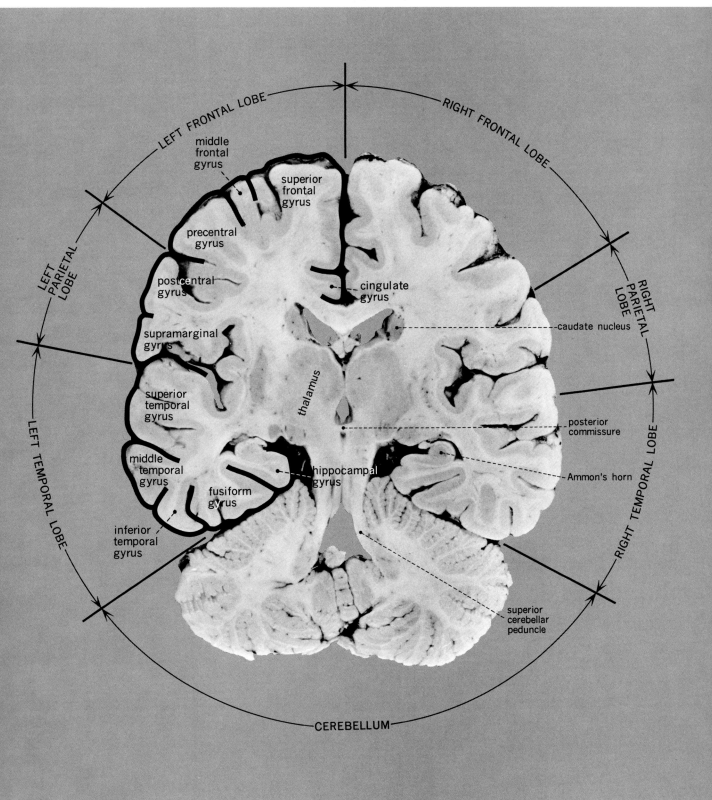

40° section, No. 11, uppersurface indicating prominent structures, lobes and gyri.

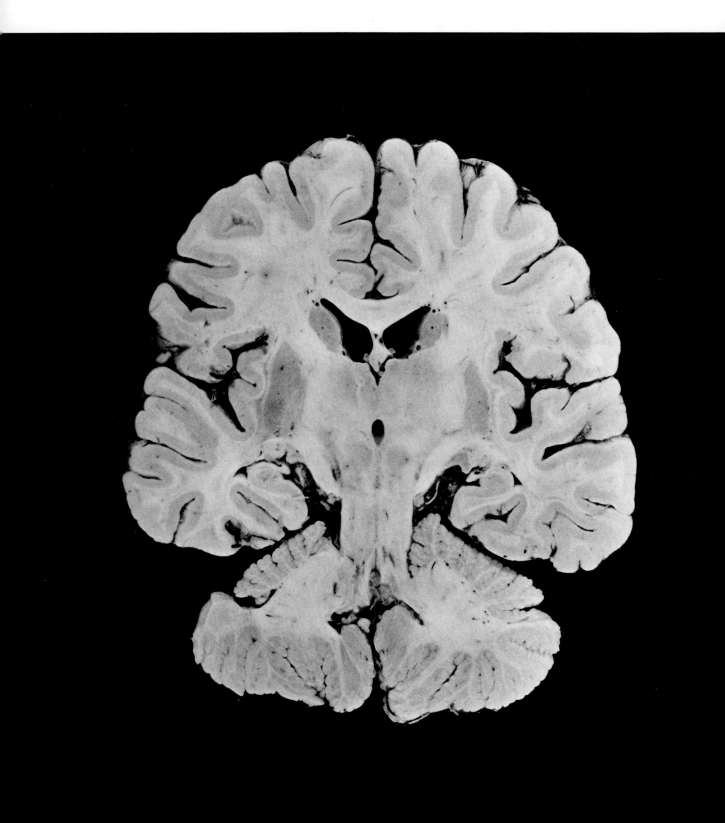

40° section, No. 12, uppersurface.

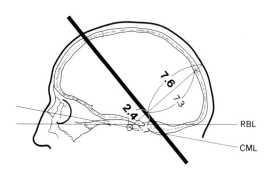

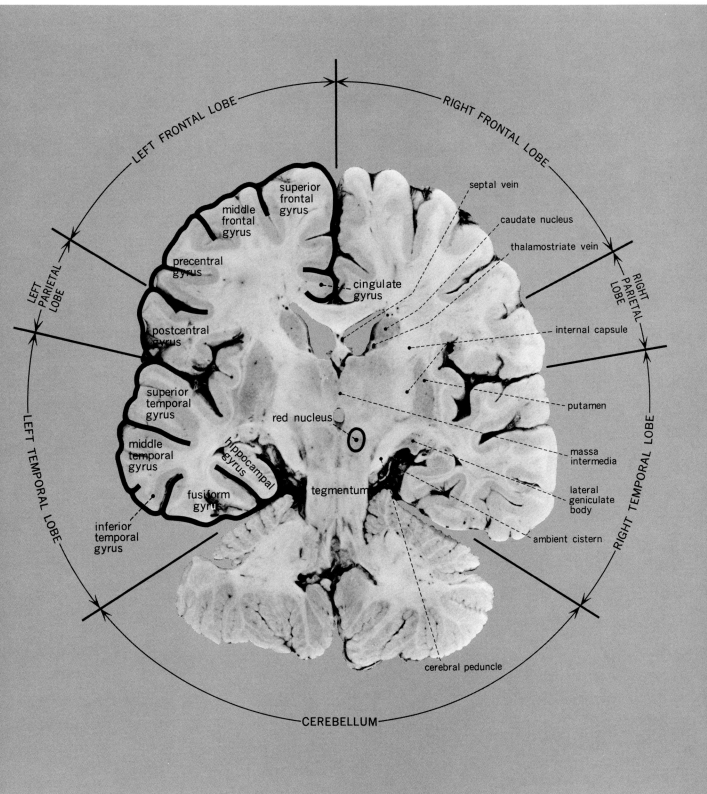

40° section, No. 12, uppersurface indicating prominent structures, lobes and gyri.

295

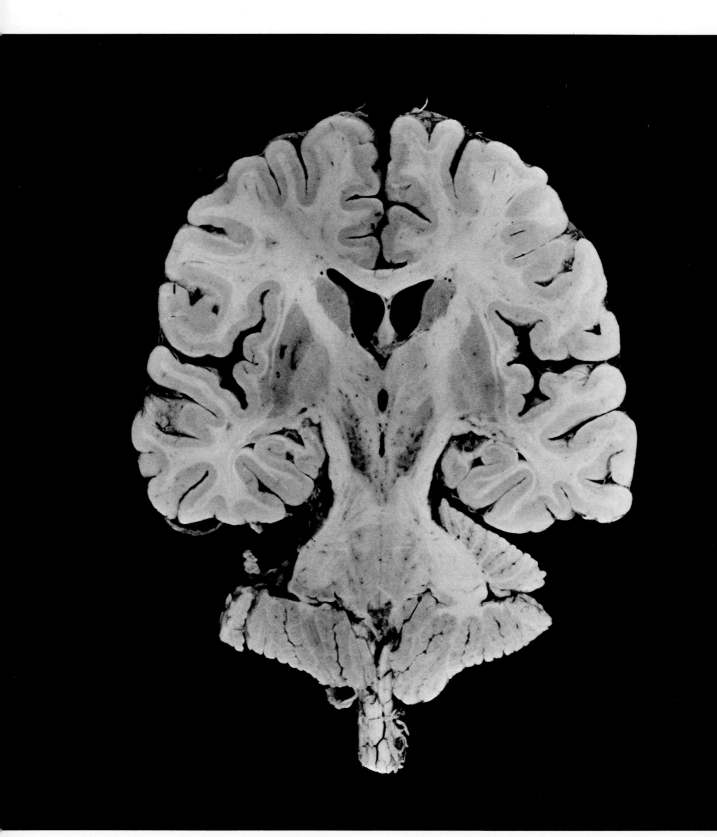

40° section, No. 13, uppersurface.

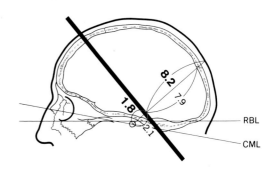

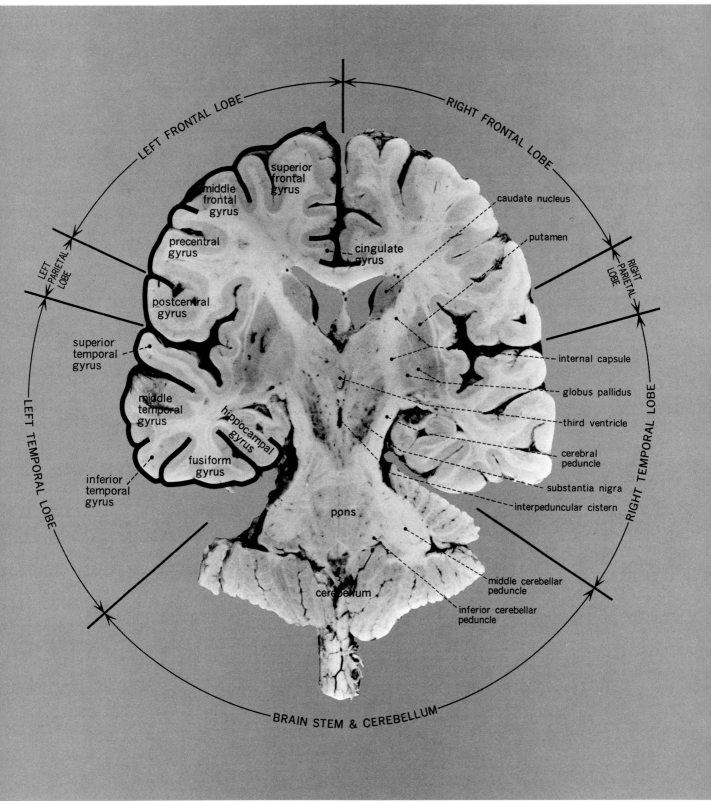

RBL

CML

8.2 7.9

1.8 2.1

LEFT FRONTAL LOBE

RIGHT FRONTAL LOBE

LEFT PARIETAL LOBE

RIGHT PARIETAL LOBE

LEFT TEMPORAL LOBE

RIGHT TEMPORAL LOBE

BRAIN STEM & CEREBELLUM

superior frontal gyrus

middle frontal gyrus

precentral gyrus

postcentral gyrus

cingulate gyrus

caudate nucleus

putamen

internal capsule

globus pallidus

third ventricle

cerebral peduncle

substantia nigra

interpeduncular cistern

superior temporal gyrus

middle temporal gyrus

hippocampal gyrus

fusiform gyrus

inferior temporal gyrus

pons

cerebellum

middle cerebellar peduncle

inferior cerebellar peduncle

40° section, No. 13, uppersurface indicating prominent structures, lobes and gyri.

297

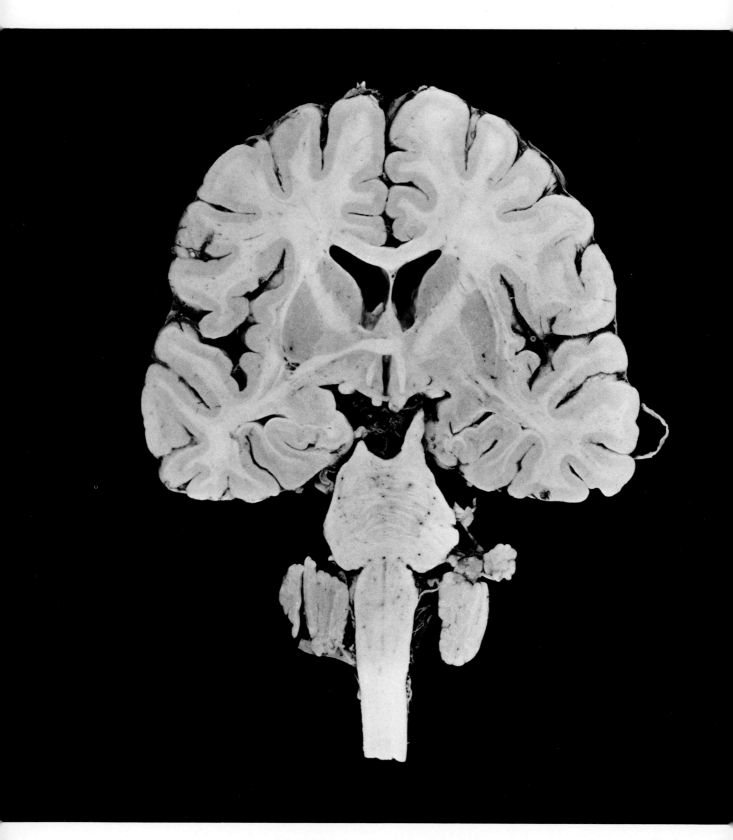

40° section, No. 14, uppersurface.

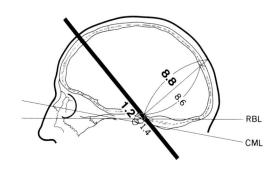

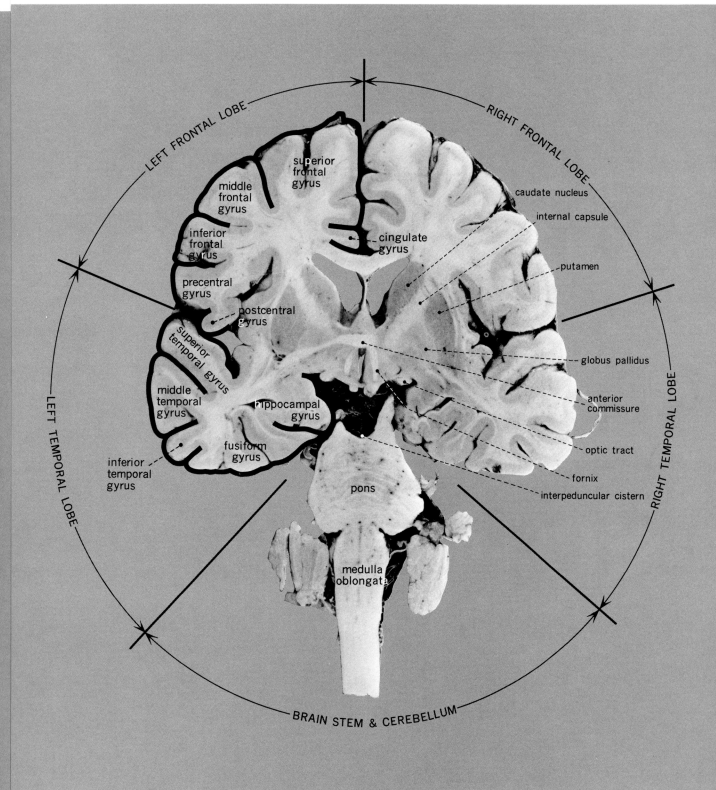

40° section, No. 14, uppersurface indicating prominent structures, lobes and gyri.

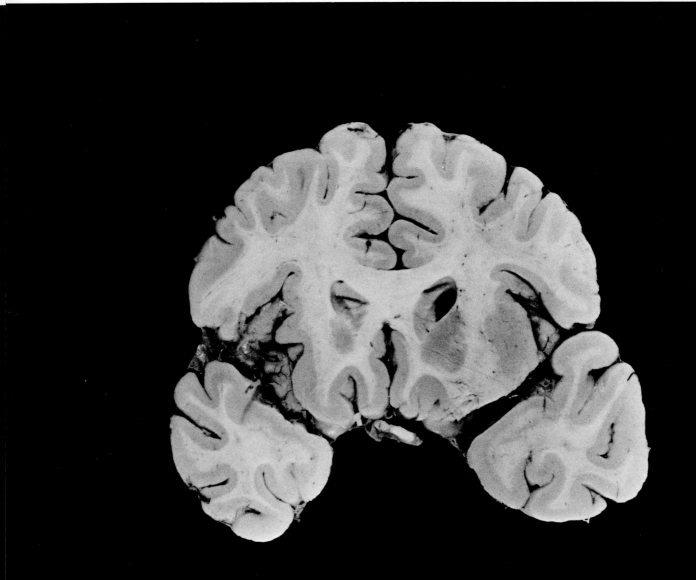

40° section, No. 16, uppersurface.

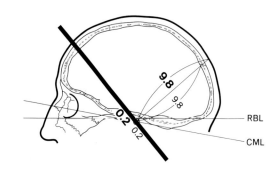

RBL

CML

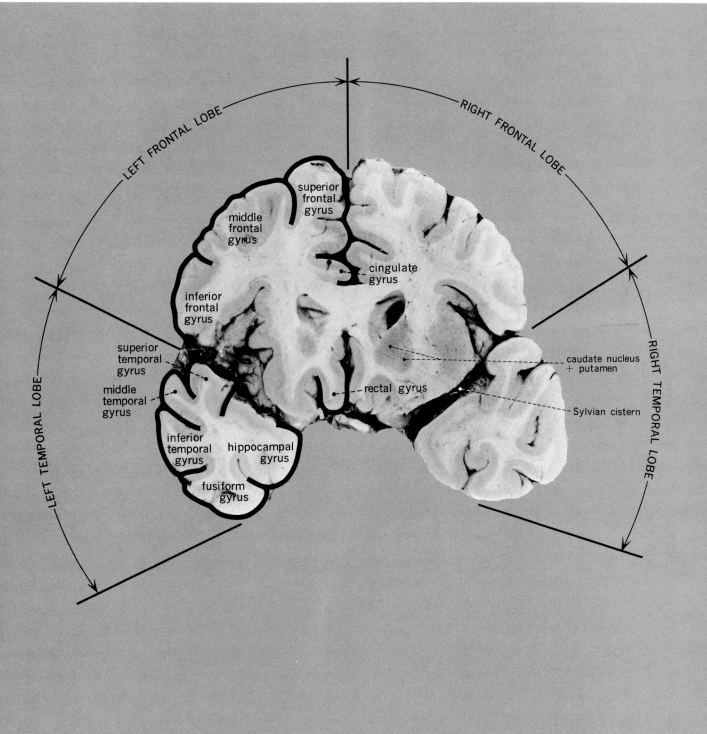

40° section, No. 16, uppersurface indicating prominent structures, lobes and gyri.

40°- 17

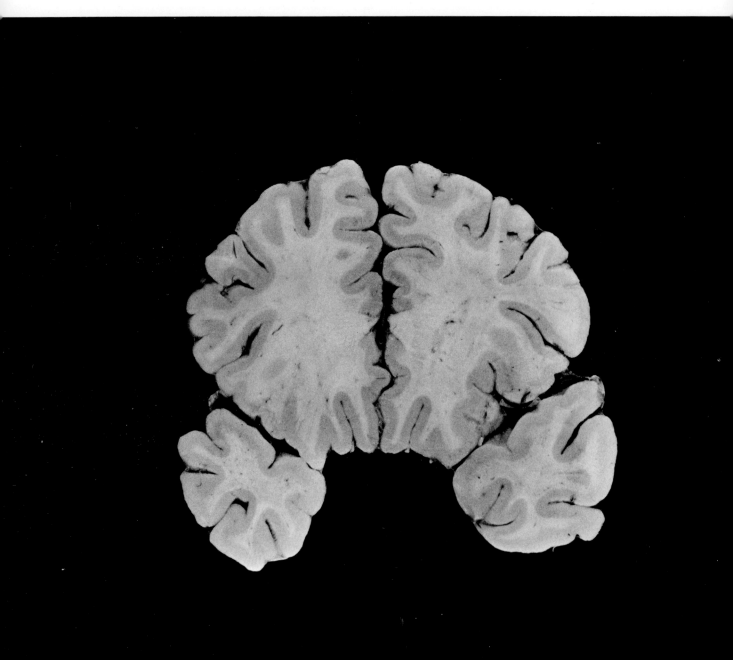

40° section, No. 17, uppersurface.

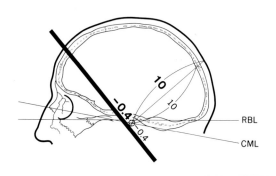

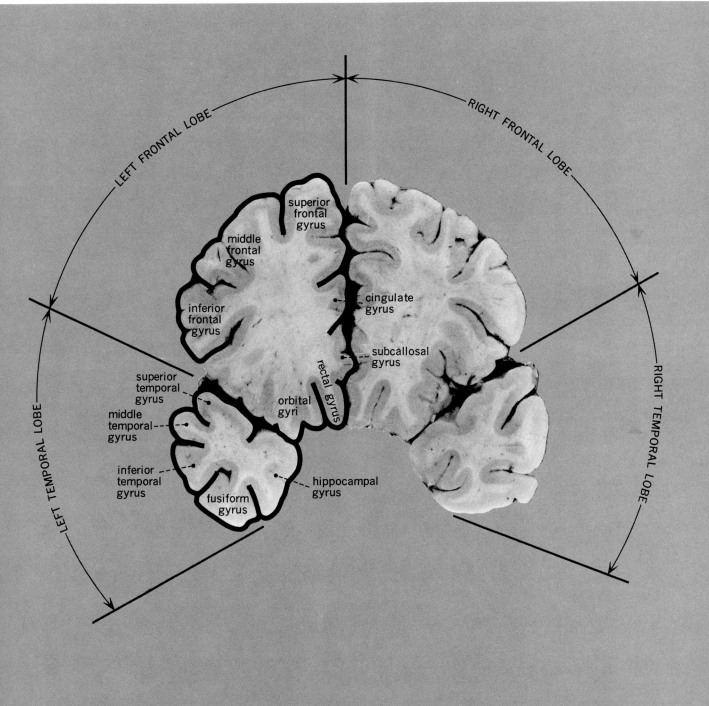

40° section, No. 17, uppersurface indicating prominent lobes and gyri.

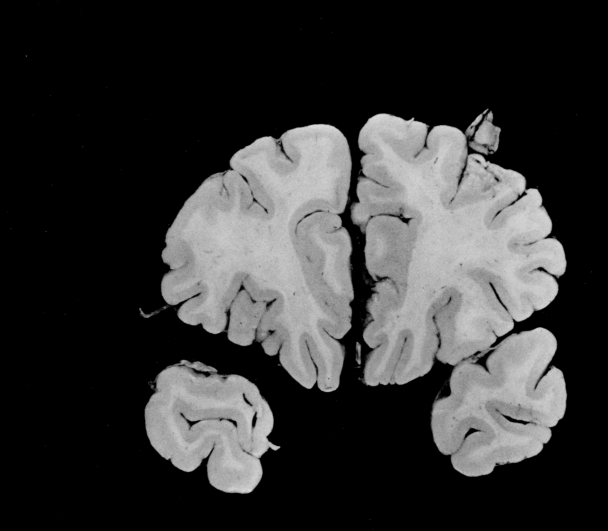

40° section, No. 18, uppersurface.

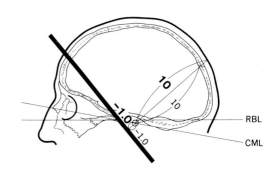

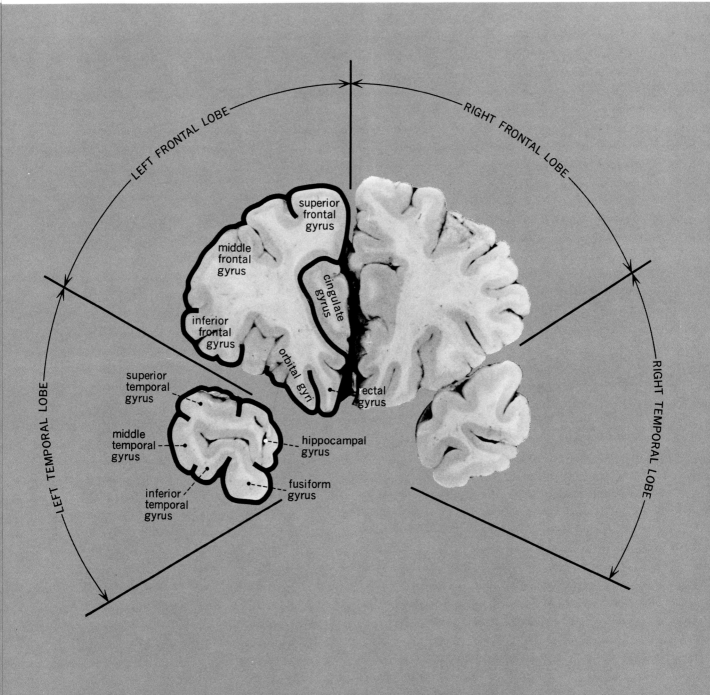

superior
frontal
gyrus

middle
frontal
gyrus

inferior
frontal
gyrus

cingulate
gyrus

orbital gyri

rectal
gyrus

superior
temporal
gyrus

middle
temporal
gyrus

inferior
temporal
gyrus

hippocampal
gyrus

fusiform
gyrus

LEFT FRONTAL LOBE

RIGHT FRONTAL LOBE

LEFT TEMPORAL LOBE

RIGHT TEMPORAL LOBE

RBL

CML

40° section, No. 18, uppersurface indicating prominent lobes and gyri.

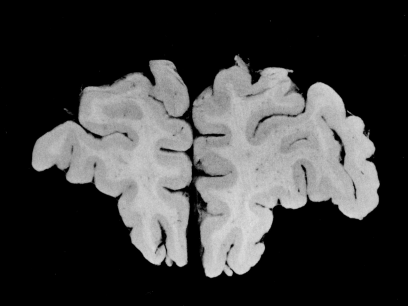

40° section, No. 20, uppersurface.

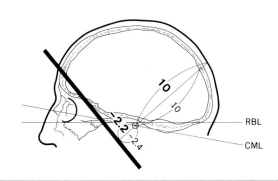

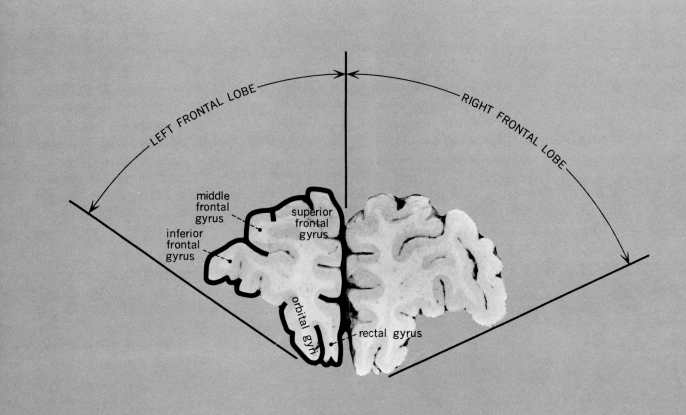

LEFT FRONTAL LOBE

RIGHT FRONTAL LOBE

middle
frontal
gyrus

superior
frontal
gyrus

inferior
frontal
gyrus

orbital gyri

rectal gyrus

40° section, No. 20, uppersurface indicating prominent lobes and gyri.

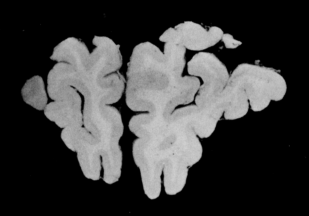

40° section, No. 21, uppersurface.

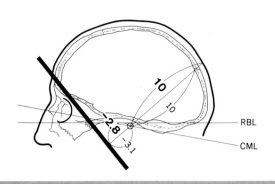

RBL

CML

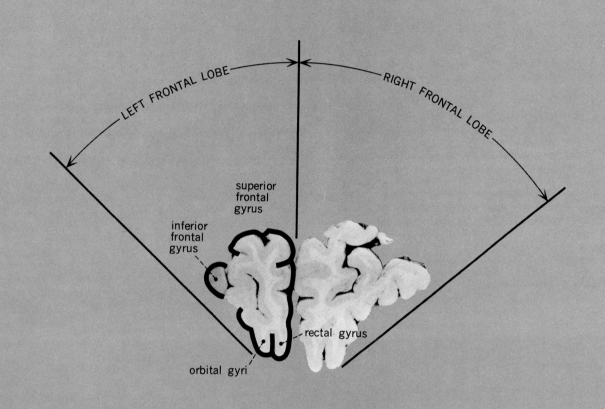

40° section, No. 21, uppersurface indicating prominent lobes and gyri.

313

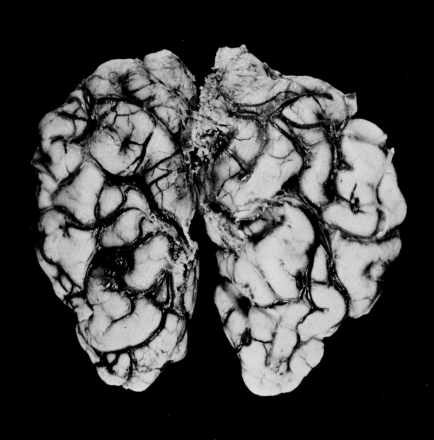

50° section, No. 1, uppersurface.

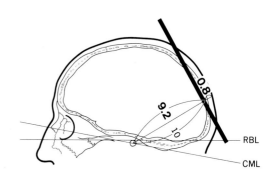

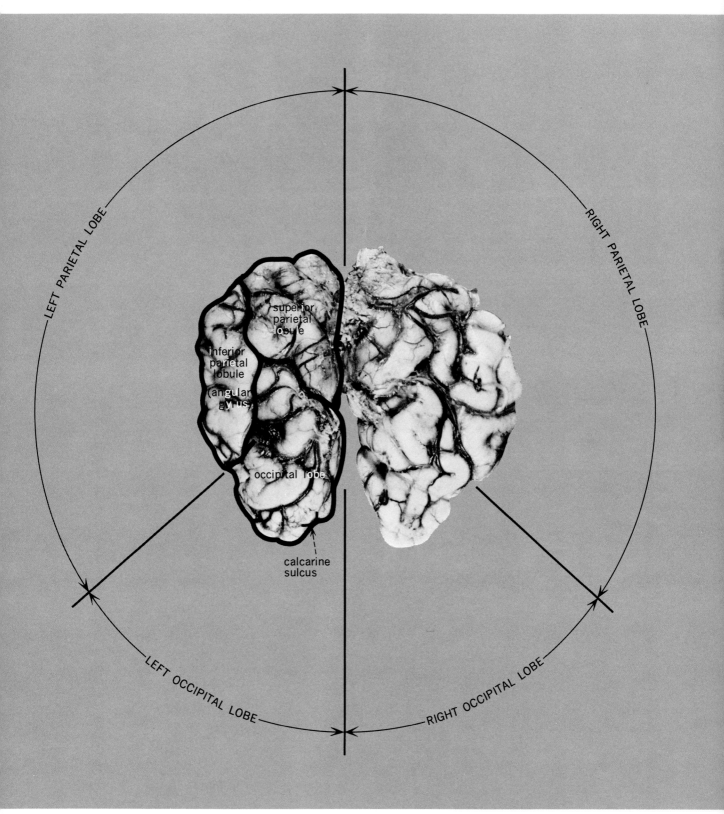

50° section, No. 1, uppersurface indicating prominent lobes and gyri.

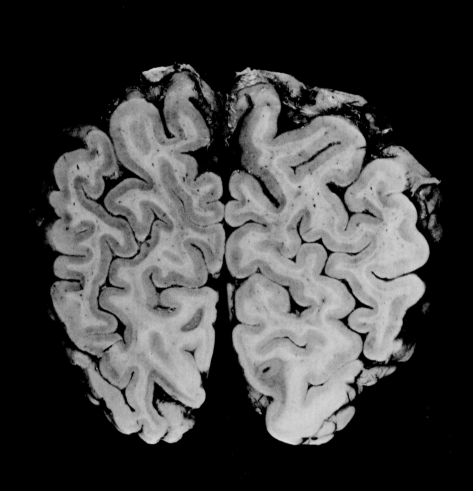

50° section, No. 2, uppersurface.

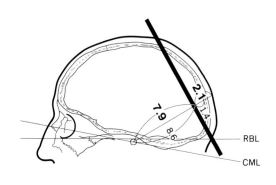

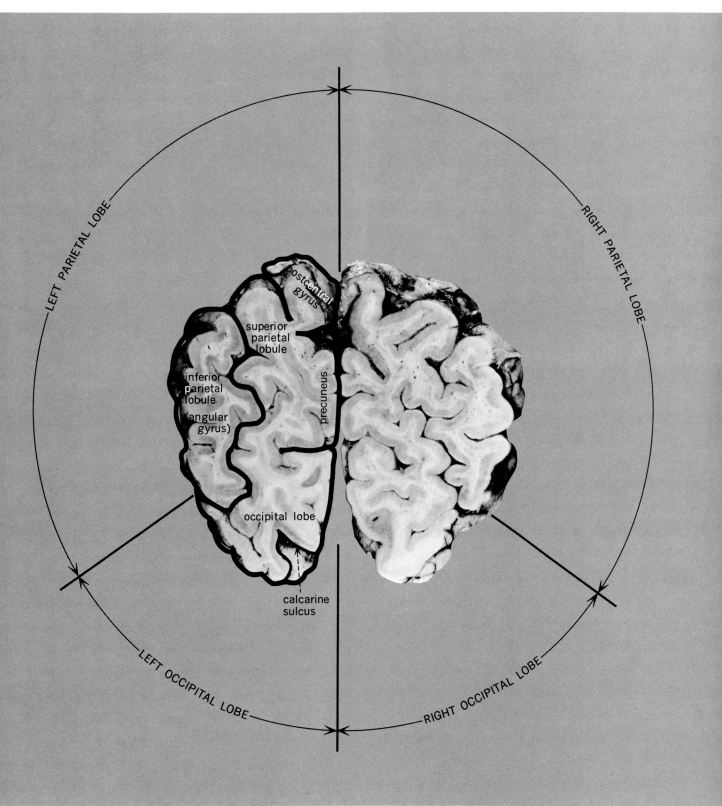

50° section, No. 2, uppersurface indicating prominent lobes and gyri.

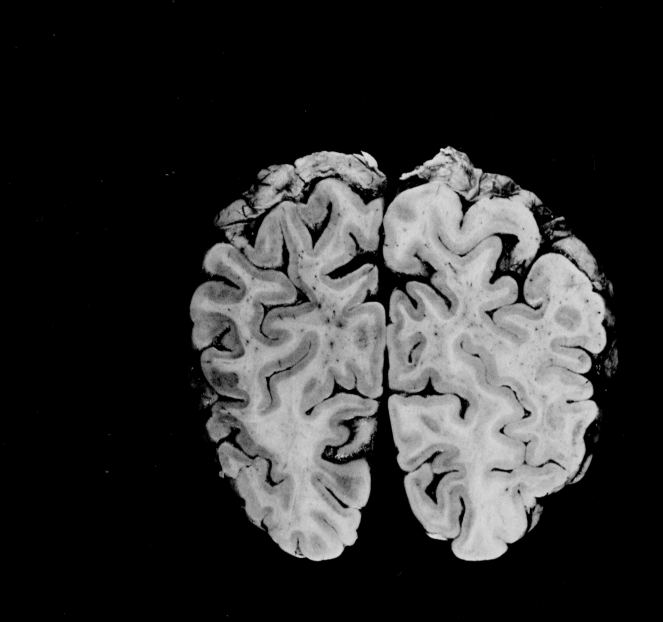

50° section, No. 3, uppersurface.

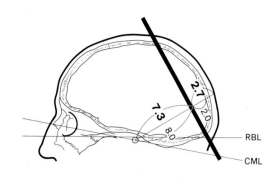

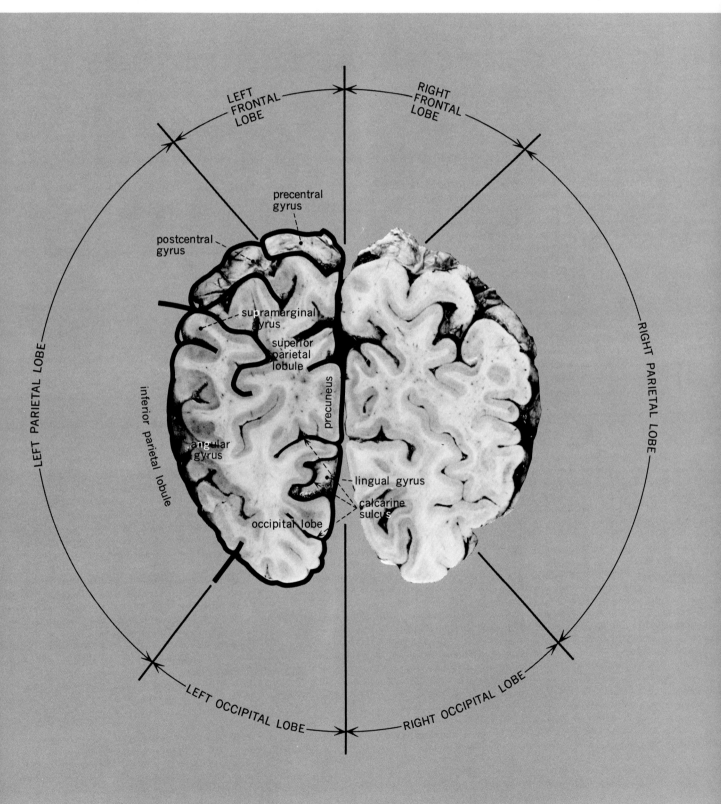

50° section, No. 3, uppersurface indicating prominent lobes and gyri.

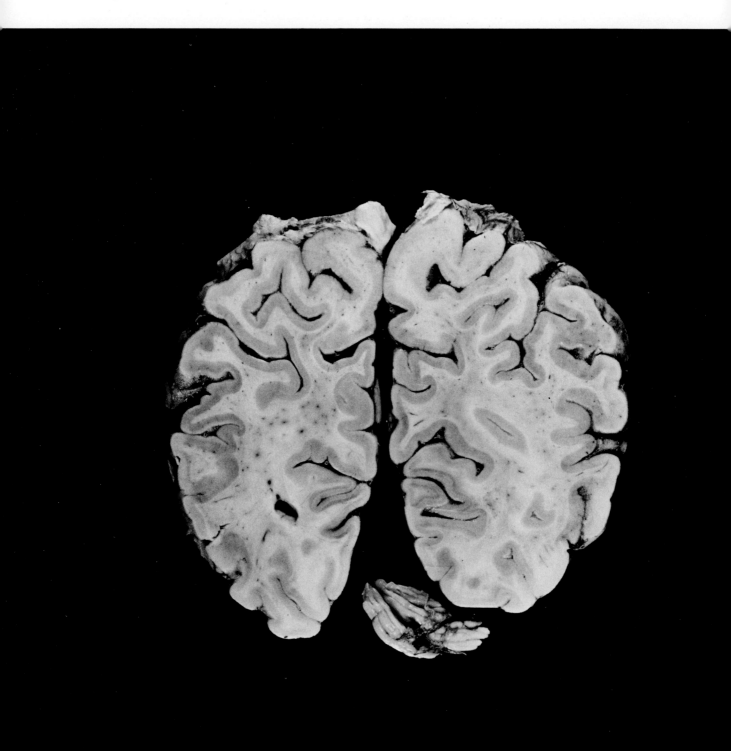

50° section, No. 4, uppersurface.

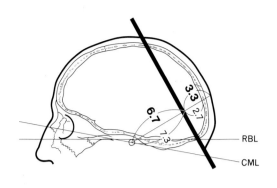

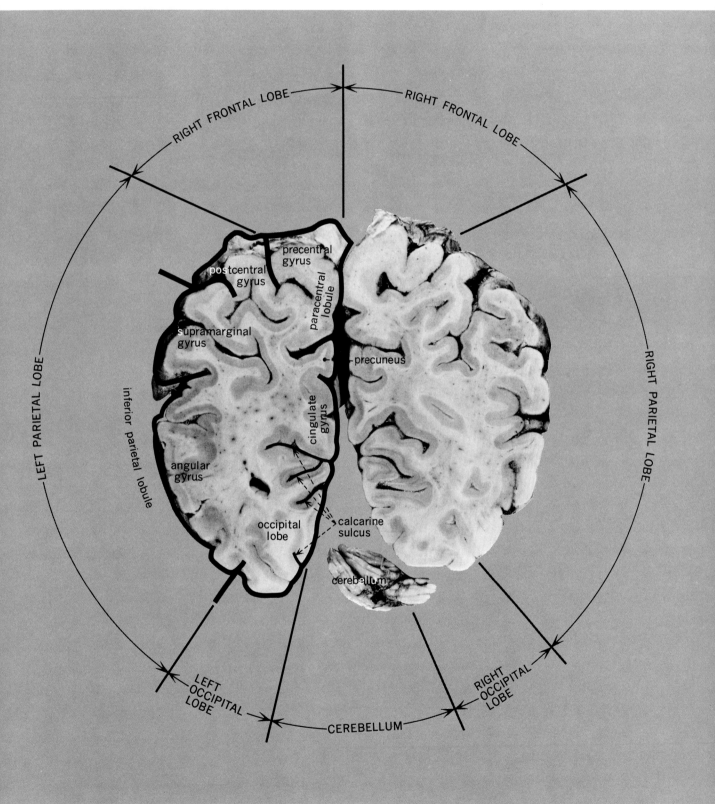

50° section, No. 4, uppersurface indicating prominent lobes and gyri.

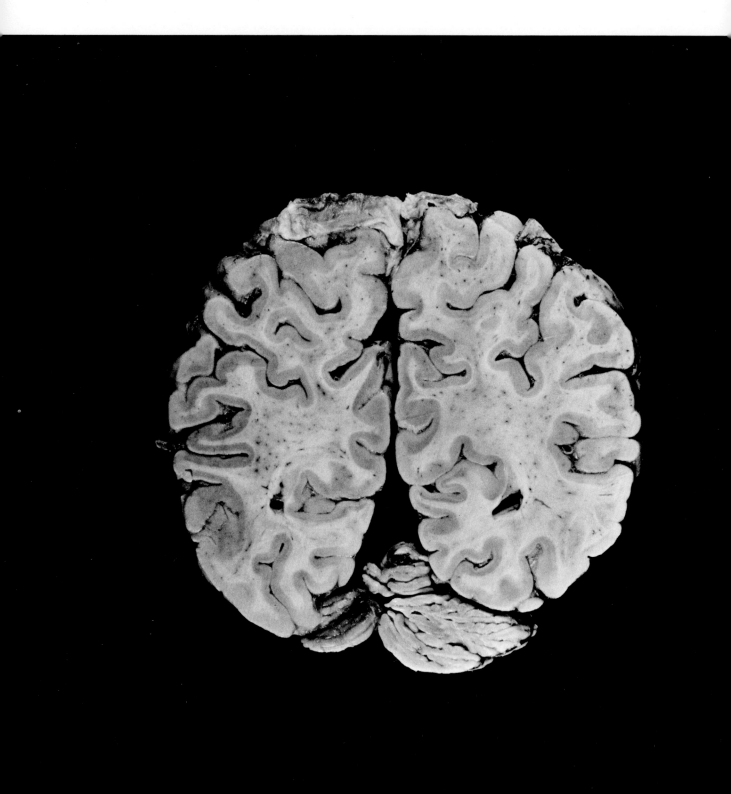

50° section, No. 5, uppersurface.

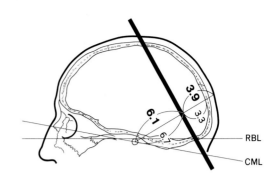

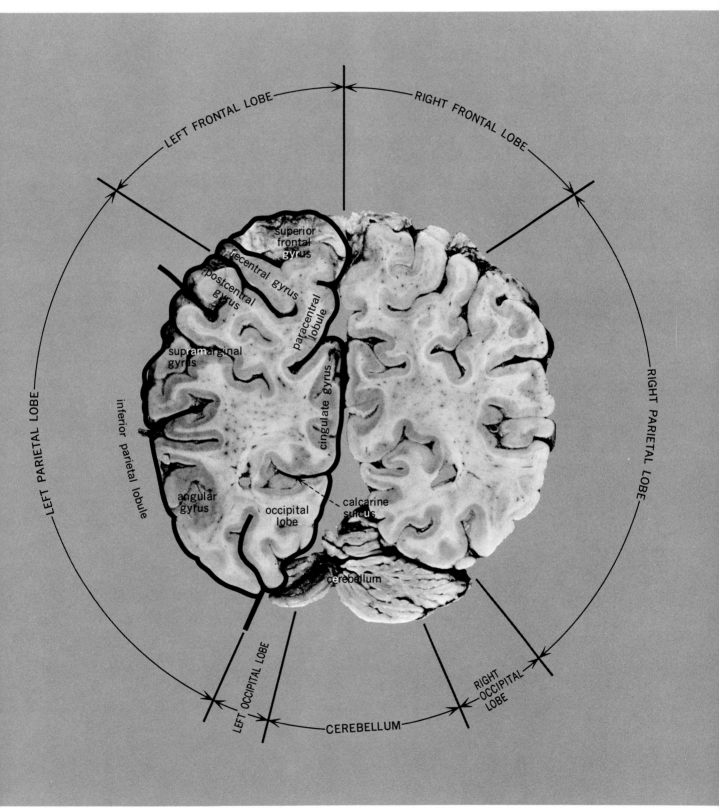

50° section, No. 5, uppersurface indicating prominent lobes and gyri.

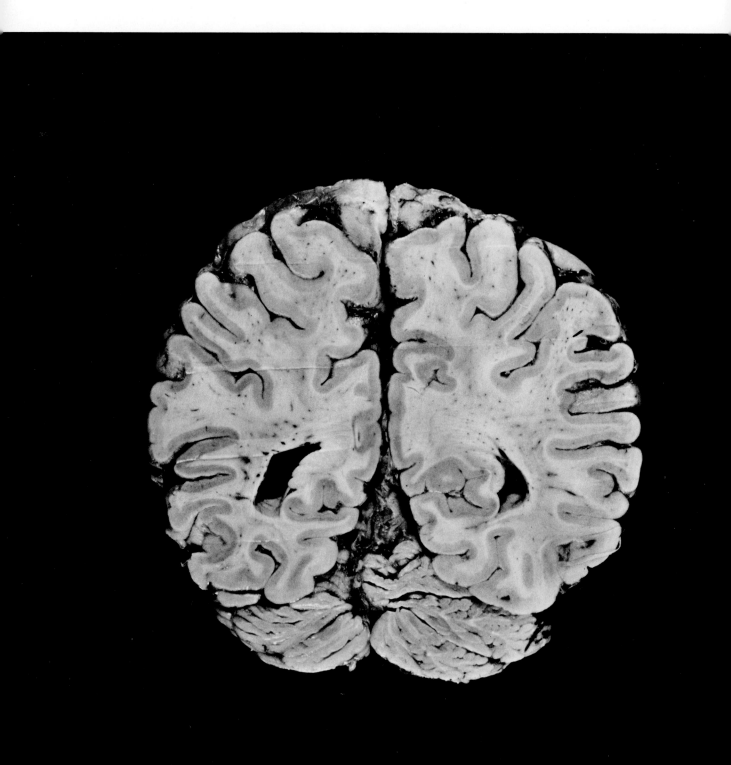

50° section, No. 6, uppersurface.

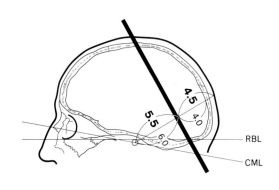

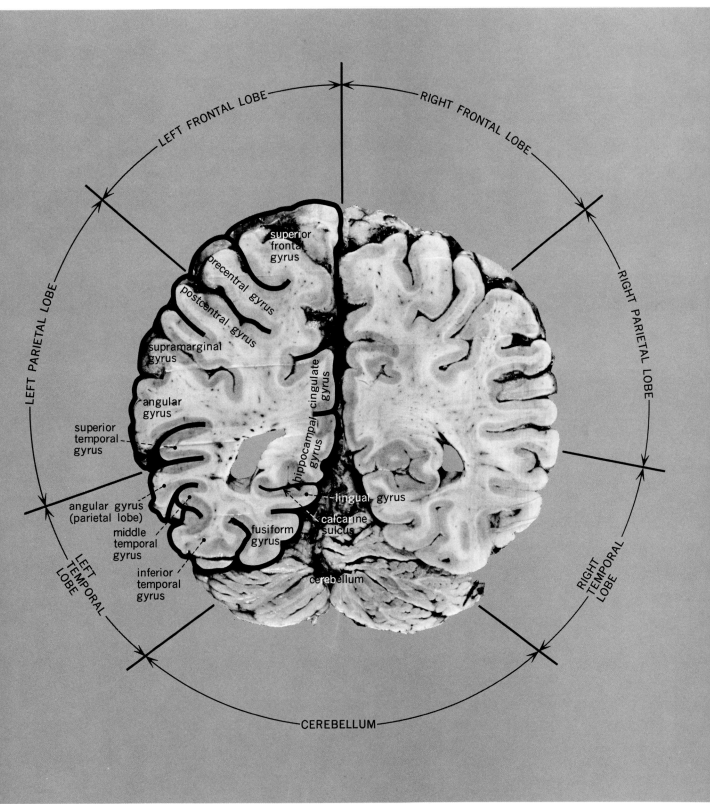

50° section, No. 6, uppersurface indicating prominent lobes and gyri.

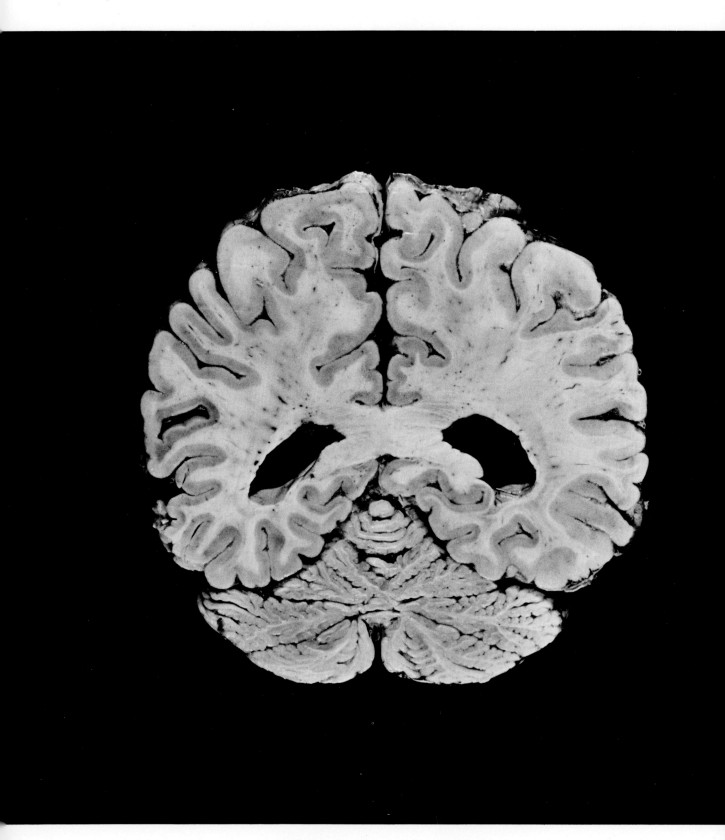

50° section, No. 7, uppersurface.

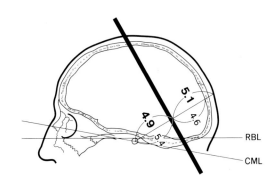

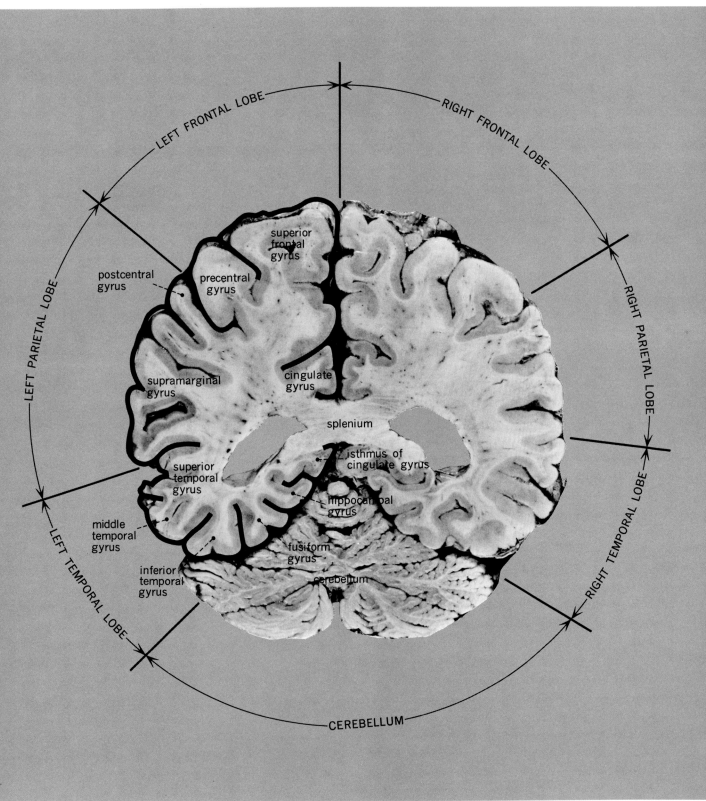

50° section, No. 7, uppersurface indicating prominent lobes and gyri.

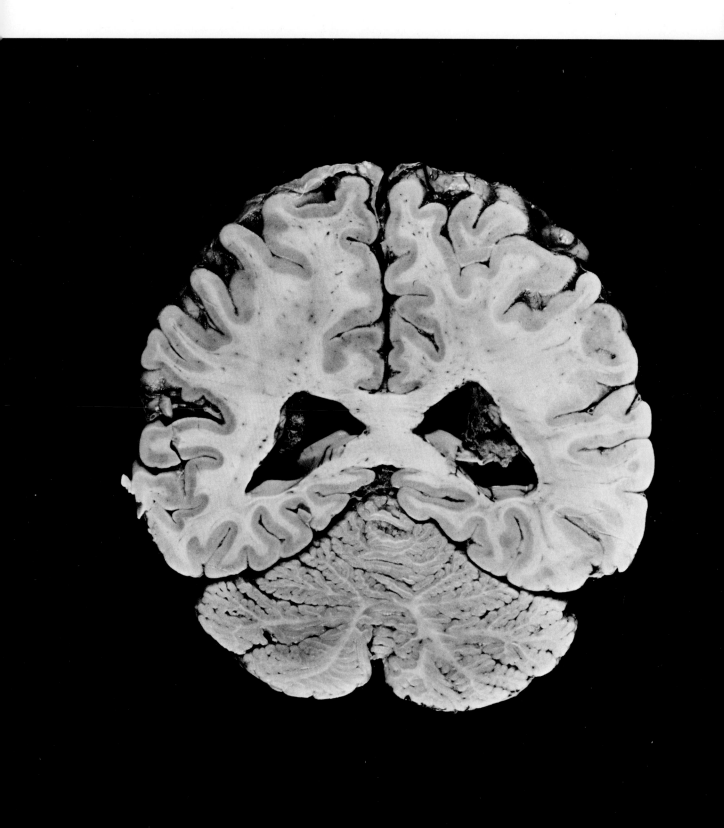

50° section, No. 8, uppersurface.

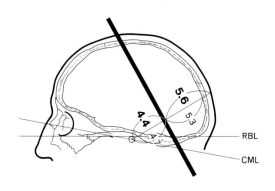

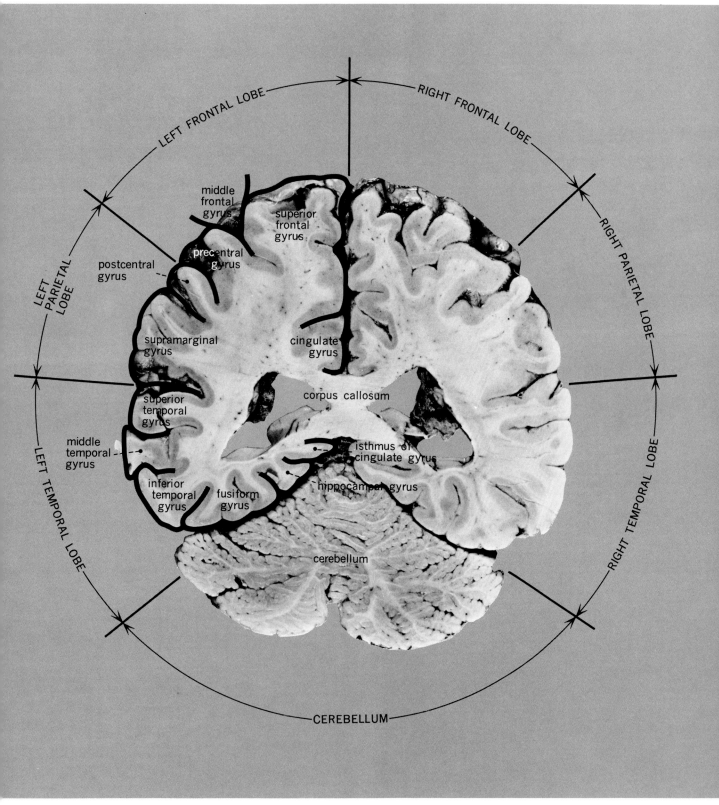

50° section, No. 8, uppersurface indicating prominent lobes and gyri.

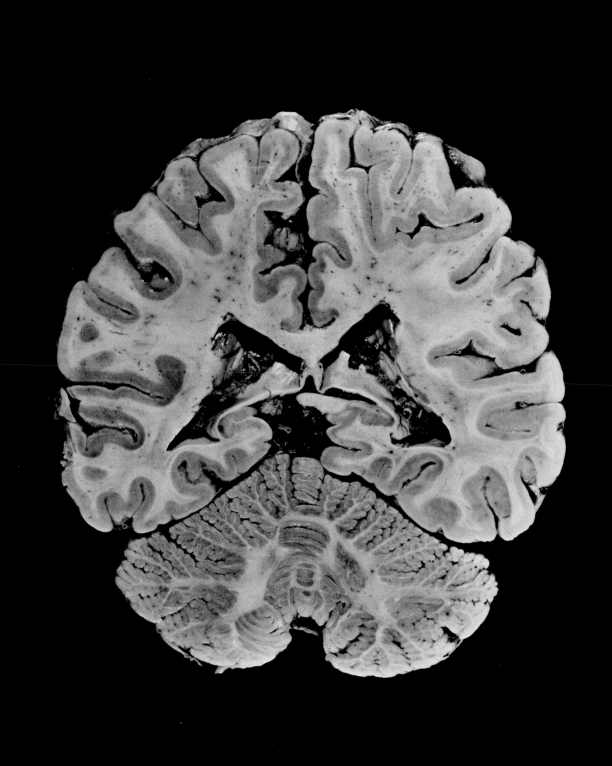

50° section, No. 9, uppersurface.

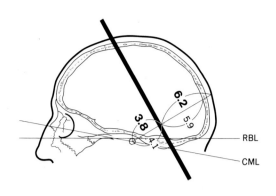

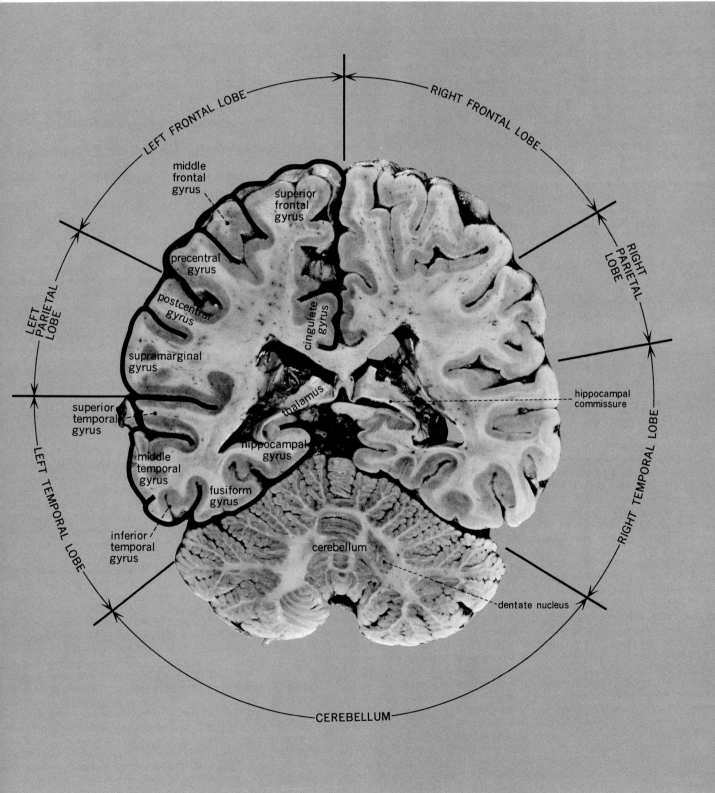

RBL

CML

LEFT FRONTAL LOBE

RIGHT FRONTAL LOBE

RIGHT PARIETAL LOBE

LEFT PARIETAL LOBE

middle frontal gyrus

superior frontal gyrus

precentral gyrus

postcentral gyrus

cingulate gyrus

supramarginal gyrus

thalamus

hippocampal commissure

superior temporal gyrus

hippocampal gyrus

middle temporal gyrus

fusiform gyrus

cerebellum

RIGHT TEMPORAL LOBE

LEFT TEMPORAL LOBE

inferior temporal gyrus

dentate nucleus

CEREBELLUM

50° section, No. 9, uppersurface indicating prominent structures, lobes and gyri.

50°- 10

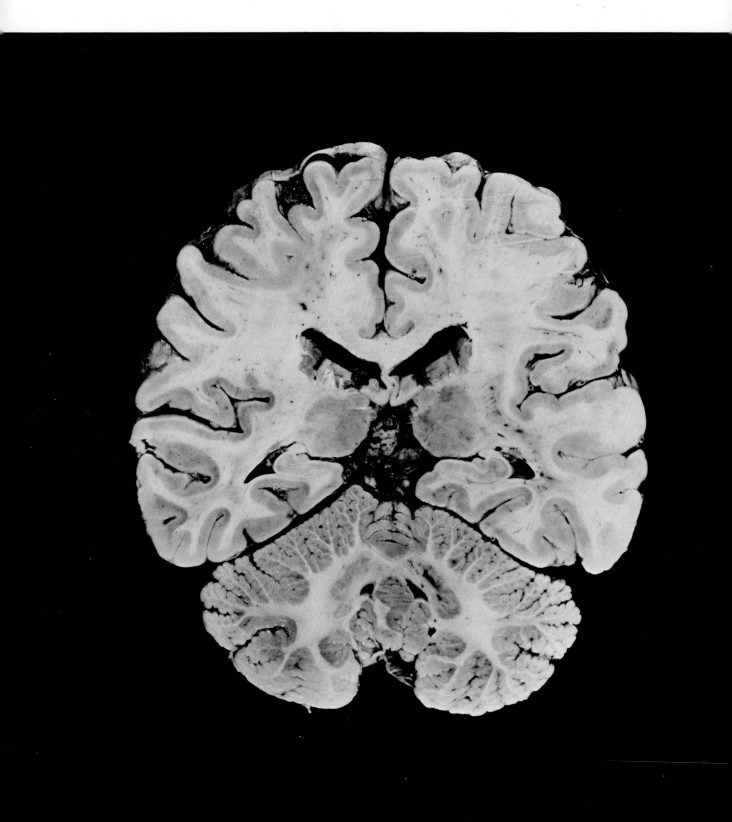

50° section, No. 10, uppersurface.

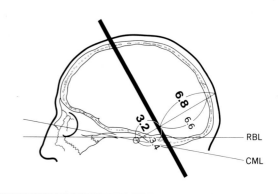

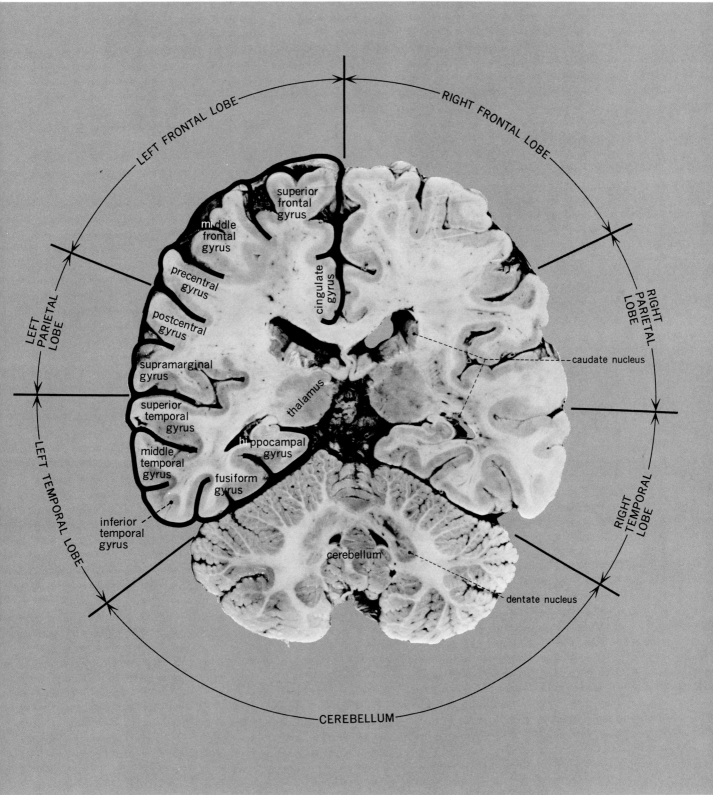

50° section, No. 10, uppersurface indicating prominent structures, lobes and gyri.

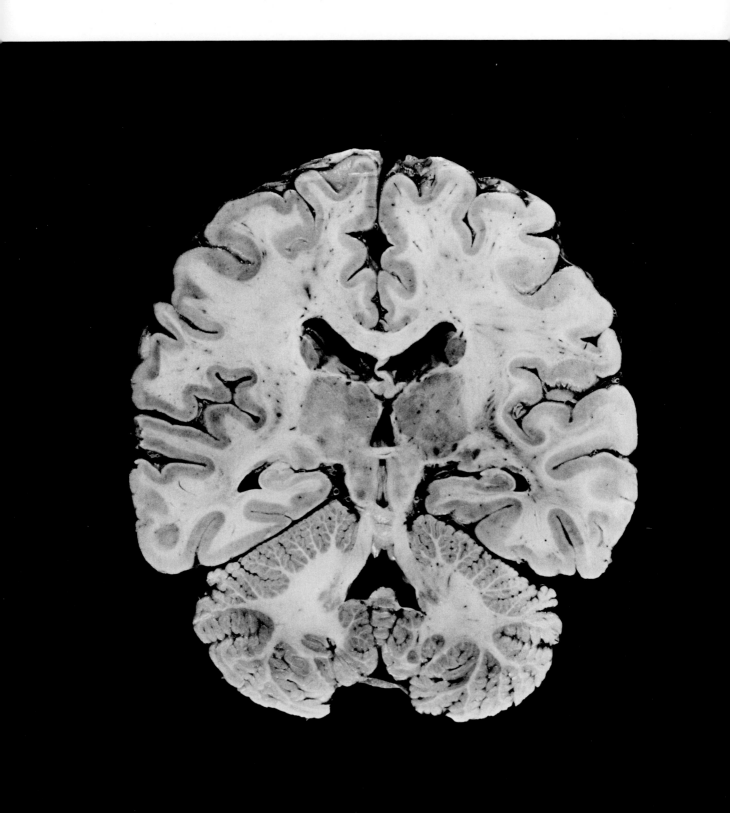

50° section, No. 11, uppersurface.

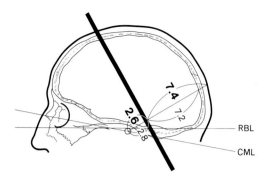

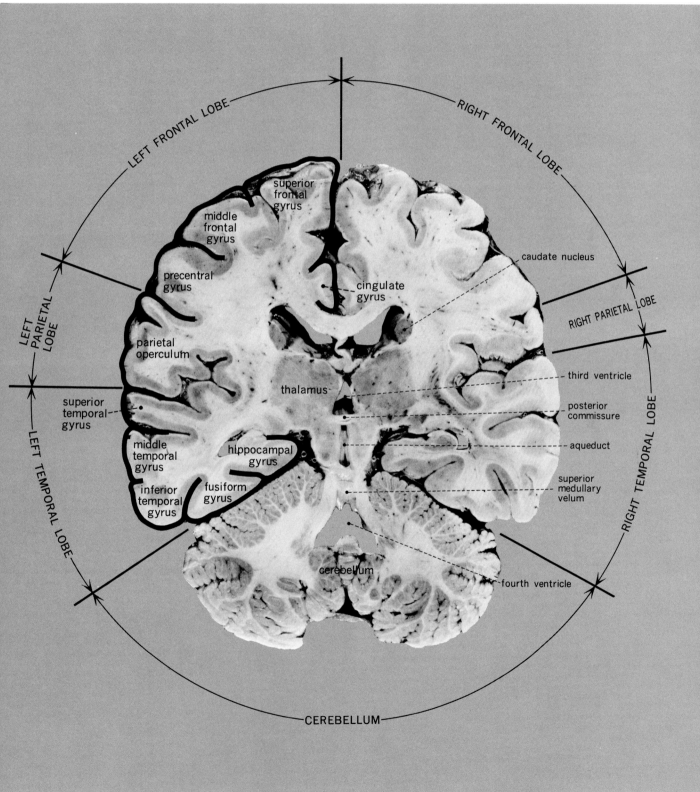

50° section, No. 11, uppersurface indicating prominent structures, lobes and gyri.

50°- 12

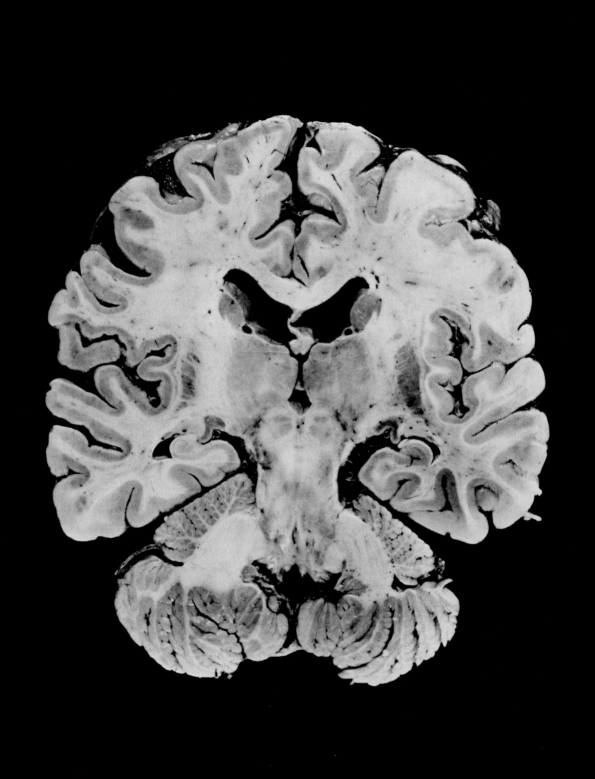

50° section, No. 12, uppersurface.

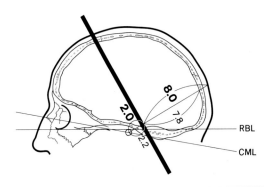

RBL
CML
8.0
7.8
2.0
2.2

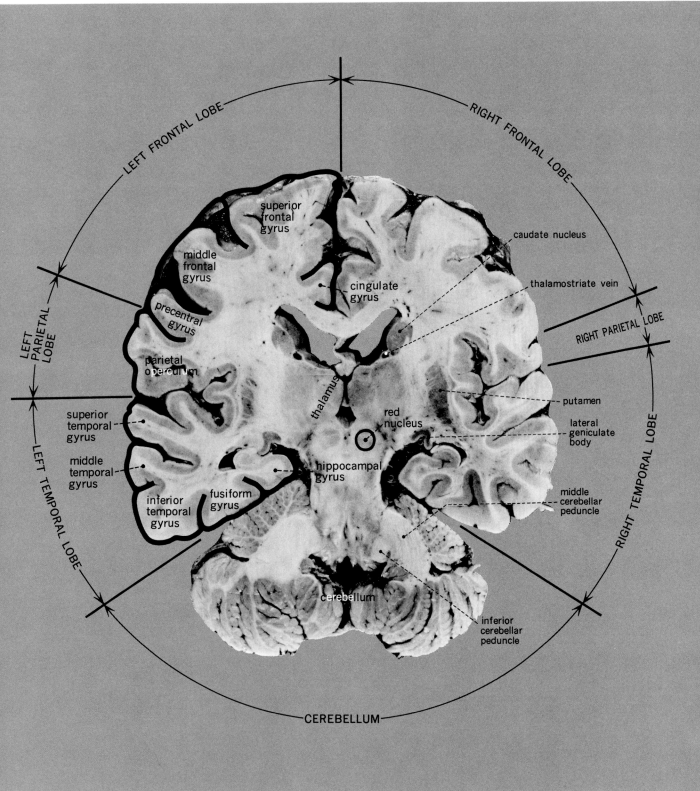

LEFT FRONTAL LOBE

RIGHT FRONTAL LOBE

superior
frontal
gyrus

middle
frontal
gyrus

precentral
gyrus

parietal
operculum

caudate nucleus

thalamostriate vein

cingulate
gyrus

RIGHT PARIETAL LOBE

LEFT
PARIETAL
LOBE

superior
temporal
gyrus

middle
temporal
gyrus

inferior
temporal
gyrus

fusiform
gyrus

thalamus

red
nucleus

hippocampal
gyrus

putamen

lateral
geniculate
body

middle
cerebellar
peduncle

RIGHT TEMPORAL LOBE

LEFT TEMPORAL LOBE

cerebellum

inferior
cerebellar
peduncle

CEREBELLUM

50° section, No. 12, uppersurface indicating prominent structures, lobes and gyri.

337

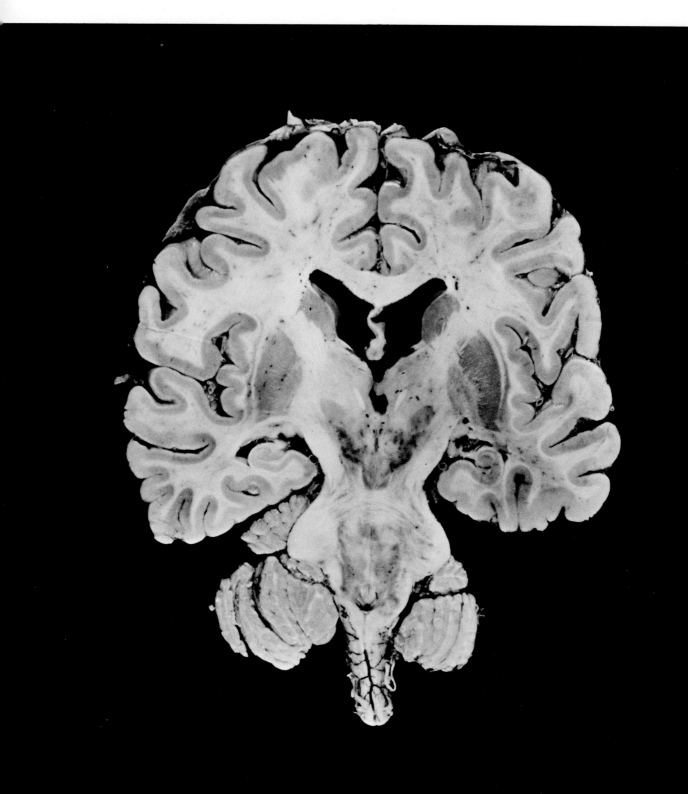

50° section, No. 13, uppersurface.

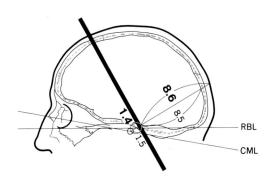

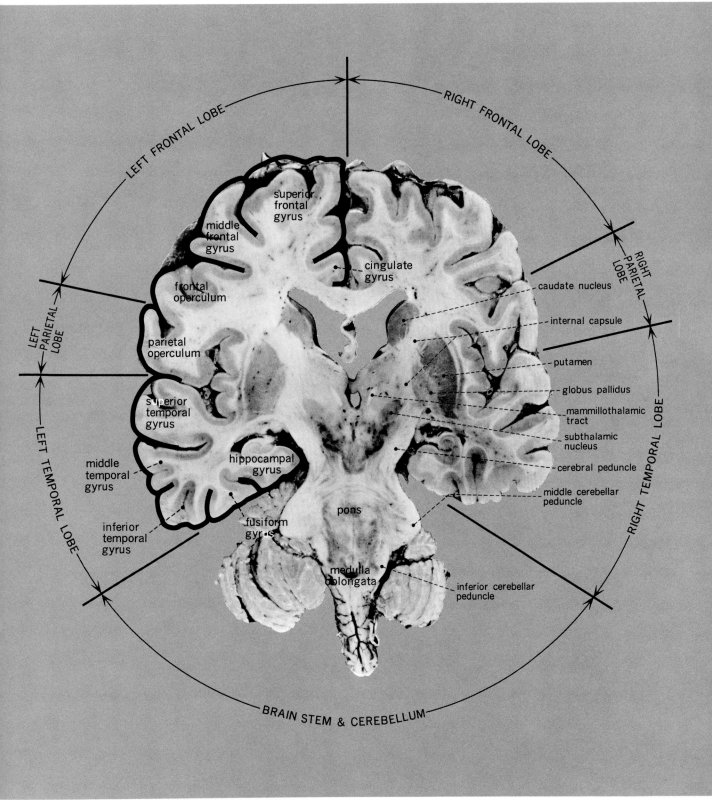

LEFT FRONTAL LOBE

RIGHT FRONTAL LOBE

RIGHT PARIETAL LOBE

LEFT PARIETAL LOBE

RIGHT TEMPORAL LOBE

LEFT TEMPORAL LOBE

BRAIN STEM & CEREBELLUM

superior frontal gyrus

middle frontal gyrus

frontal operculum

cingulate gyrus

caudate nucleus

internal capsule

parietal operculum

putamen

globus pallidus

superior temporal gyrus

mammillothalamic tract

subthalamic nucleus

hippocampal gyrus

cerebral peduncle

middle temporal gyrus

middle cerebellar peduncle

inferior temporal gyrus

fusiform gyrus

pons

medulla oblongata

inferior cerebellar peduncle

50° section, No. 13, uppersurface indicating prominent structures, lobes and gyri.

339

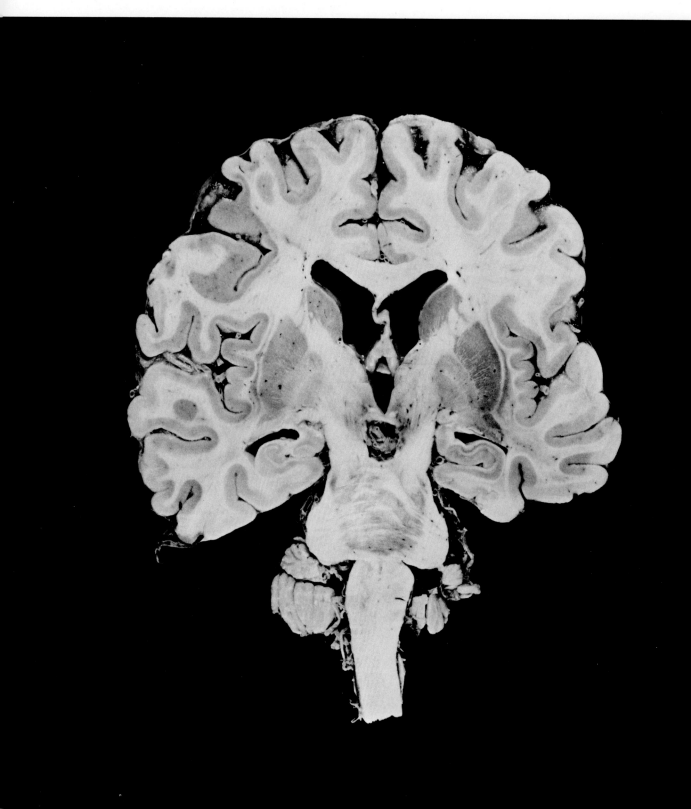

50° section, No. 14, uppersurface.

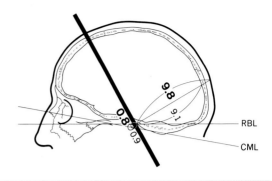

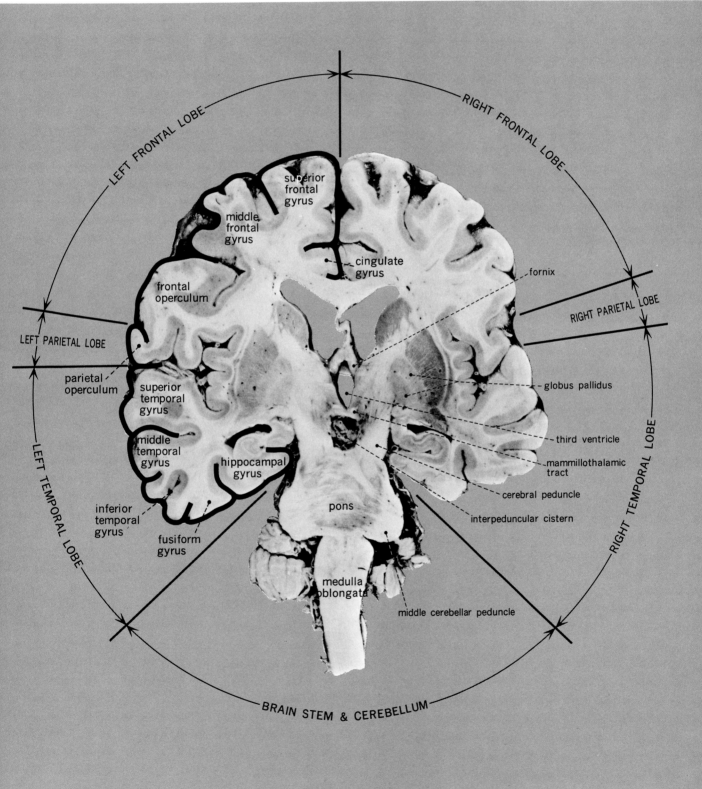

50° section, No. 14, uppersurface indicating prominent structures, lobes and gyri.

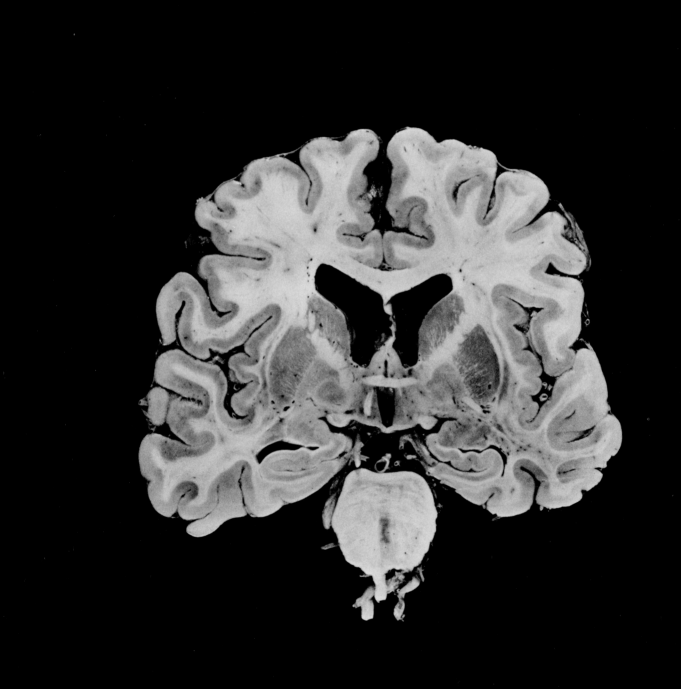

50° section, No. 15, uppersurface.

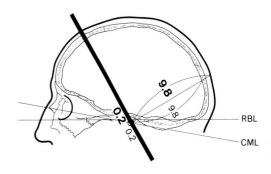

RBL

CML

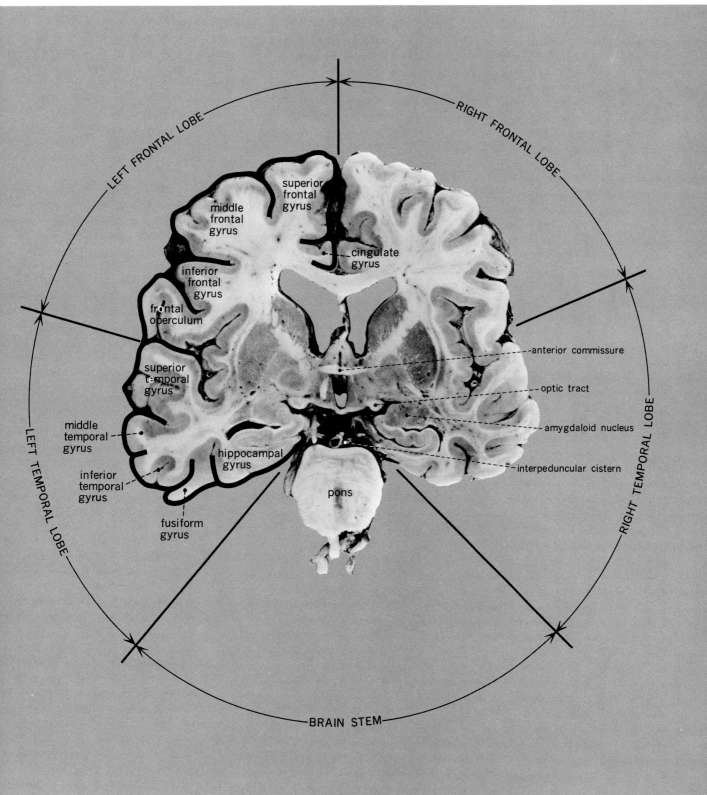

LEFT FRONTAL LOBE

RIGHT FRONTAL LOBE

superior frontal gyrus

middle frontal gyrus

cingulate gyrus

inferior frontal gyrus

frontal operculum

anterior commissure

optic tract

superior temporal gyrus

amygdaloid nucleus

interpeduncular cistern

RIGHT TEMPORAL LOBE

middle temporal gyrus

hippocampal gyrus

inferior temporal gyrus

pons

fusiform gyrus

LEFT TEMPORAL LOBE

BRAIN STEM

50° section, No. 15, uppersurface indicating prominent structures, lobes and gyri.

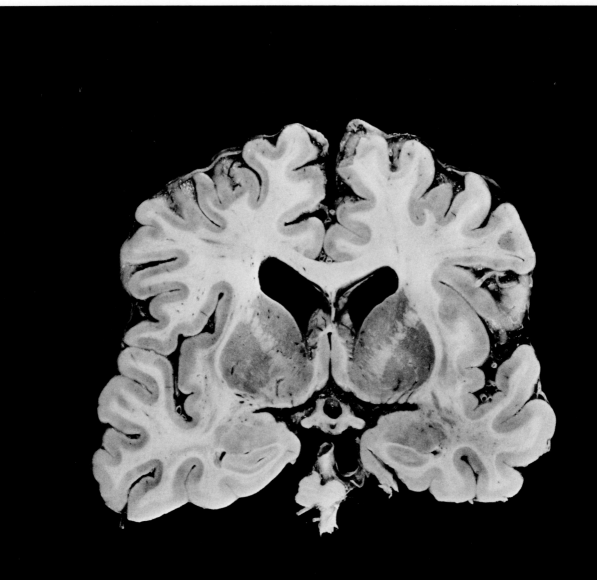

50° section, No. 16, uppersurface.

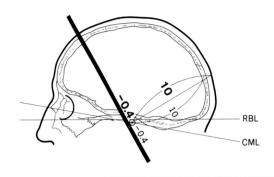

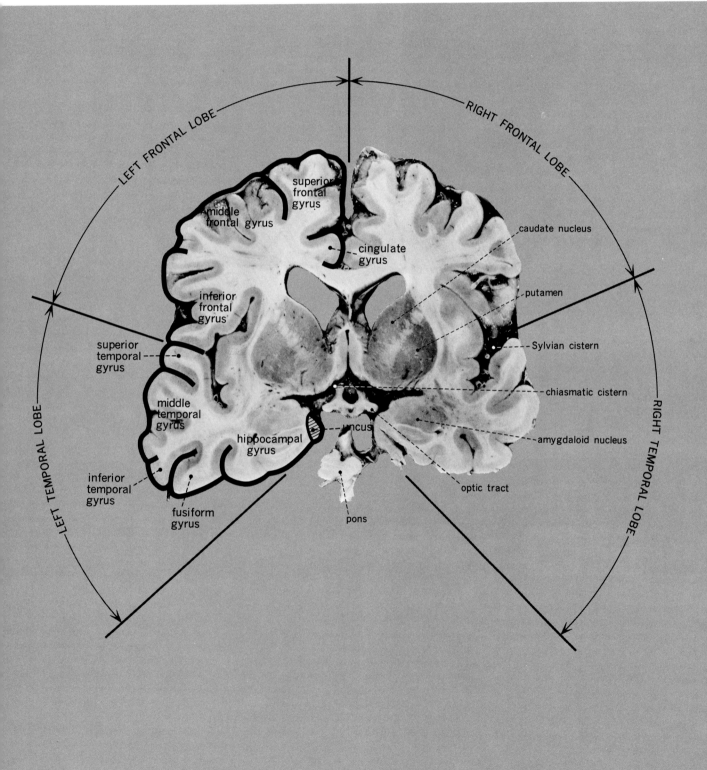

LEFT FRONTAL LOBE

RIGHT FRONTAL LOBE

superior
frontal
gyrus

middle
frontal gyrus

cingulate
gyrus

caudate nucleus

putamen

inferior
frontal
gyrus

superior
temporal
gyrus

Sylvian cistern

chiasmatic cistern

middle
temporal
gyrus

hippocampal
gyrus

uncus

amygdaloid nucleus

inferior
temporal
gyrus

optic tract

fusiform
gyrus

pons

LEFT TEMPORAL LOBE

RIGHT TEMPORAL LOBE

50° section, No. 16, uppersurface indicating prominent structures, lobes and gyri.

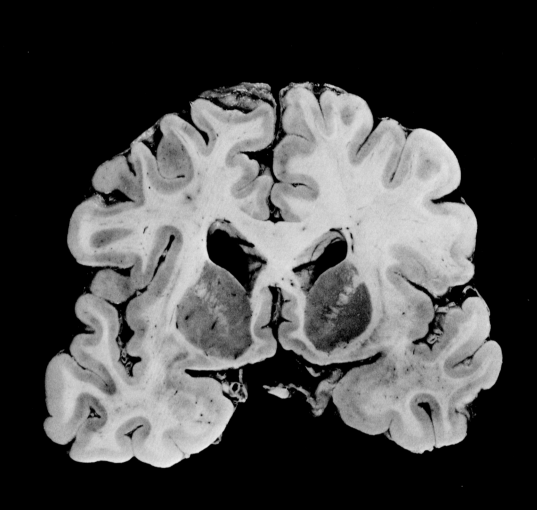

50° section, No. 17, uppersurface.

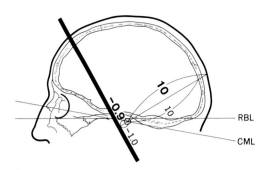

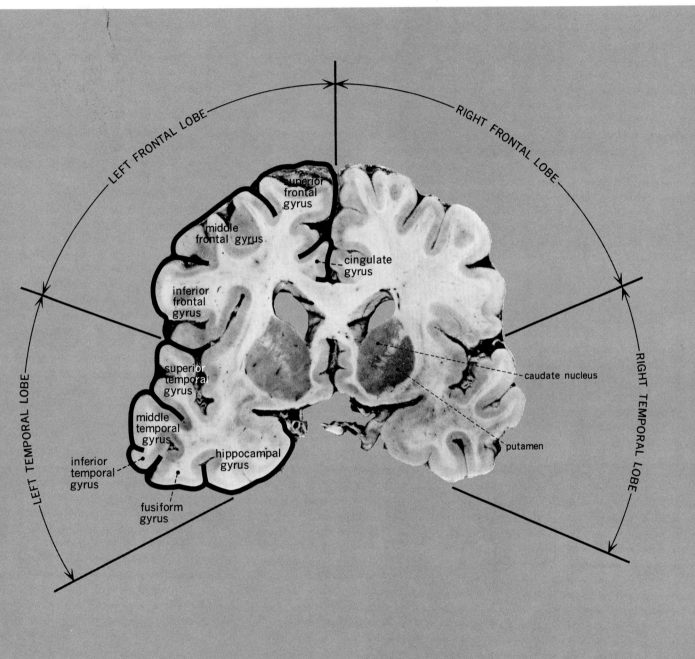

50° section, No. 17, uppersurface indicating prominent structures, lobes and gyri.

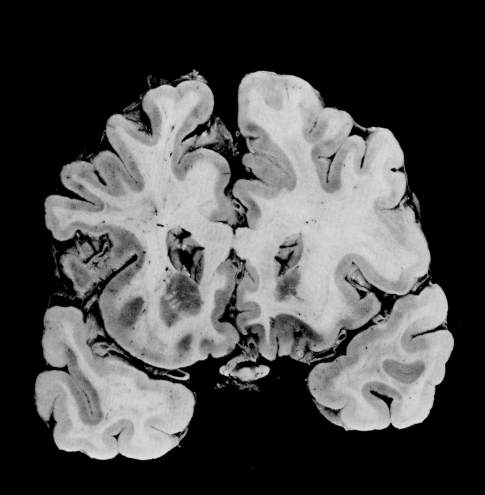

50° section, No. 18, uppersurface.

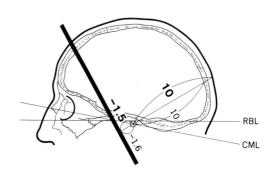

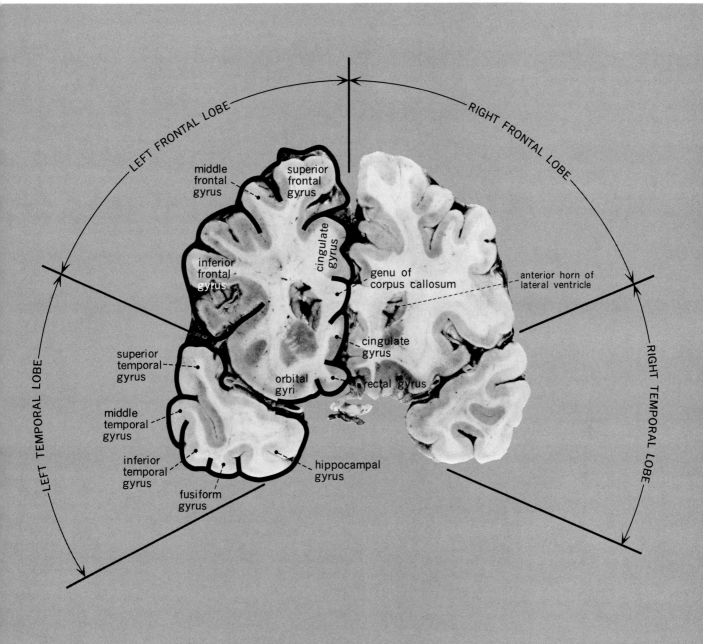

LEFT FRONTAL LOBE

RIGHT FRONTAL LOBE

LEFT TEMPORAL LOBE

RIGHT TEMPORAL LOBE

middle
frontal
gyrus

superior
frontal
gyrus

cingulate
gyrus

inferior
frontal
gyrus

genu of
corpus callosum

anterior horn of
lateral ventricle

cingulate
gyrus

superior
temporal
gyrus

orbital
gyri

rectal gyrus

middle
temporal
gyrus

inferior
temporal
gyrus

hippocampal
gyrus

fusiform
gyrus

50° section, No. 18, uppersurface indicating prominent structures, lobes and gyri.

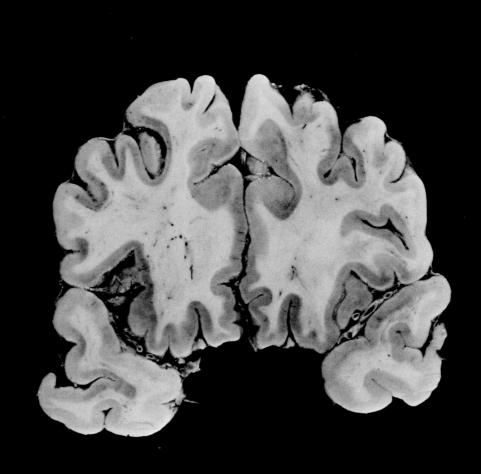

50° section, No. 19, uppersurface.

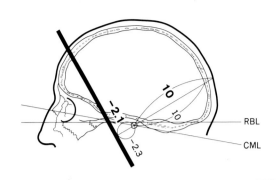

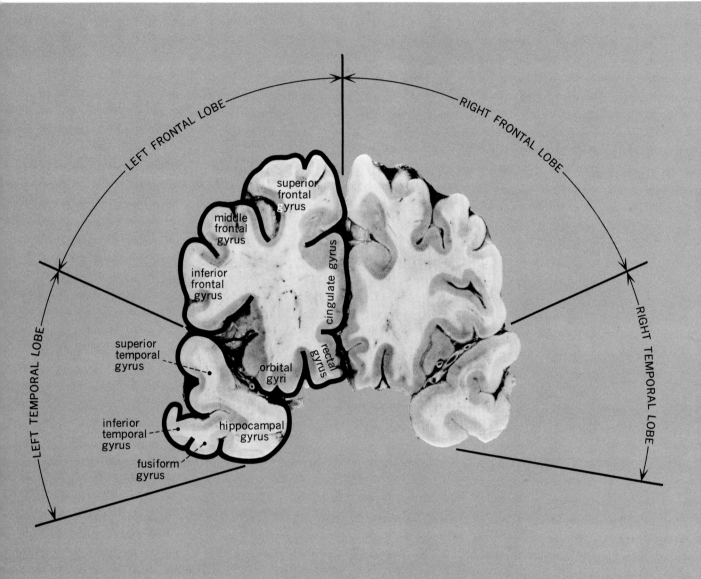

50° section, No. 19, uppersurface indicating prominent lobes and gyri.

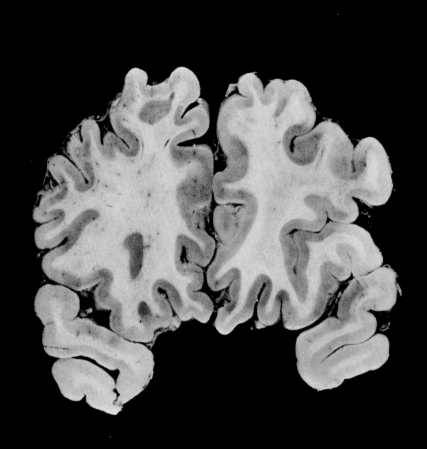

50° section, No. 20, uppersurface.

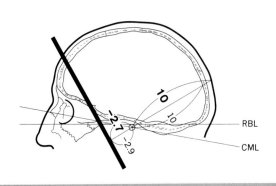

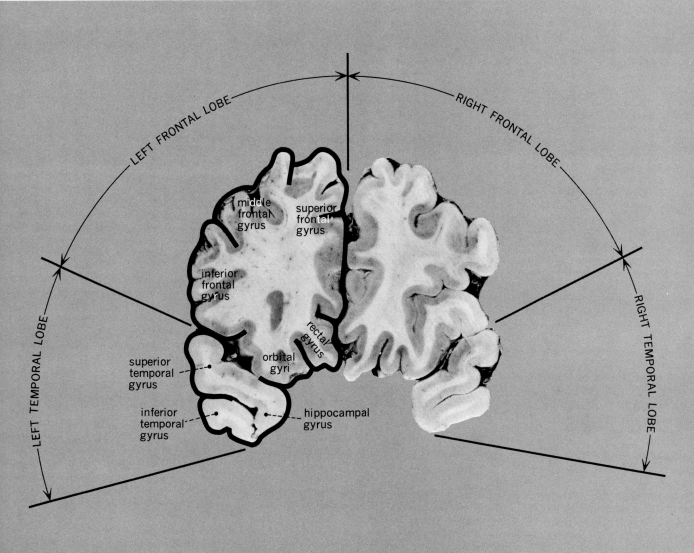

LEFT FRONTAL LOBE

RIGHT FRONTAL LOBE

LEFT TEMPORAL LOBE

RIGHT TEMPORAL LOBE

middle frontal gyrus

superior frontal gyrus

inferior frontal gyrus

rectal gyrus

orbital gyri

superior temporal gyrus

inferior temporal gyrus

hippocampal gyrus

50° section, No. 20, uppersurface indicating prominent lobes and gyri.

50°-21

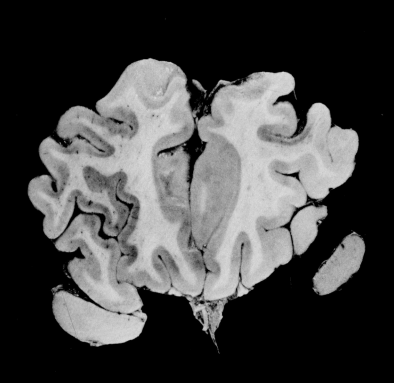

50° section, No. 21, uppersurface.

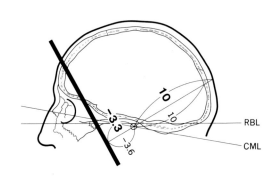

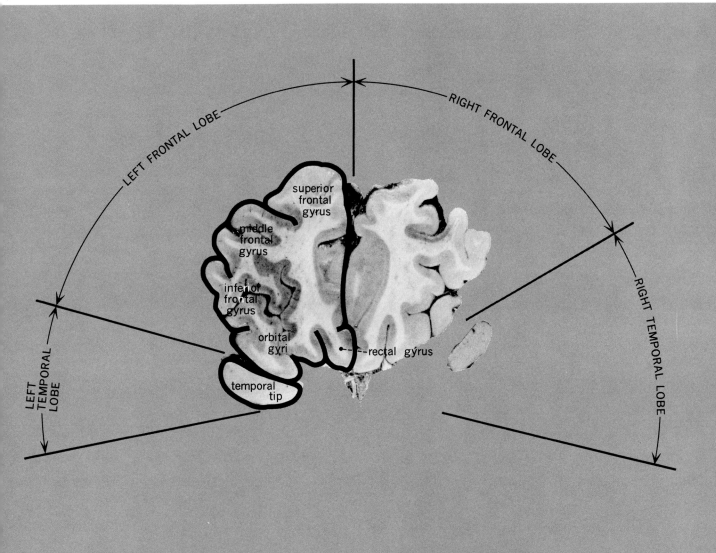

50° section, No. 21, uppersurface indicating prominent lobes and gyri.

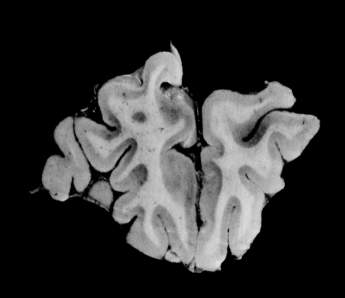

50° section, No. 22, uppersurface.

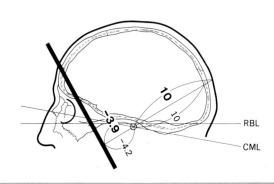

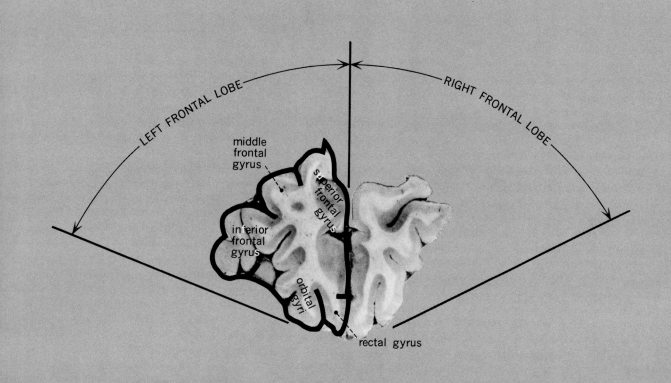

LEFT FRONTAL LOBE

RIGHT FRONTAL LOBE

middle
frontal
gyrus

superior
frontal
gyrus

inferior
frontal
gyrus

orbital
gyri

rectal gyrus

50° section, No. 22, uppersurface indicating prominent lobes and gyri.

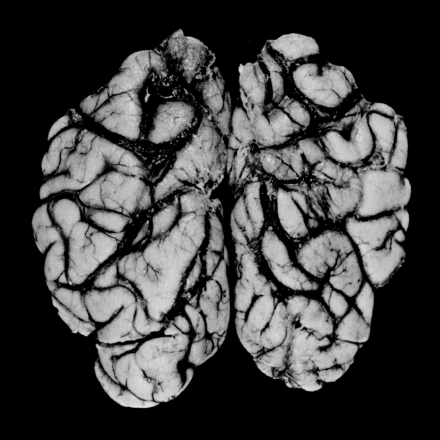

60° section, No. 1, uppersurface.

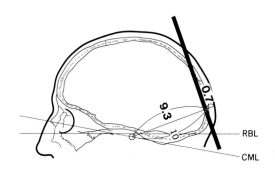

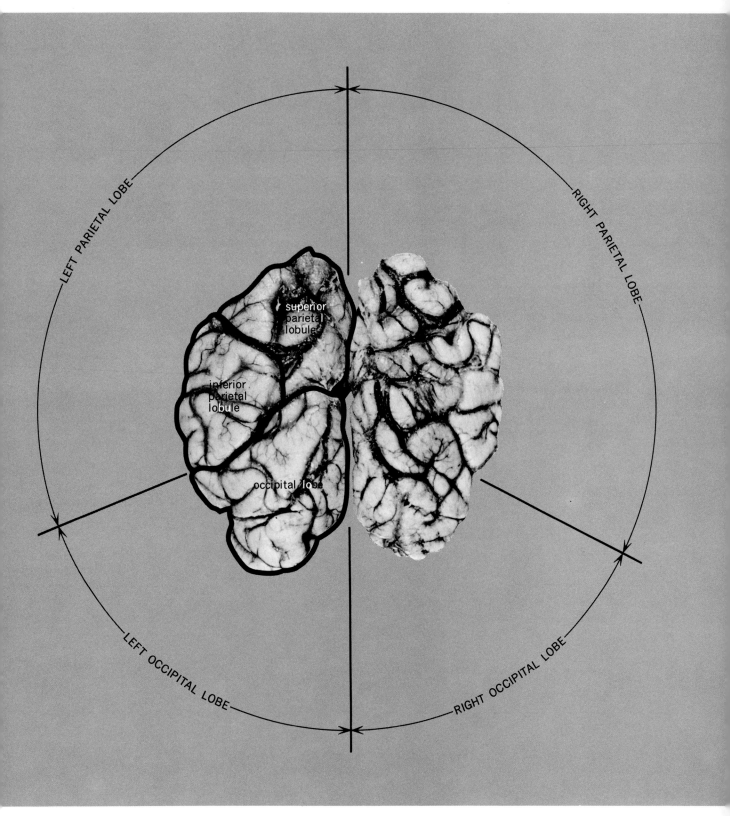

60° section, No. 1, uppersurface indicating prominent lobes and gyri.

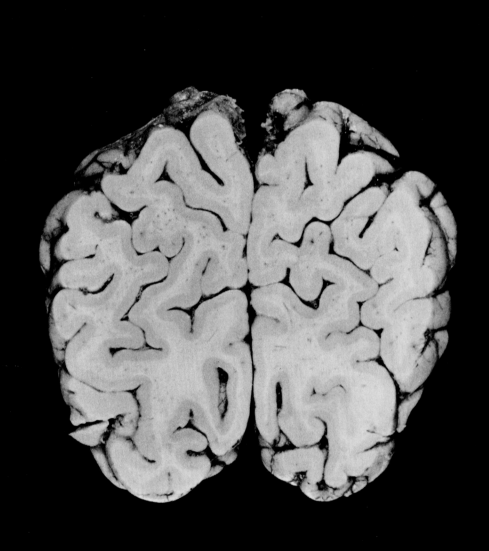

60° section, No. 2, uppersurface.

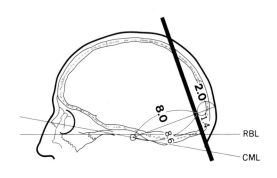

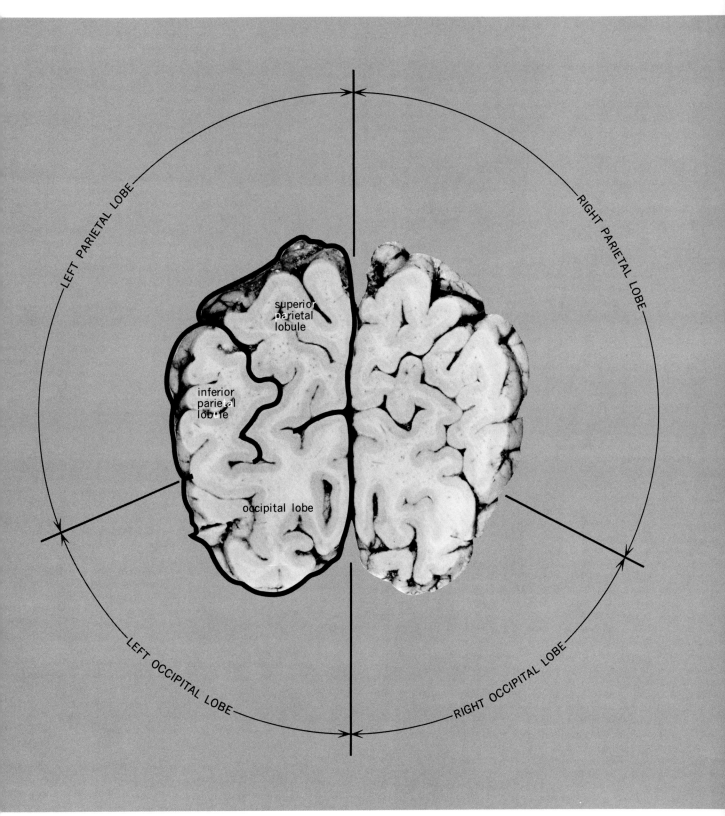

60° section, No. 2, uppersurface indicating prominent lobes and gyri.

60°-3

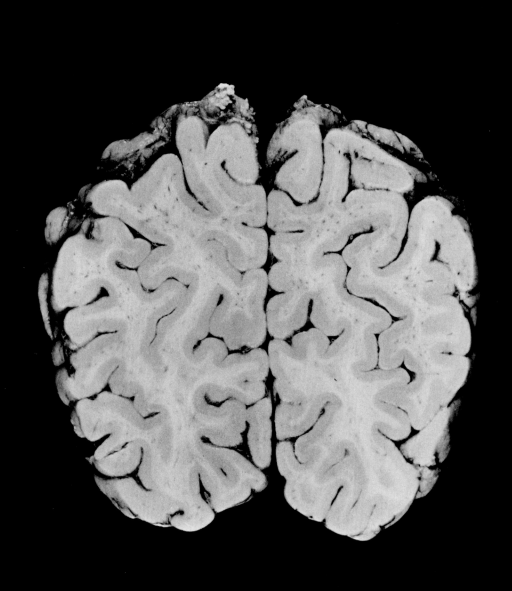

60° section, No. 3, uppersurface.

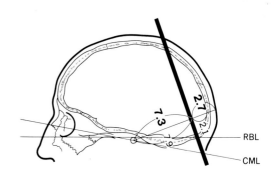

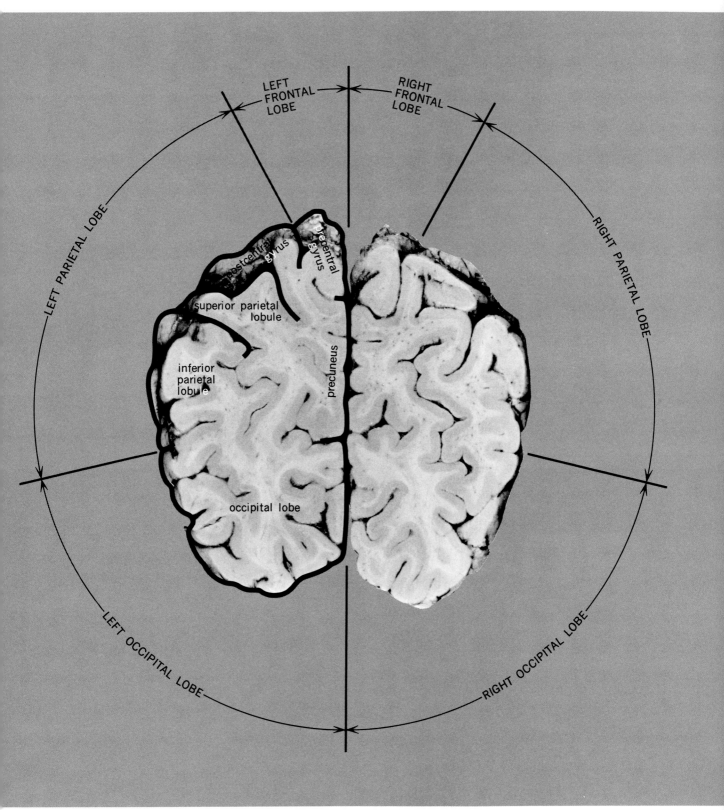

60° section, No. 3, uppersurface indicating prominent lobes and gyri.

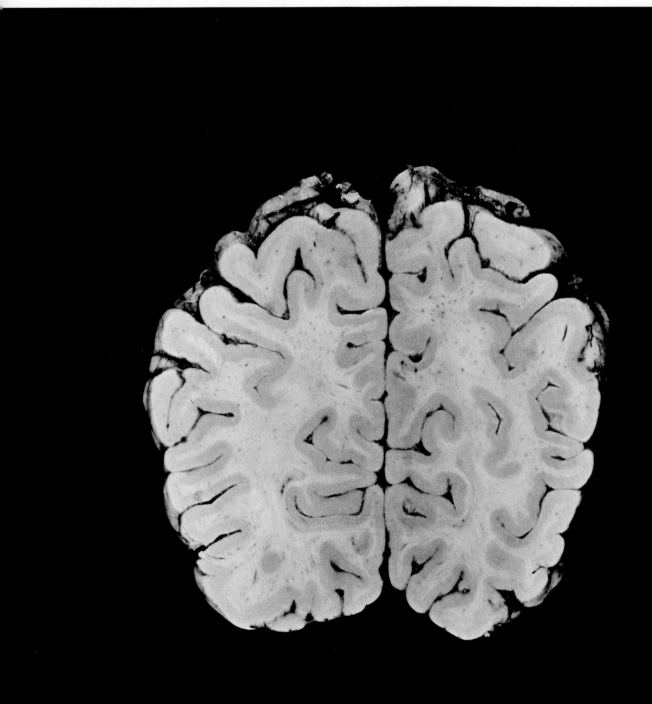

60° section, No. 4, uppersurface.

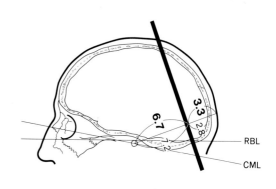

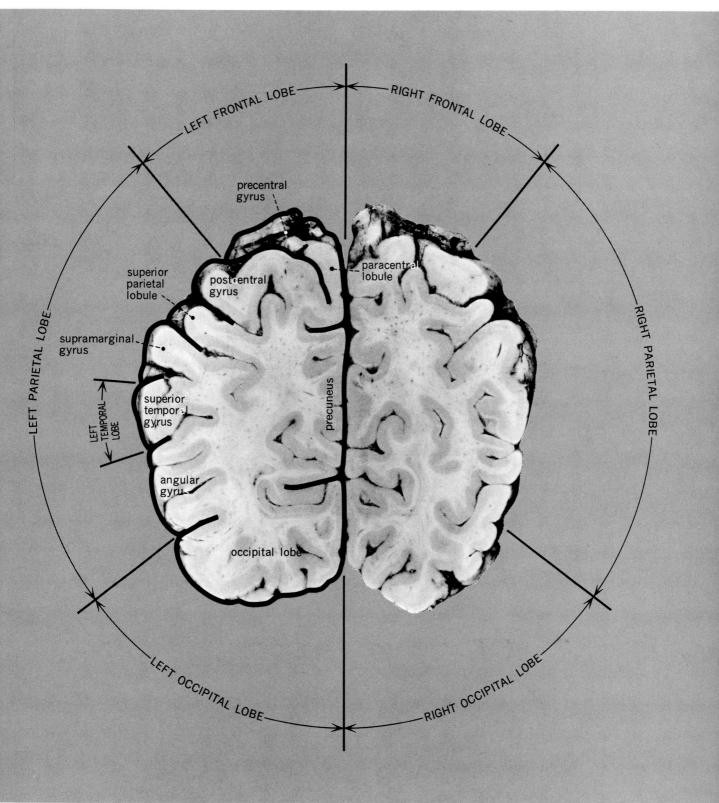

60° section, No. 4, uppersurface indicating prominent lobes and gyri.

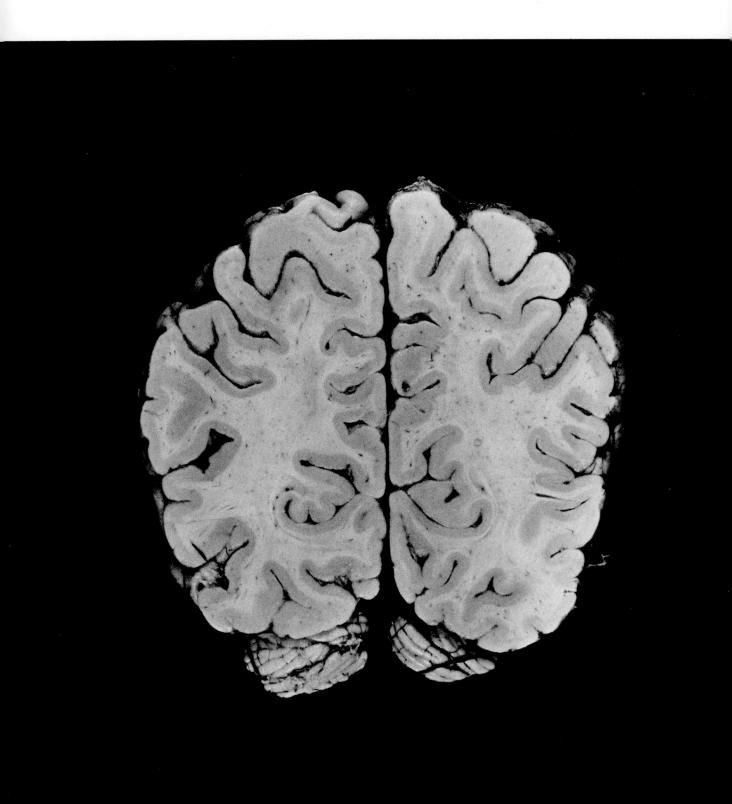

60° section, No. 5, uppersurface.

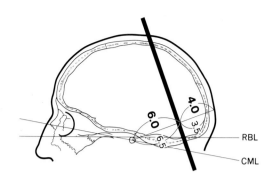

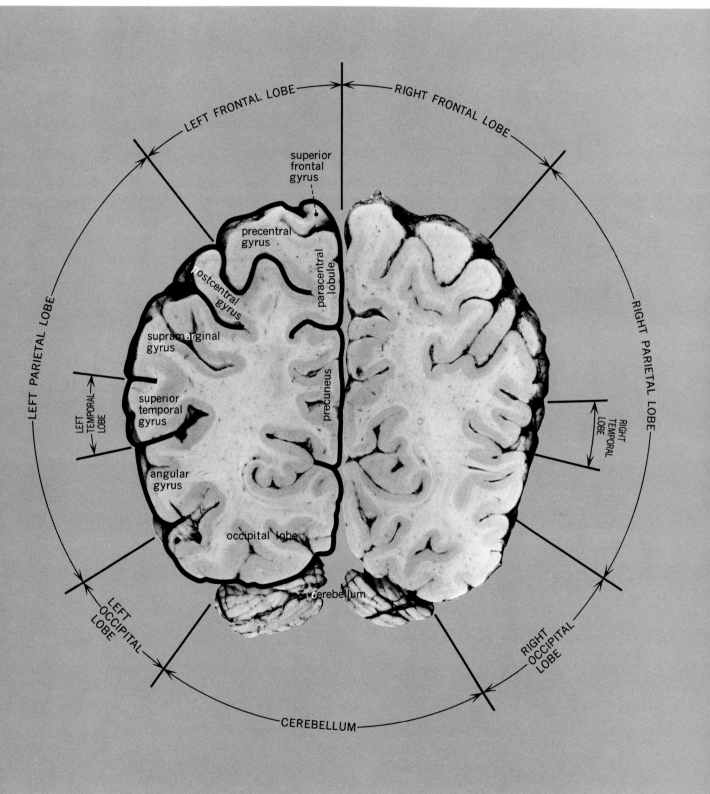

60° section, No. 5, uppersurface indicating prominent lobes and gyri.

367

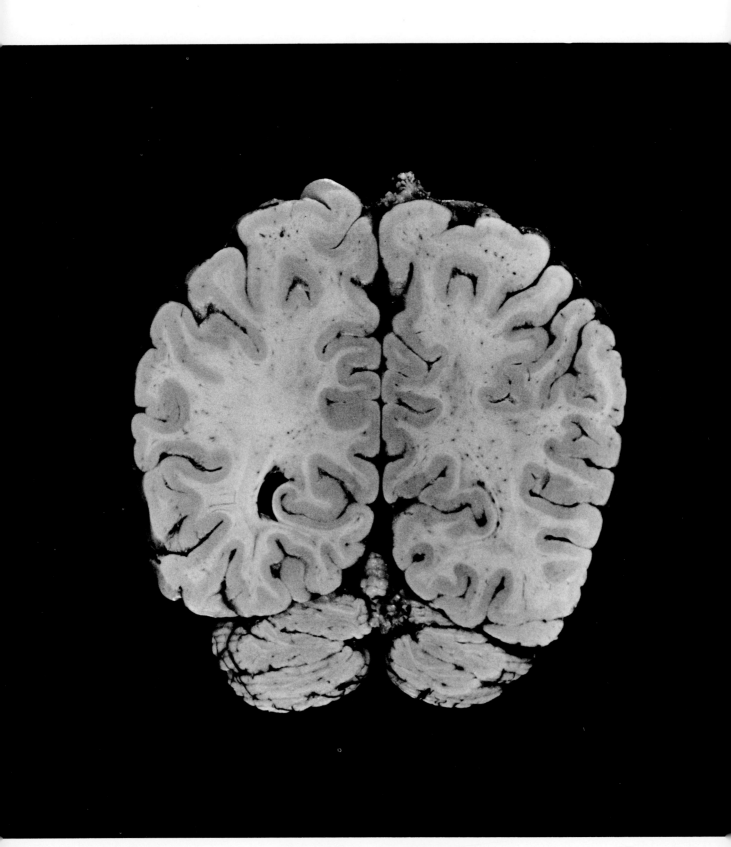

60° section, No. 6, uppersurface.

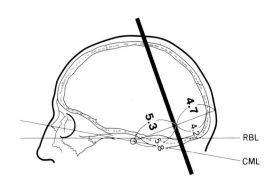

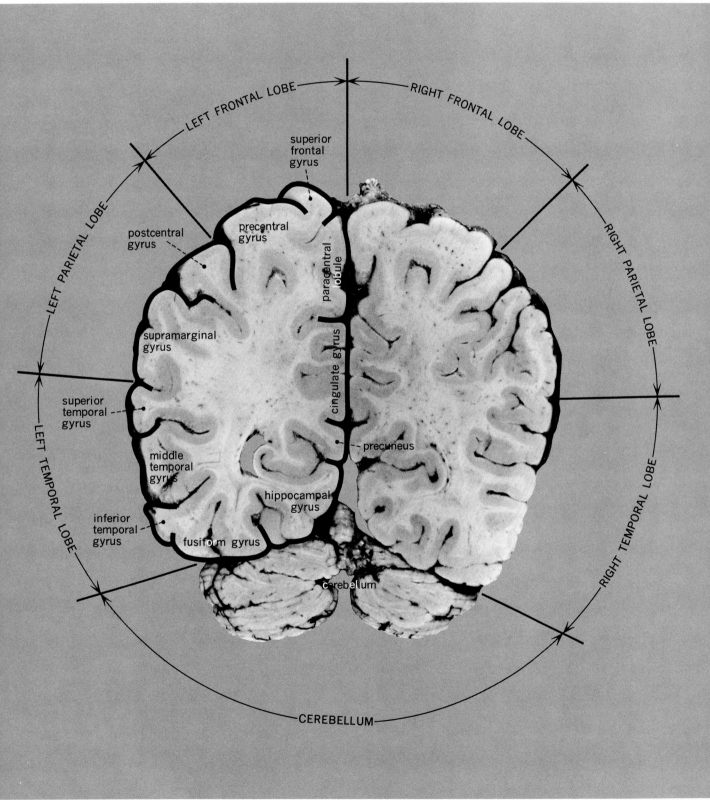

60° section, No. 6, uppersurface indicating prominent lobes and gyri.

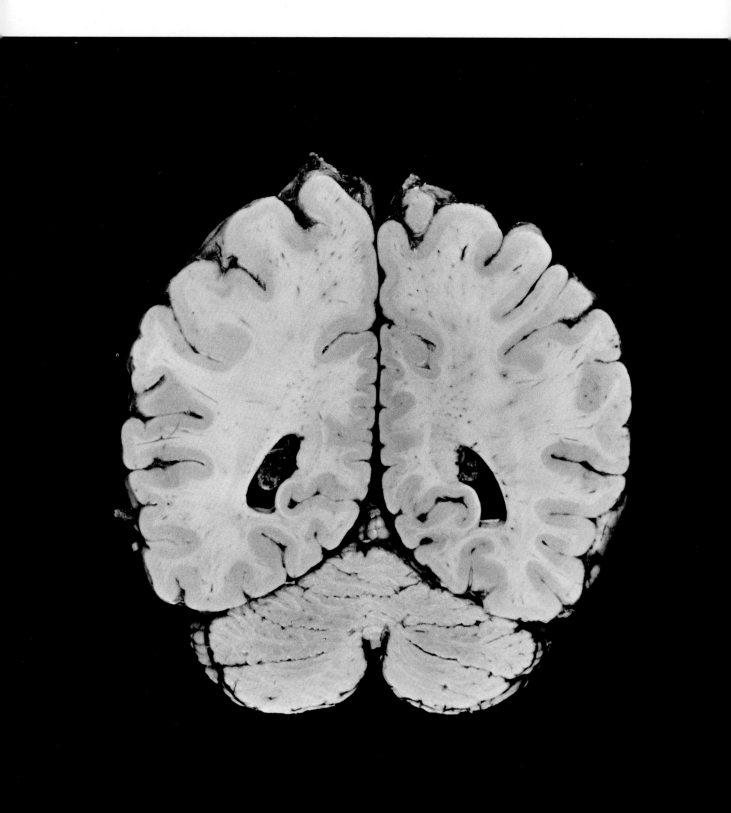

60° section, No. 7, uppersurface.

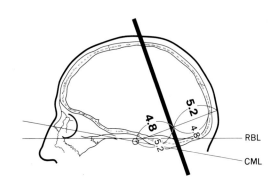

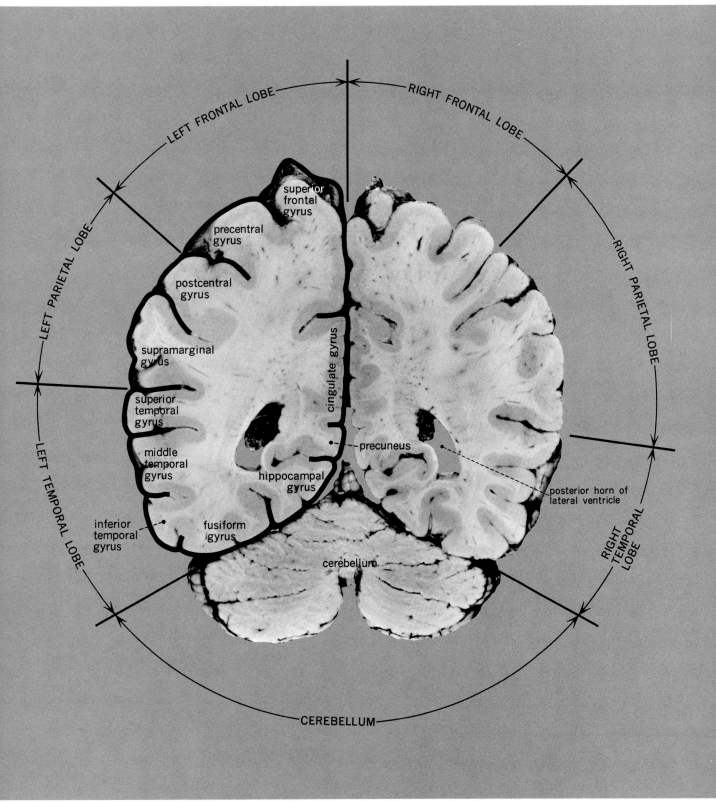

60° section, No. 7, uppersurface indicating prominent structures, lobes and gyri.

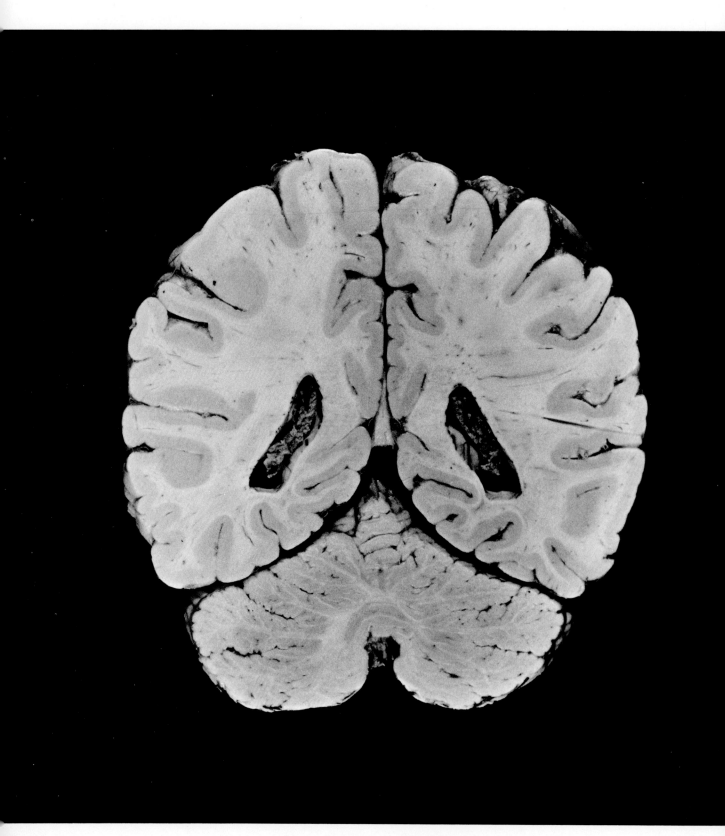

60° section, No. 8, uppersurface.

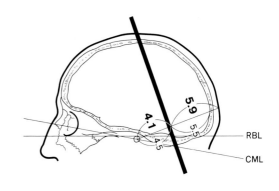

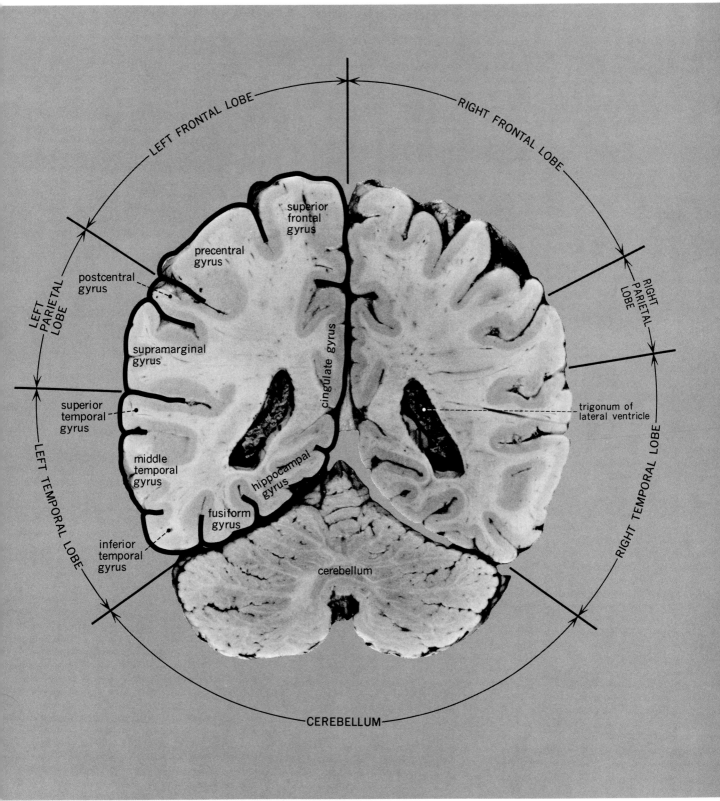

60° section, No. 8, uppersurface indicating prominent structures, lobes and gyri.

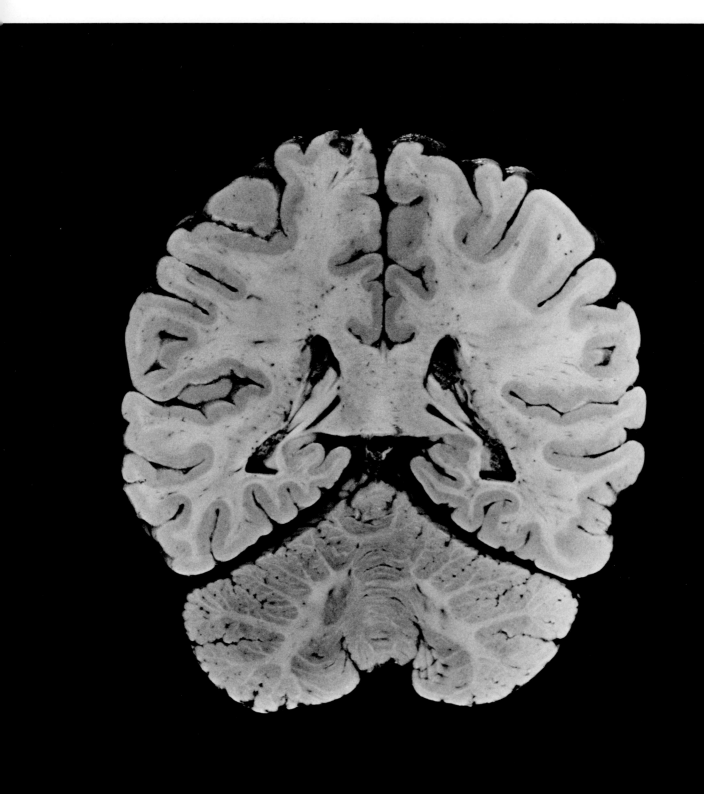

60° section, No. 9, uppersurface.

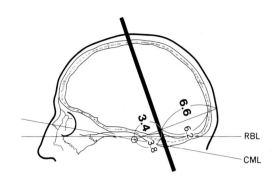

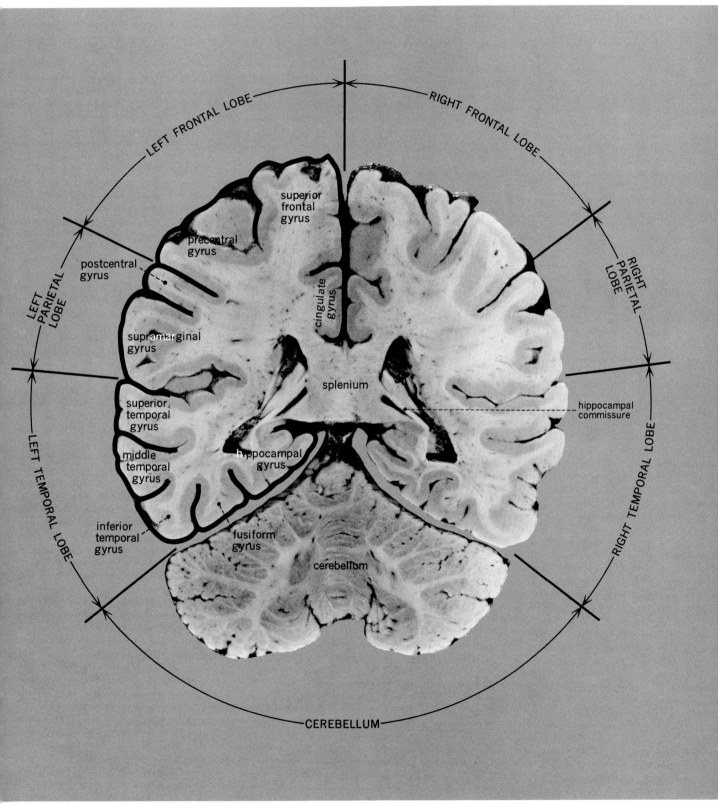

60° section, No. 9, uppersurface indicating prominent structures, lobes and gyri.

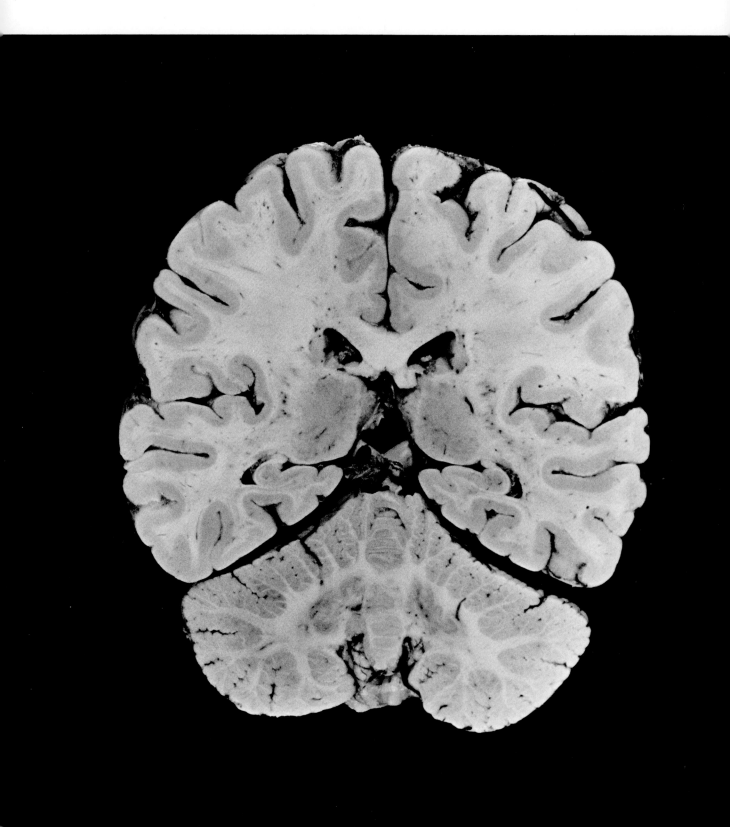

60° section, No. 10, uppersurface.

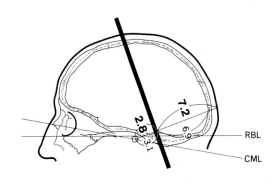

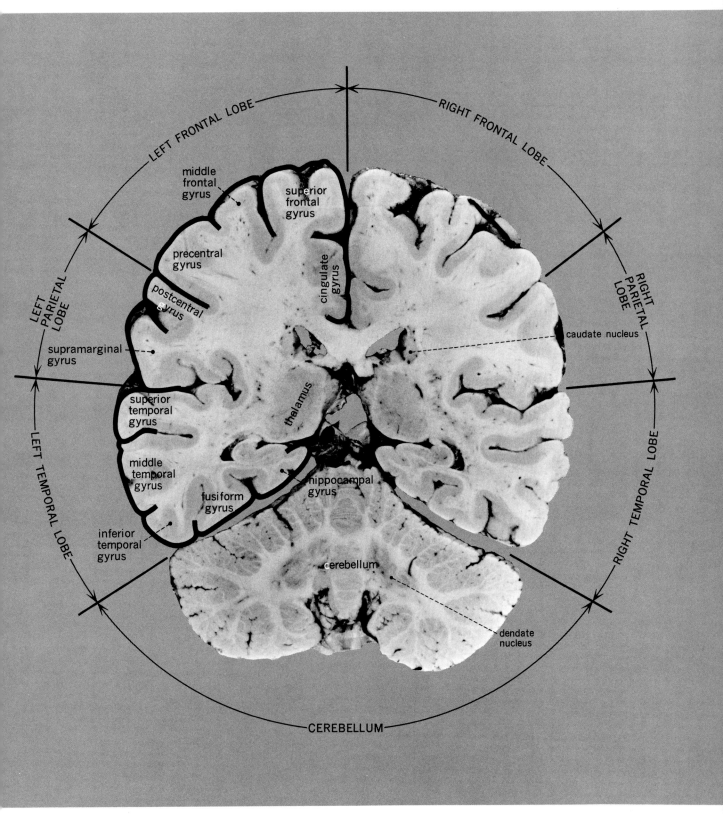

60° section, No. 10, uppersurface indicating prominent structures, lobes and gyri.

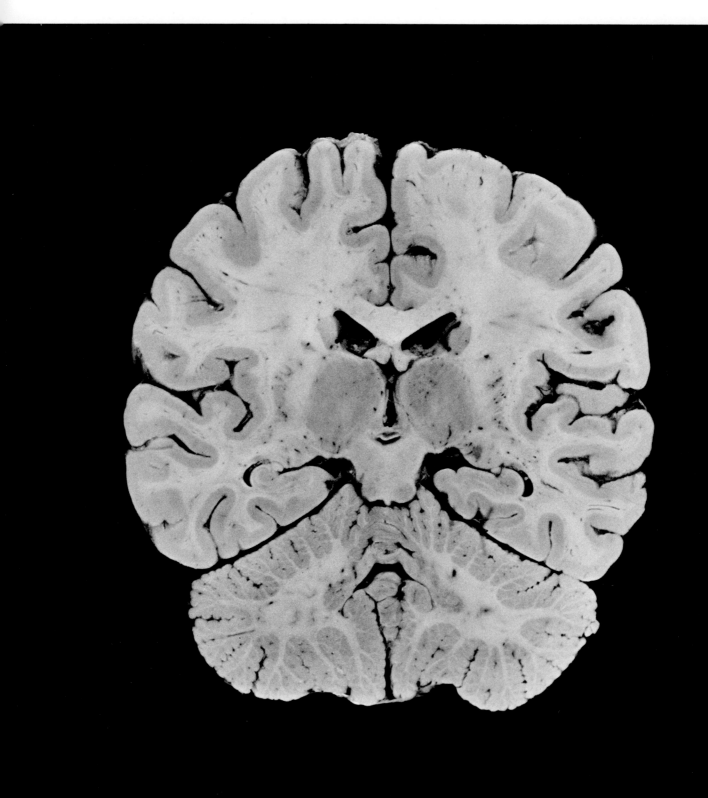

60° section, No. 11, uppersurface.

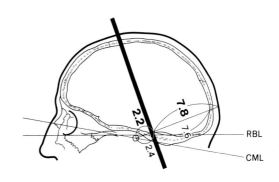

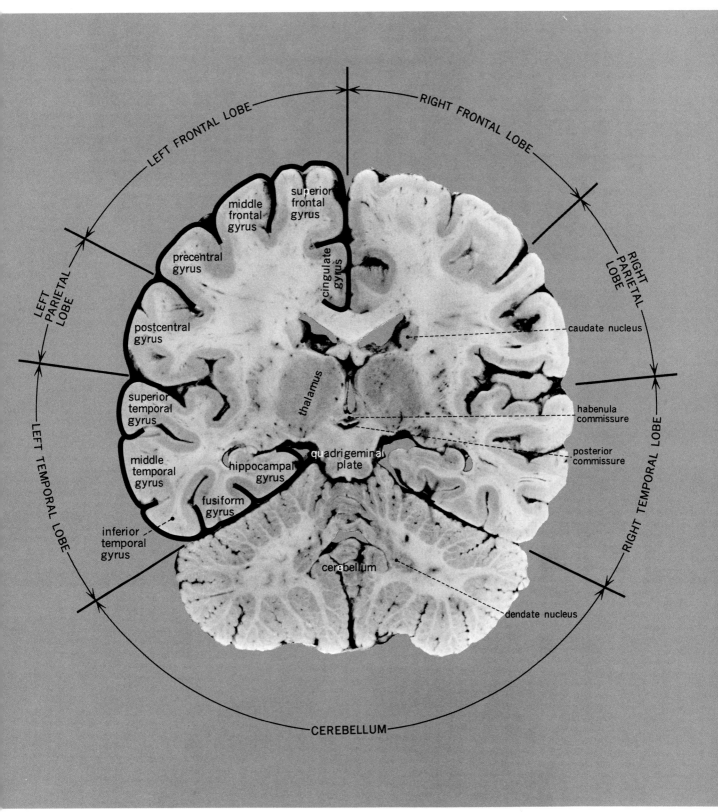

60° section, No. 11, uppersurface indicating prominent structures, lobes and gyri.

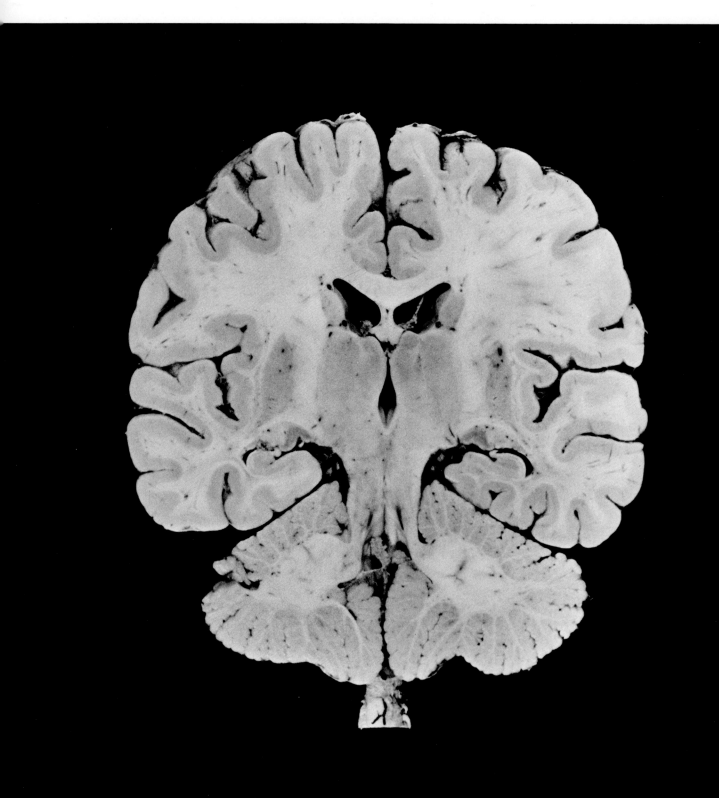

60° section, No. 12, uppersurface.

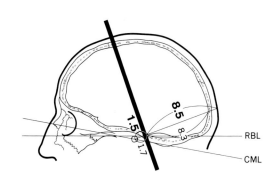

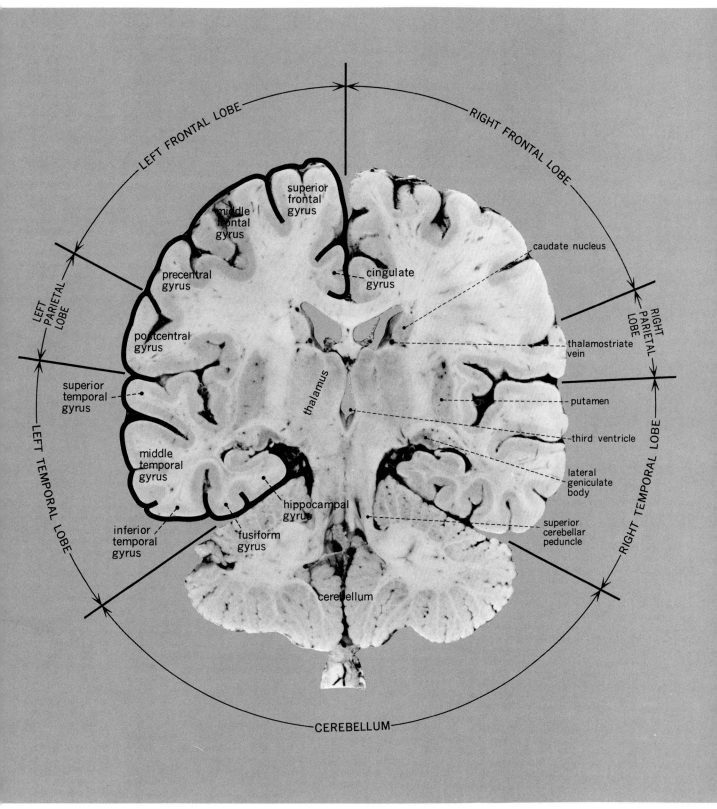

60° section, No. 12, uppersurface indicating prominent structures, lobes and gyri.

60°-13

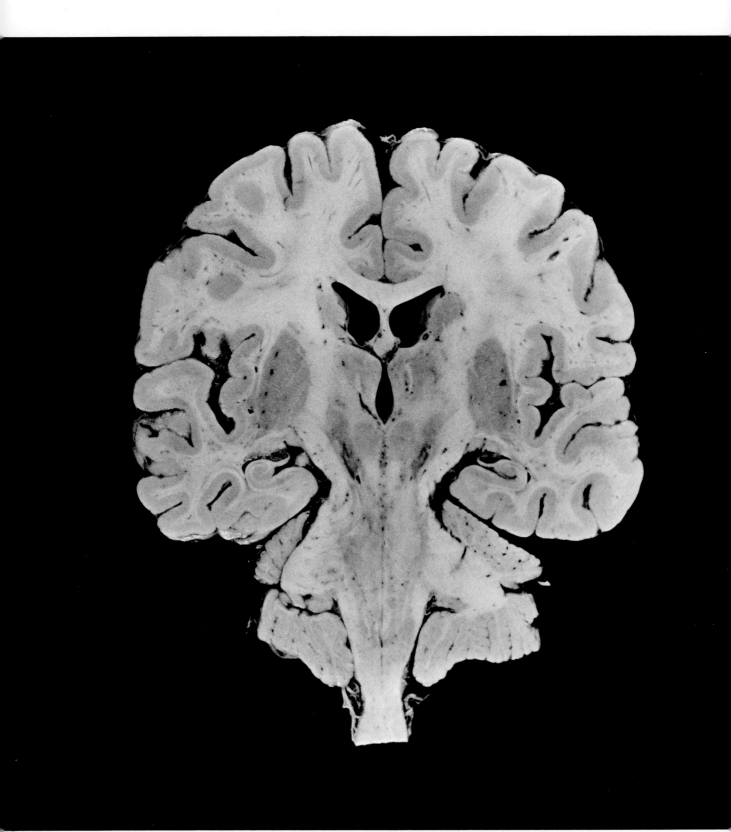

60° section, No. 13, uppersurface.

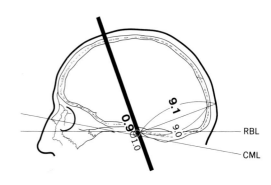

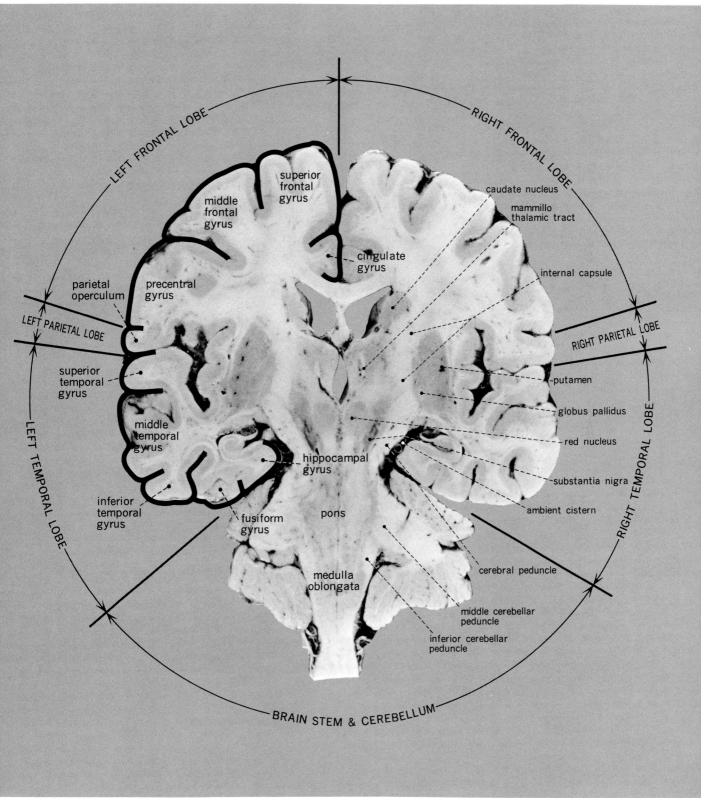

60° section, No. 13, uppersurface indicating prominent structures, lobes and gyri.

60°-14

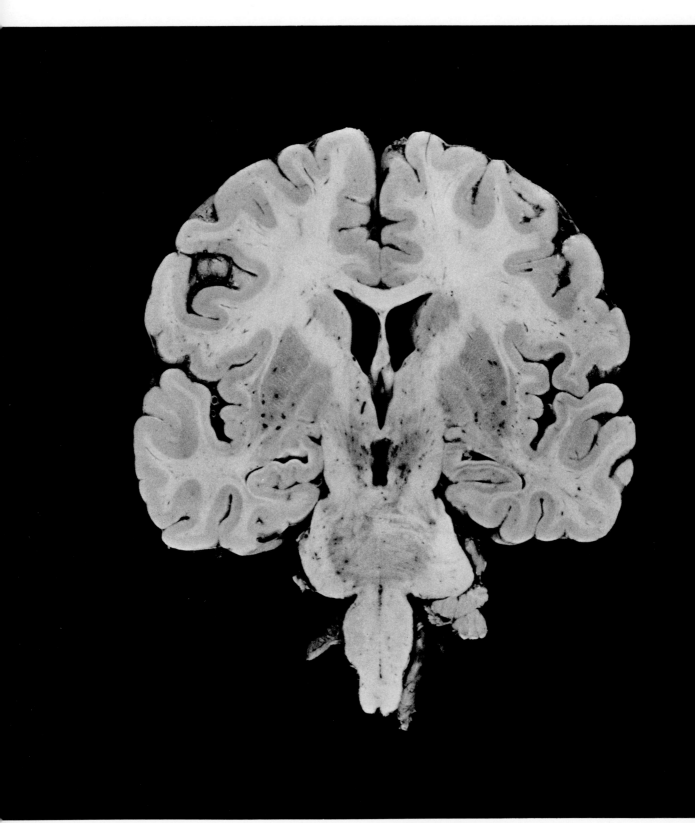

60° section, No. 14, uppersurface.

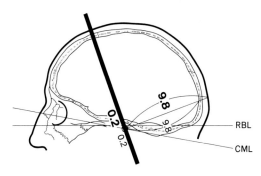

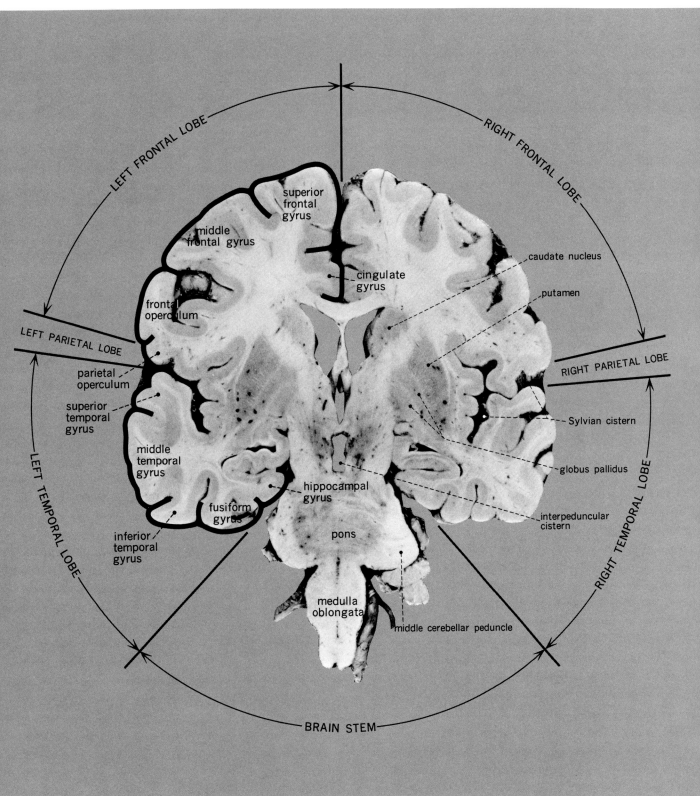

60° section, No. 14, uppersurface indicating prominent structures, lobes and gyri.

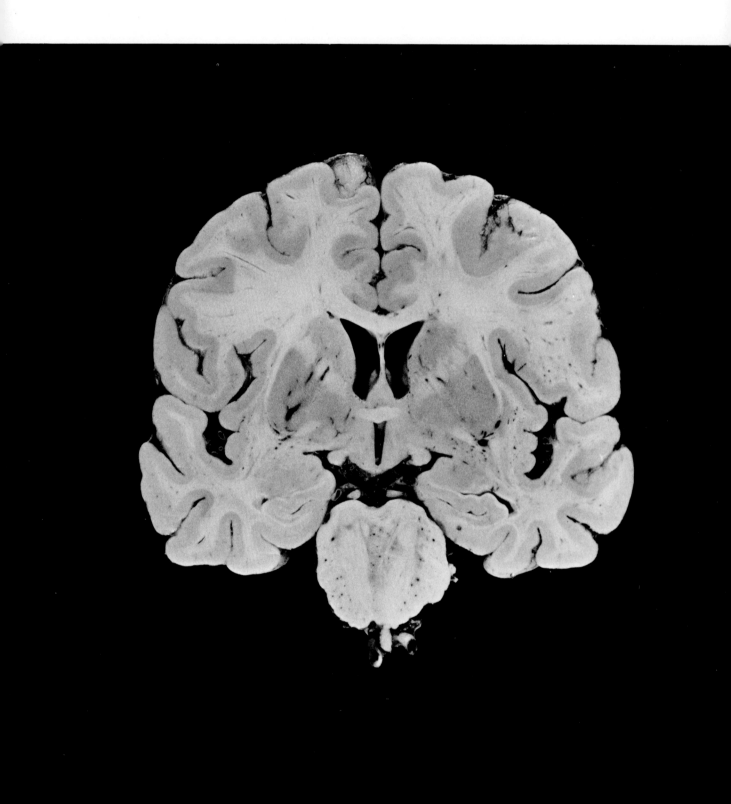

60° section, No. 15, uppersurface.

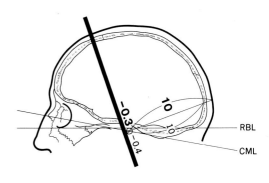

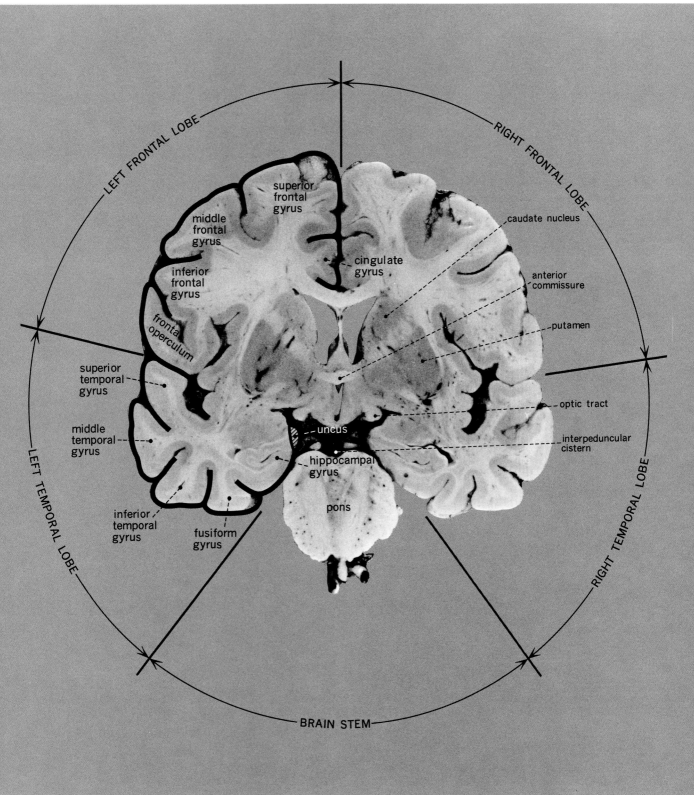

60° section, No. 15, uppersurface indicating prominent structures, lobes and gyri.

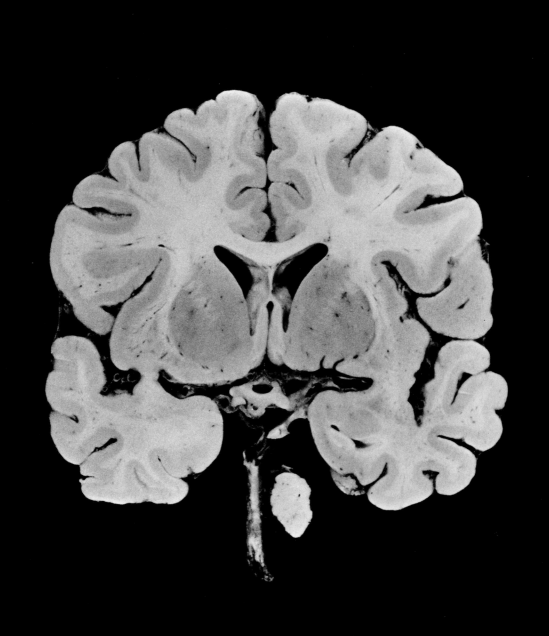

60° section, No. 16, uppersurface.

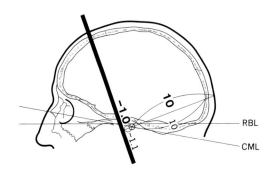

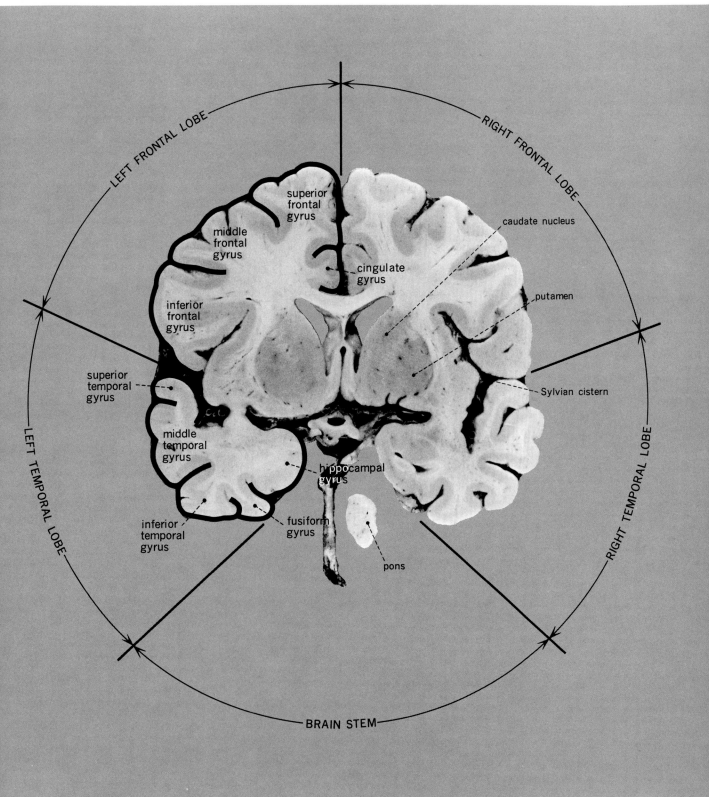

60° section, No. 16, uppersurface indicating prominent structures, lobes and gyri.

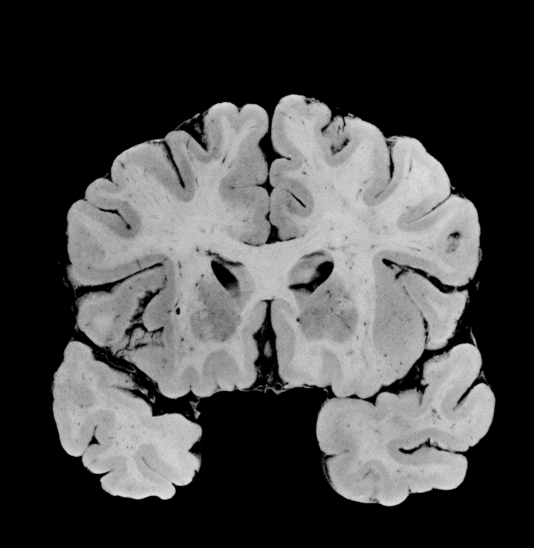

60° section, No. 17, uppersurface.

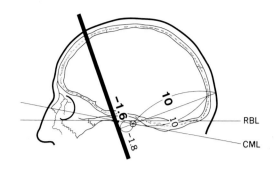

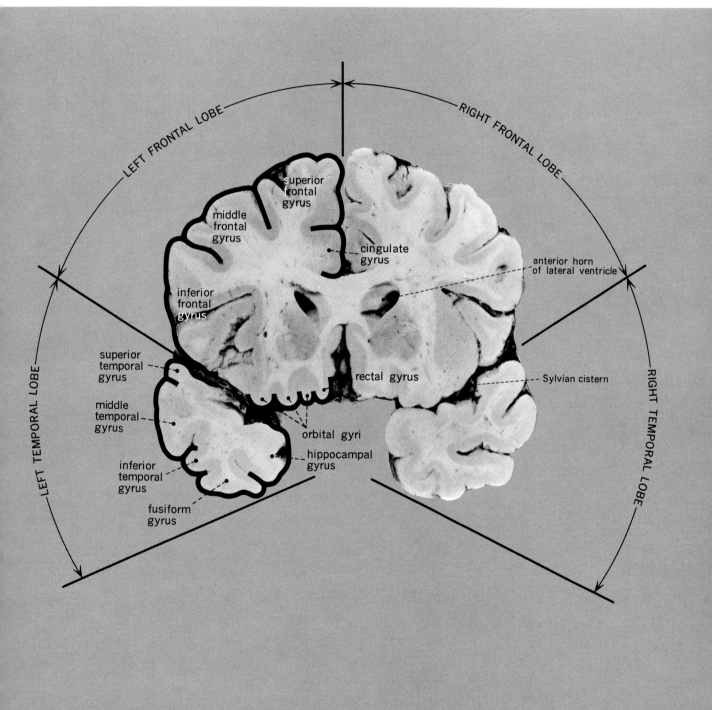

60° section, No. 17, uppersurface indicating prominent lobes and gyri.

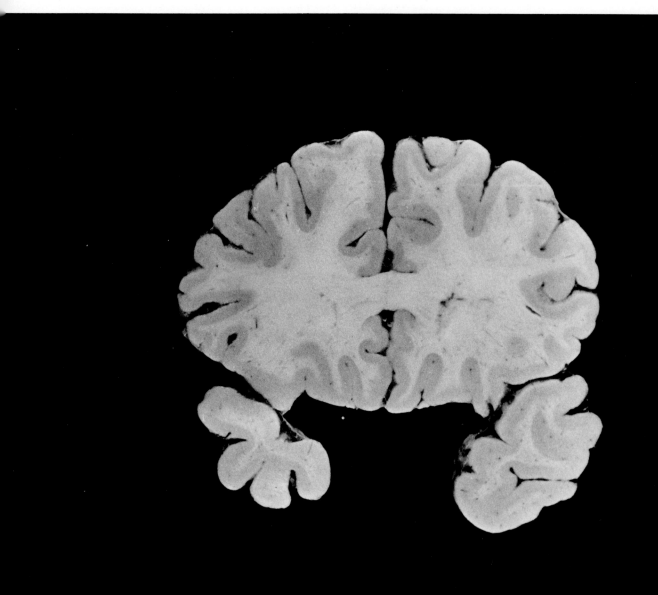

60° section, No. 18, uppersurface.

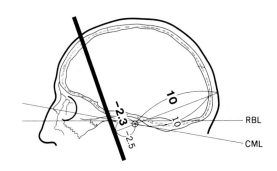

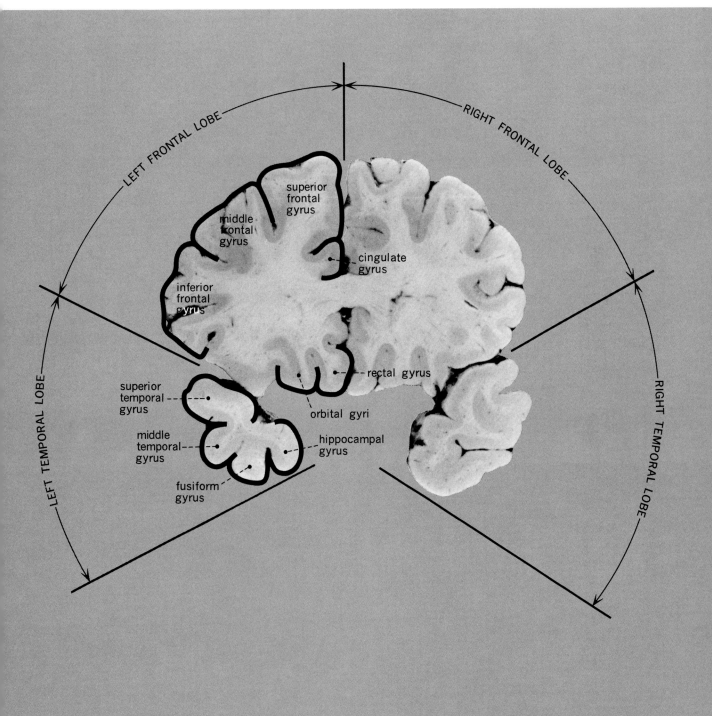

60° section, No. 18, uppersurface indicating prominent lobes and gyri.

Labels in figure:
- LEFT FRONTAL LOBE
- RIGHT FRONTAL LOBE
- LEFT TEMPORAL LOBE
- RIGHT TEMPORAL LOBE
- superior frontal gyrus
- middle frontal gyrus
- inferior frontal gyrus
- cingulate gyrus
- rectal gyrus
- orbital gyri
- superior temporal gyrus
- middle temporal gyrus
- fusiform gyrus
- hippocampal gyrus
- RBL
- CML

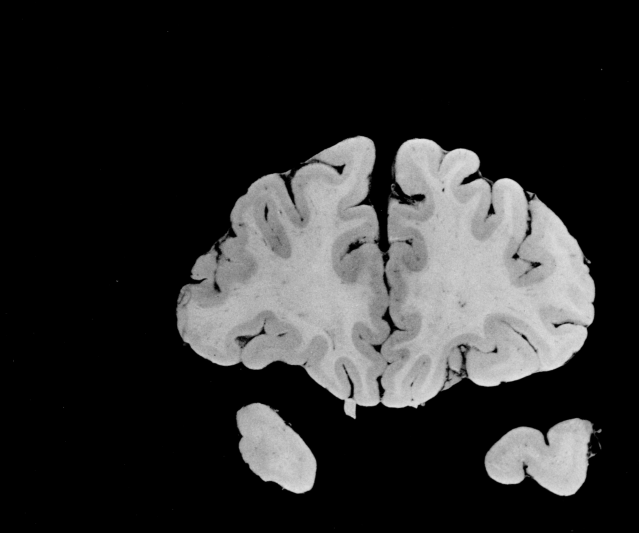

60° section, No. 19, uppersurface.

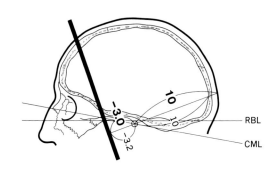

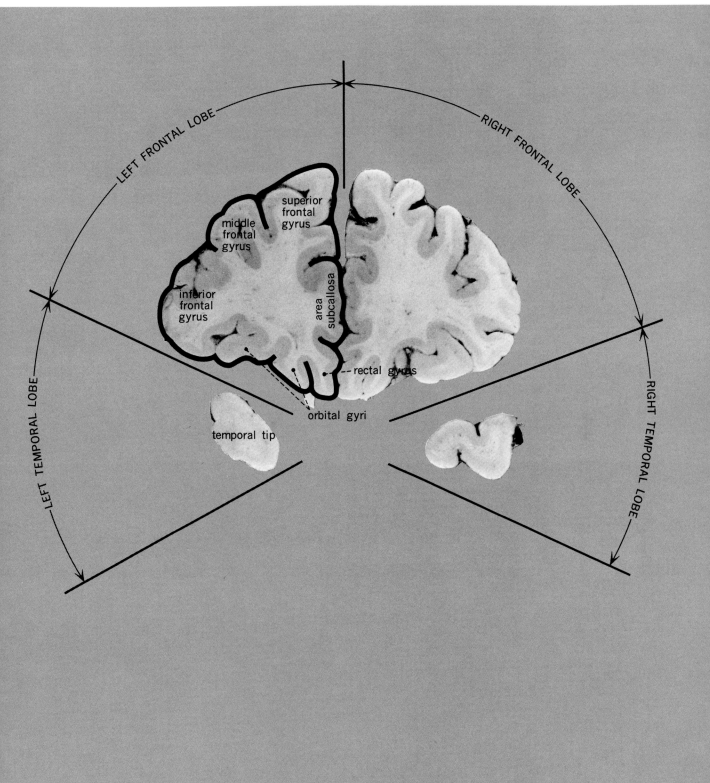

60° section, No. 19, uppersurface indicating prominent lobes and gyri.

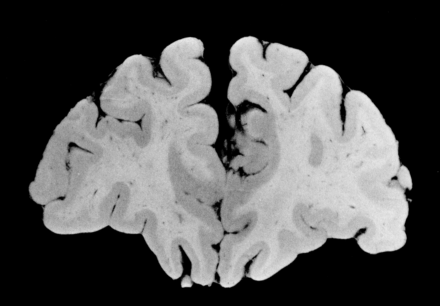

60° section, No. 20, uppersurface.

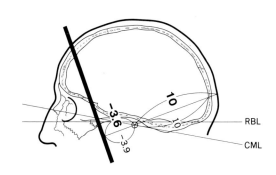

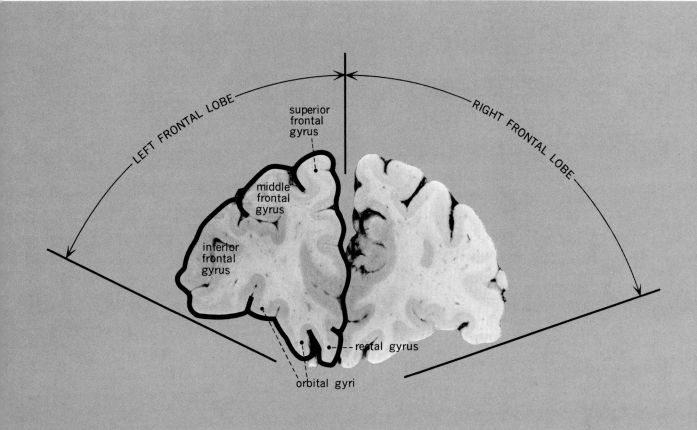

LEFT FRONTAL LOBE

RIGHT FRONTAL LOBE

superior frontal gyrus

middle frontal gyrus

inferior frontal gyrus

orbital gyri

rectal gyrus

60° section, No. 20, uppersurface indicating prominent lobes and gyri.

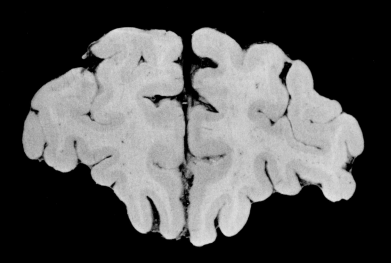

60° section, No. 21, uppersurface.

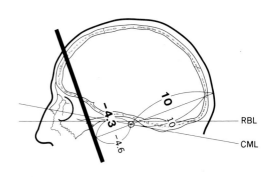

RBL

CML

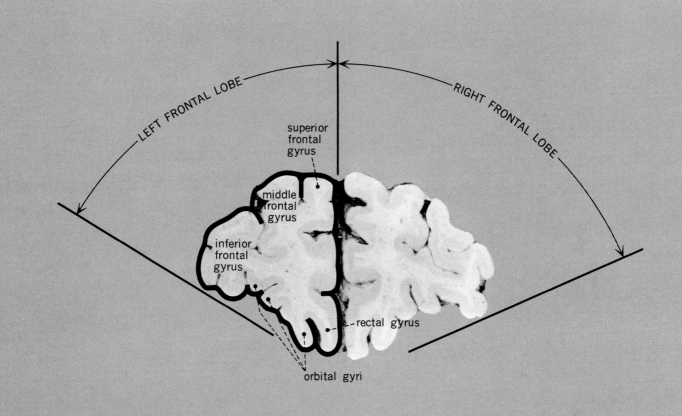

60° section, No. 21, uppersurface indicating prominent lobes and gyri.

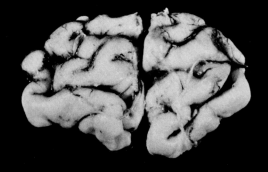

80° section, No. 1, uppersurface.

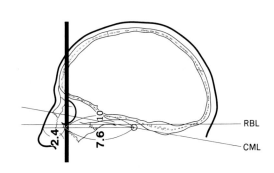

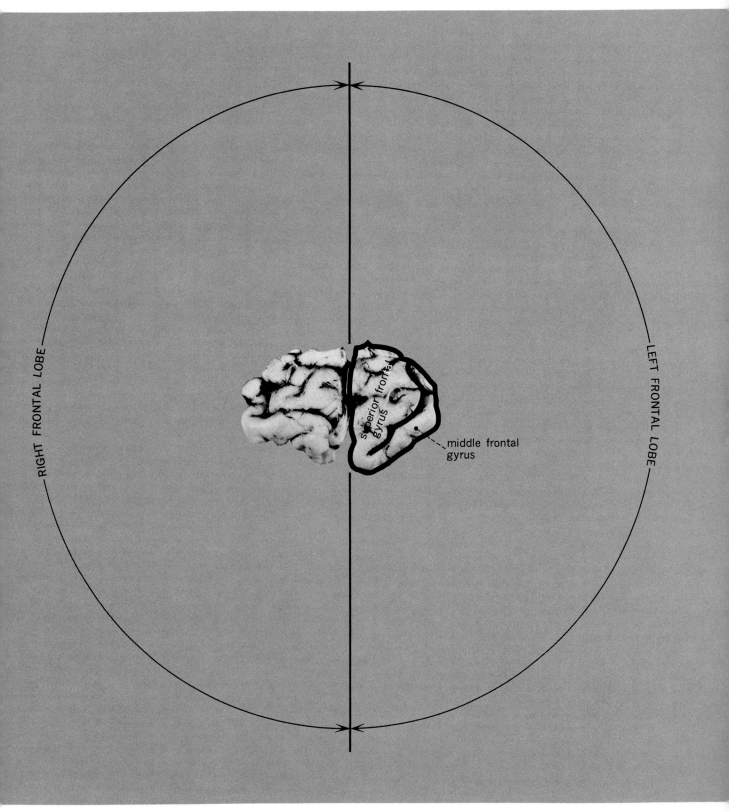

RIGHT FRONTAL LOBE

LEFT FRONTAL LOBE

superior frontal gyrus

middle frontal gyrus

80° section, No. 1, uppersurface indicating prominent lobes and gyri.

80°-2

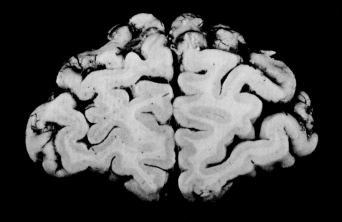

80° section, No. 2, uppersurface.

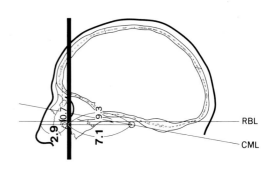

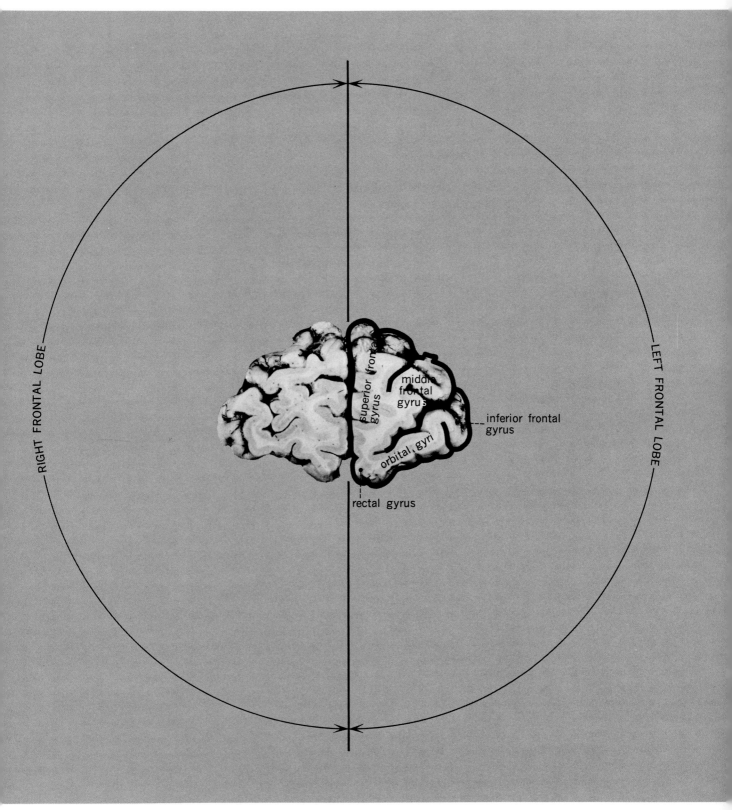

80° section, No. 2, uppersurface indicating prominent lobes and gyri.

80°-3

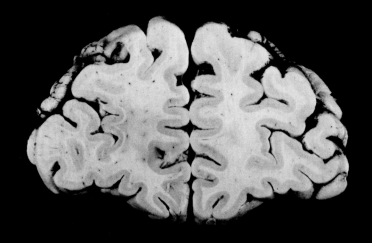

80° section, No. 3, uppersurface.

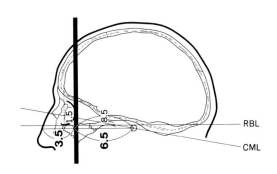

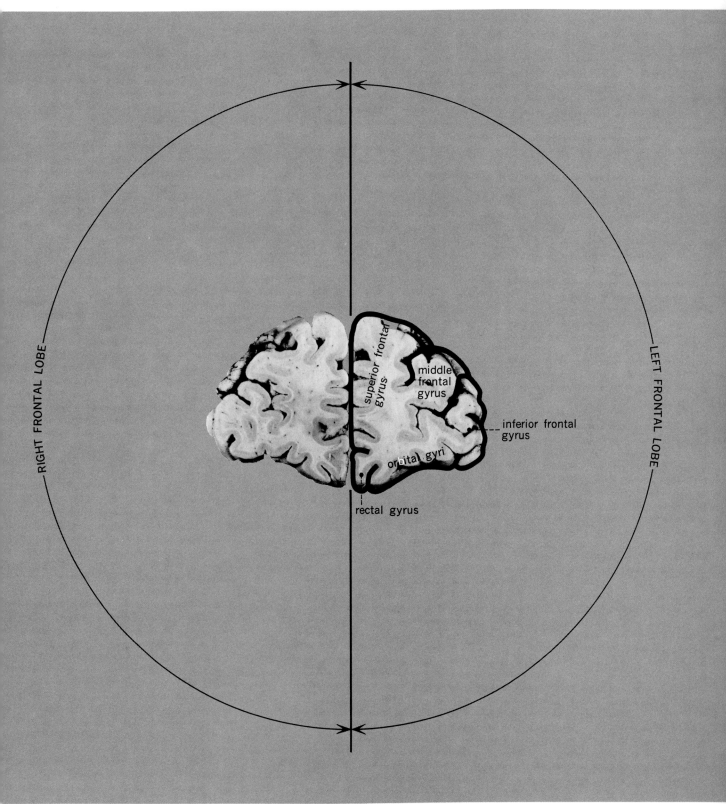

RIGHT FRONTAL LOBE

LEFT FRONTAL LOBE

superior frontal gyrus

middle frontal gyrus

inferior frontal gyrus

orbital gyri

rectal gyrus

80° section, No. 3, uppersurface indicating prominent lobes and gyri.

80°-4

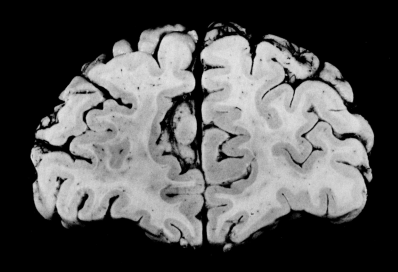

80° section, No. 4, uppersurface.

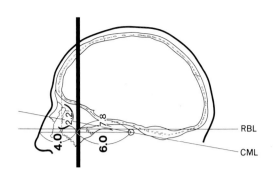

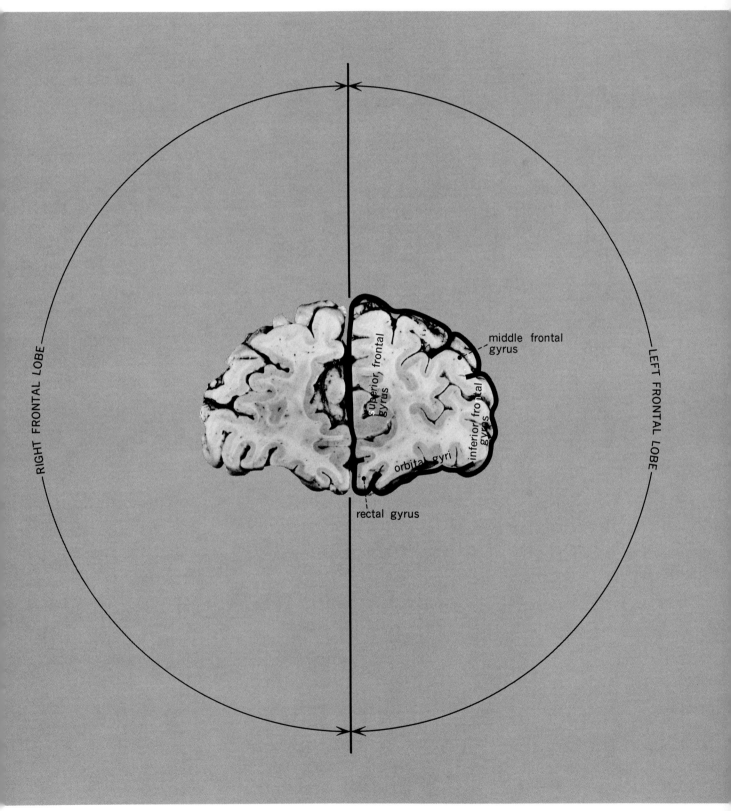

RIGHT FRONTAL LOBE

LEFT FRONTAL LOBE

middle frontal gyrus

superior frontal gyrus

inferior frontal gyrus

orbital gyri

inferior frontal gyrus

rectal gyrus

80° section, No. 4, uppersurface indicating prominent lobes and gyri.

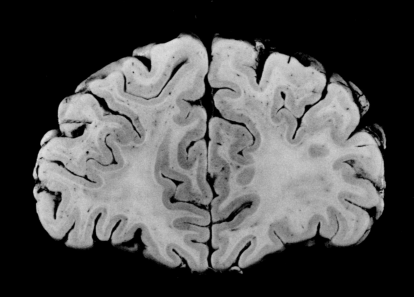

80° section, No. 5, uppersurface.

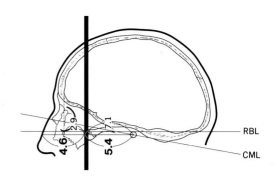

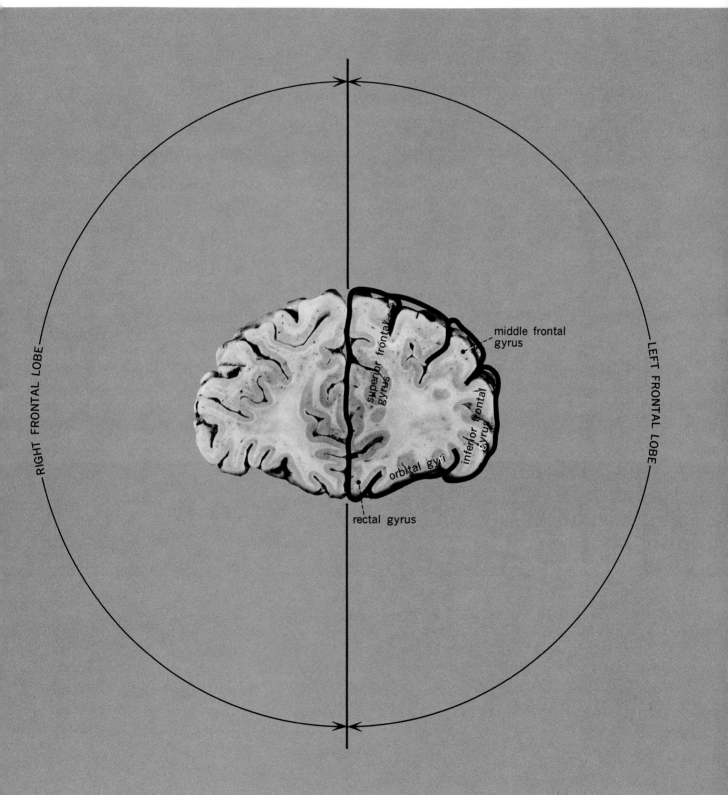

RIGHT FRONTAL LOBE

LEFT FRONTAL LOBE

superior frontal gyrus

middle frontal gyrus

inferior frontal gyrus

orbital gyri

rectal gyrus

80° section, No. 5, uppersurface indicating prominent lobes and gyri.

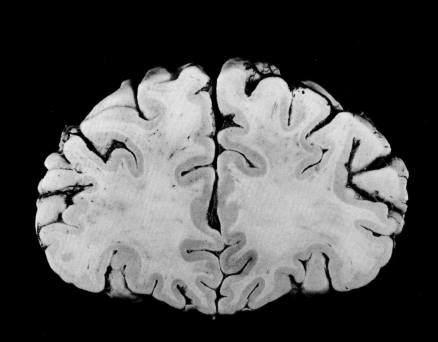

80° section, No. 6, uppersurface.

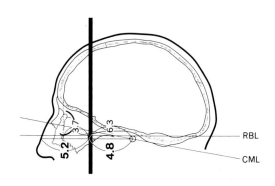

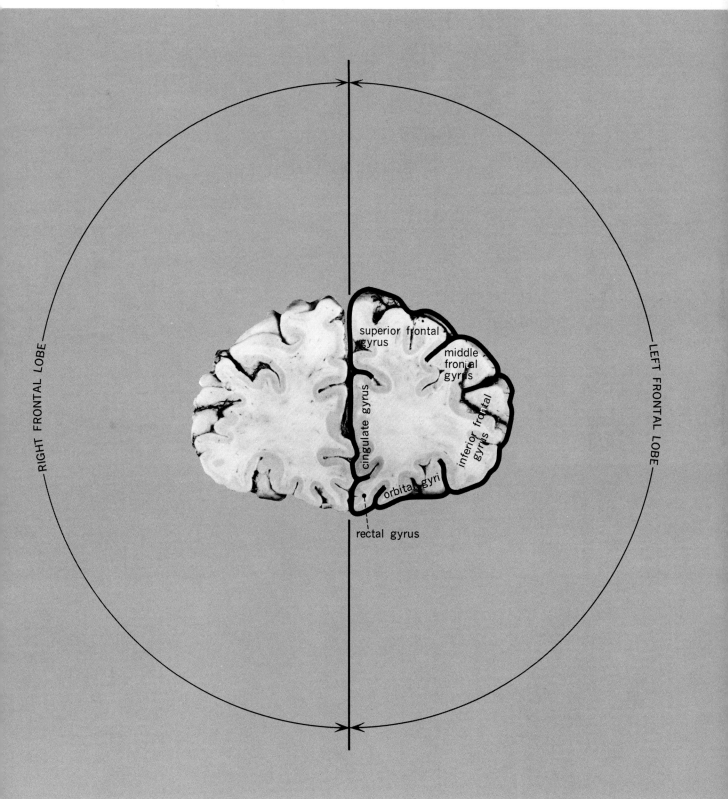

80° section, No. 6, uppersurface indicating prominent lobes and gyri.

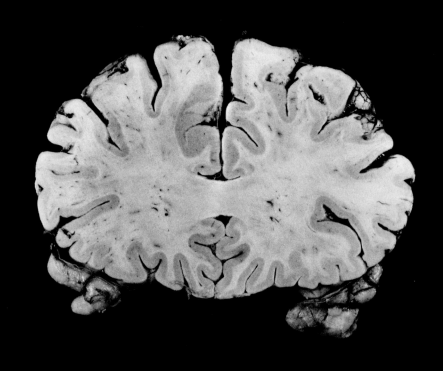

80° section, No. 7, uppersurface.

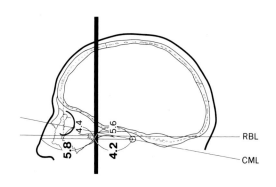

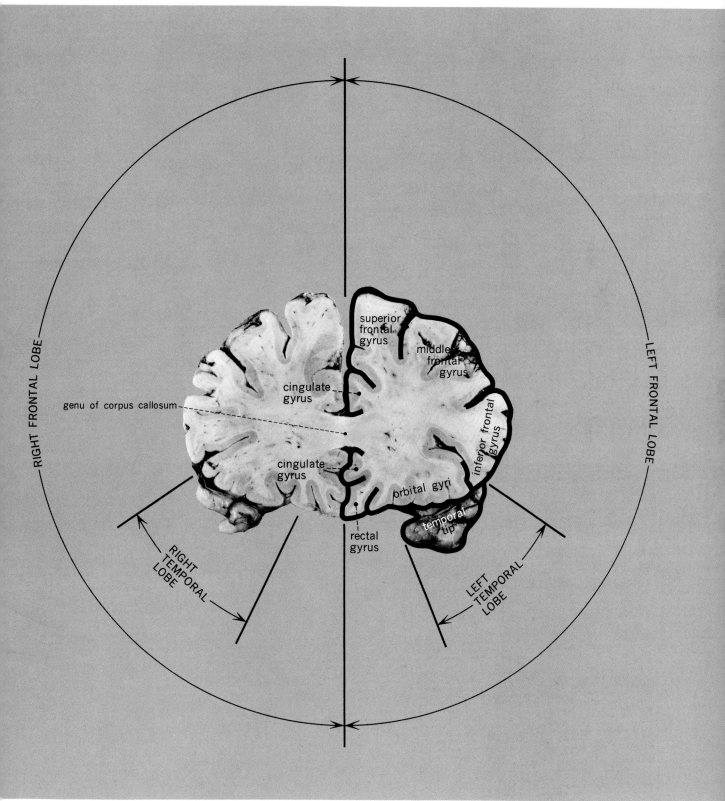

80° section, No. 7, uppersurface indicating prominent structures, lobes and gyri.

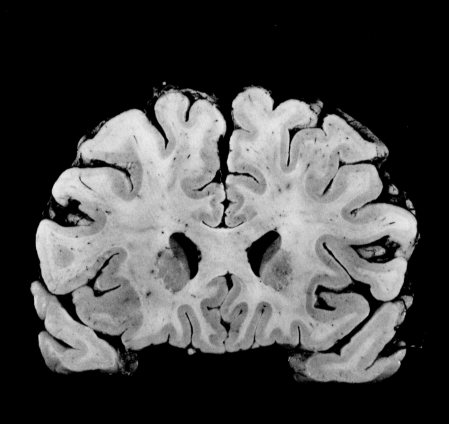

80° section, No. 8, uppersurface.

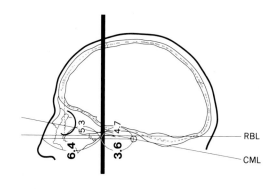

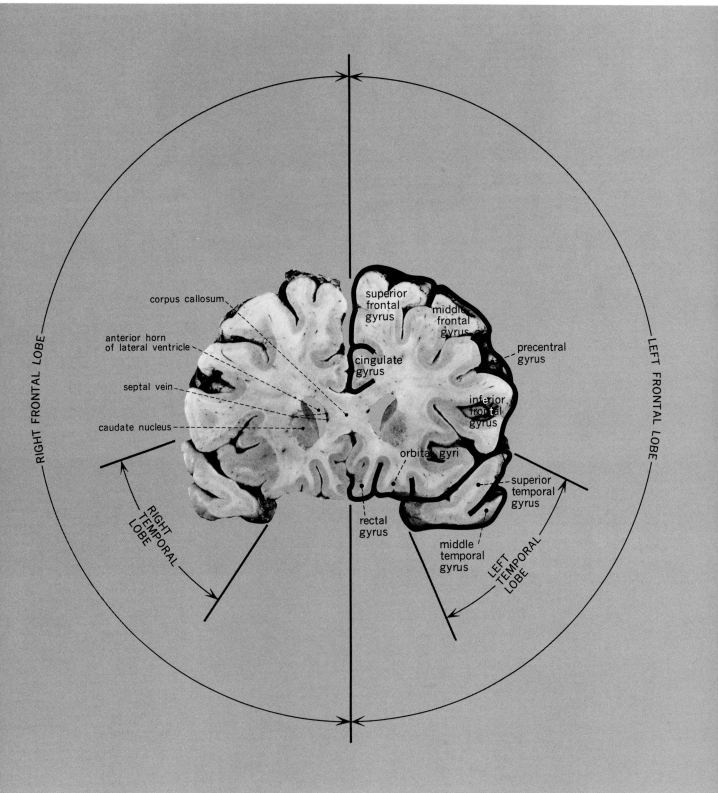

80° section, No. 8, uppersurface indicating prominent structures, lobes and gyri.

80°- 9

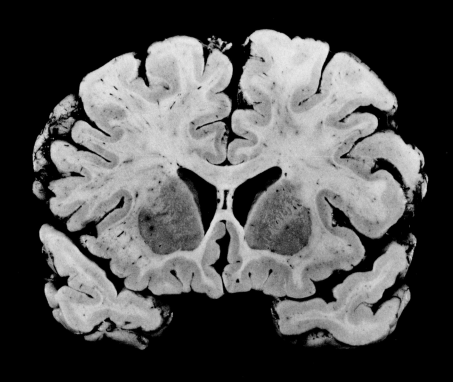

80° section, No. 9, uppersurface.

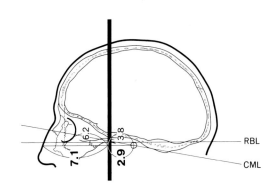

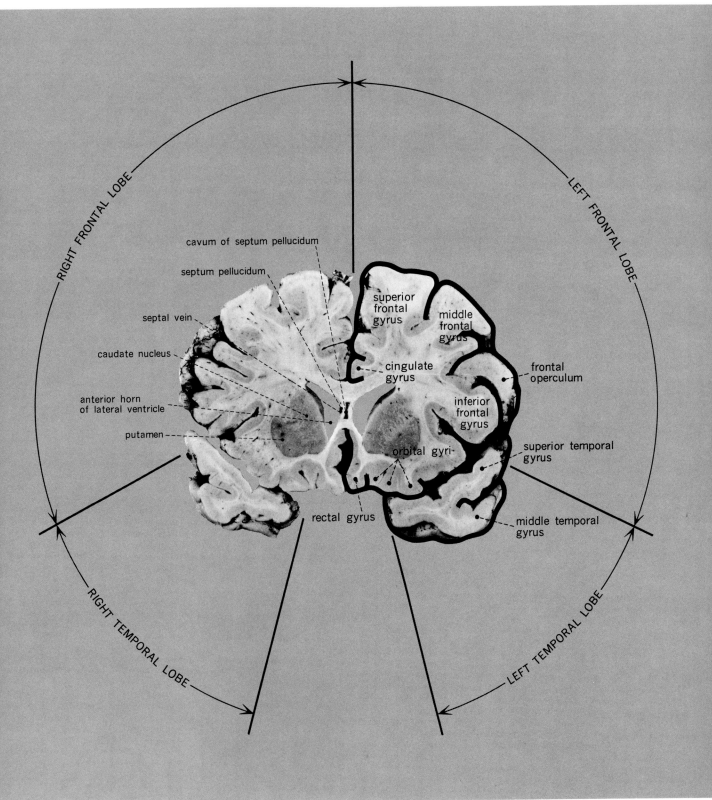

Figure labels:
- RIGHT FRONTAL LOBE
- LEFT FRONTAL LOBE
- RIGHT TEMPORAL LOBE
- LEFT TEMPORAL LOBE
- cavum of septum pellucidum
- septum pellucidum
- septal vein
- caudate nucleus
- anterior horn of lateral ventricle
- putamen
- superior frontal gyrus
- middle frontal gyrus
- cingulate gyrus
- frontal operculum
- inferior frontal gyrus
- orbital gyri
- superior temporal gyrus
- rectal gyrus
- middle temporal gyrus

80° section, No. 9, uppersurface indicating prominent structures, lobes and gyri.

417

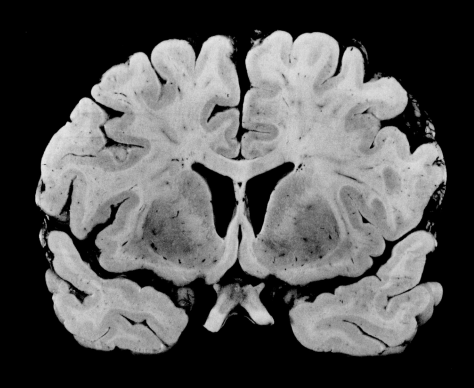

80° section, No. 10, uppersurface.

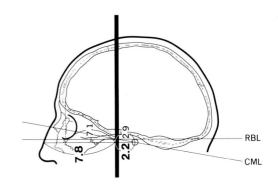

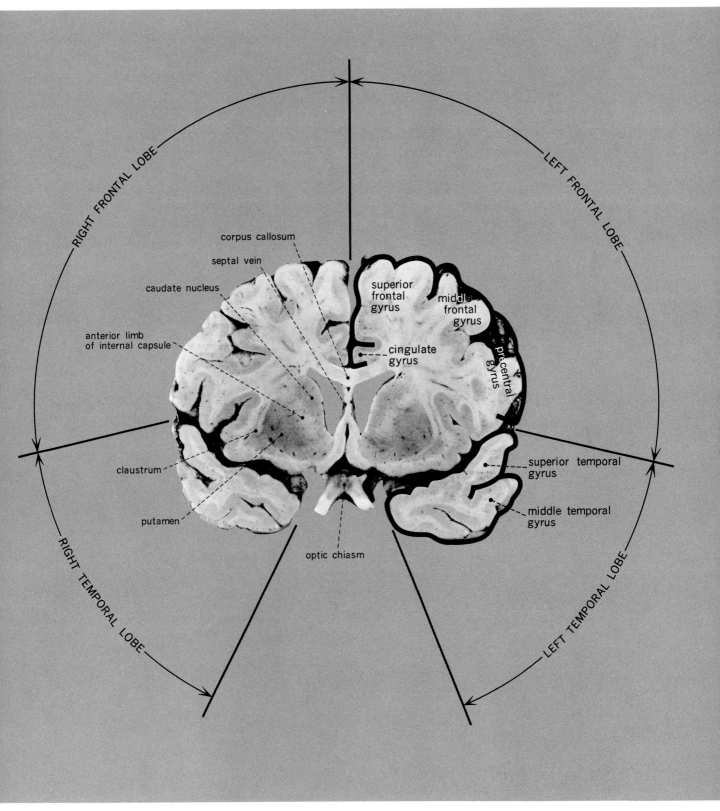

RIGHT FRONTAL LOBE

LEFT FRONTAL LOBE

corpus callosum

septal vein

caudate nucleus

superior
frontal
gyrus

middle
frontal
gyrus

anterior limb
of internal capsule

cingulate
gyrus

pre-central
gyrus

claustrum

superior temporal
gyrus

middle temporal
gyrus

putamen

RIGHT TEMPORAL LOBE

optic chiasm

LEFT TEMPORAL LOBE

80° section, No. 10, uppersurface indicating prominent structures, lobes and gyri.

419

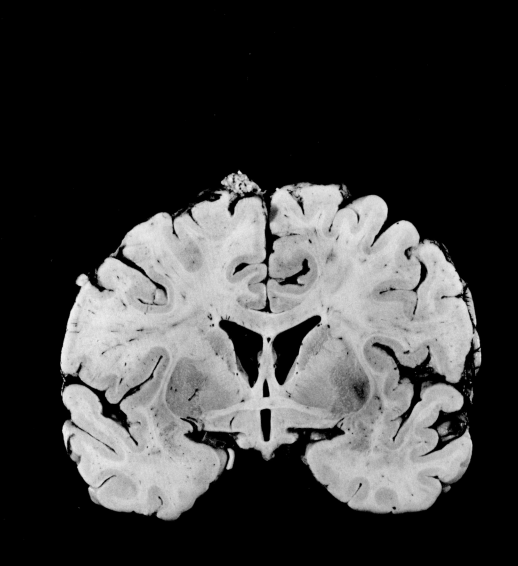

80° section, No. 11, uppersurface.

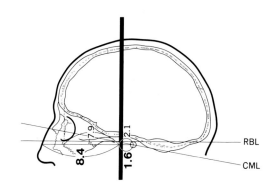

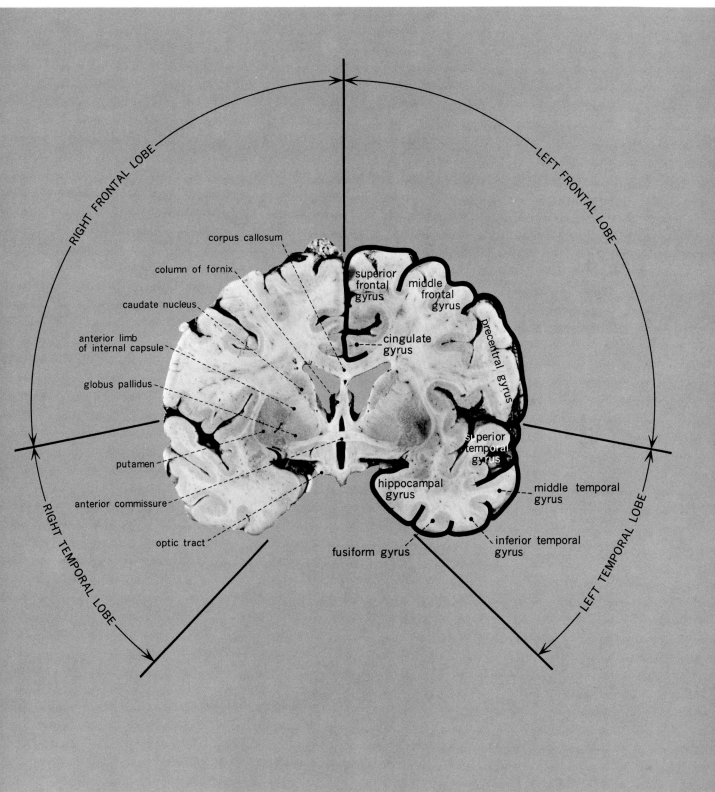

corpus callosum

column of fornix

caudate nucleus

anterior limb
of internal capsule

globus pallidus

putamen

anterior commissure

optic tract

RIGHT FRONTAL LOBE

LEFT FRONTAL LOBE

superior
frontal
gyrus

middle
frontal
gyrus

cingulate
gyrus

precentral gyrus

superior
temporal
gyrus

hippocampal
gyrus

middle temporal
gyrus

inferior temporal
gyrus

fusiform gyrus

RIGHT TEMPORAL LOBE

LEFT TEMPORAL LOBE

80° section, No. 11, uppersurface indicating prominent structures, lobes and gyri.

80°- 12

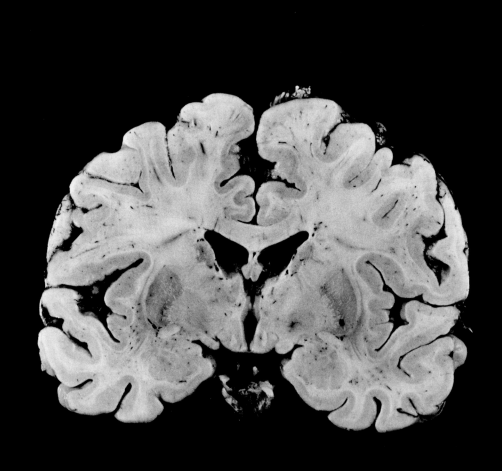

80° section, No. 12, uppersurface.

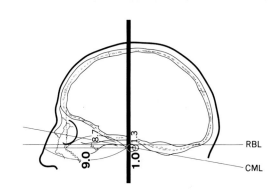

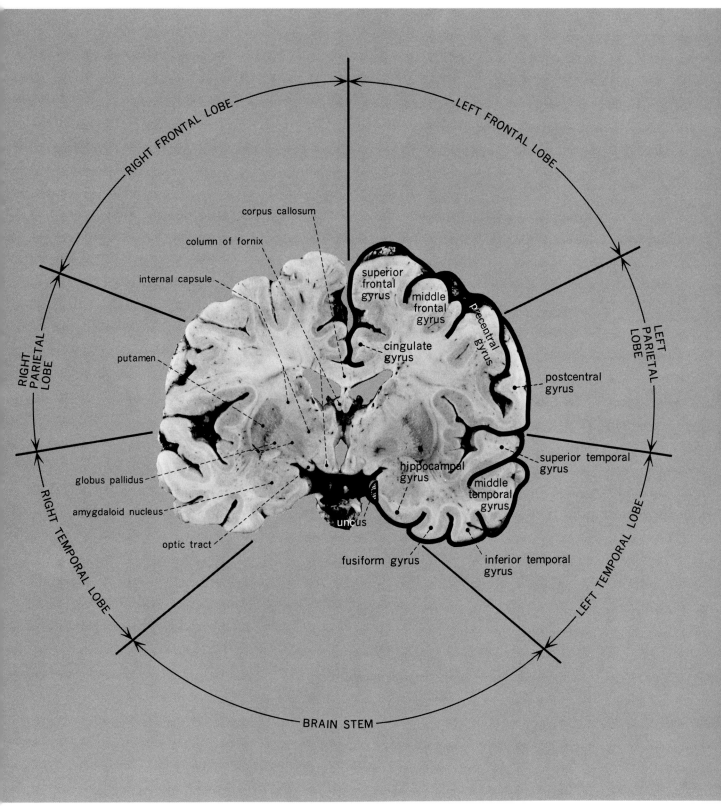

80° section, No. 12, uppersurface indicating prominent structures, lobes and gyri.

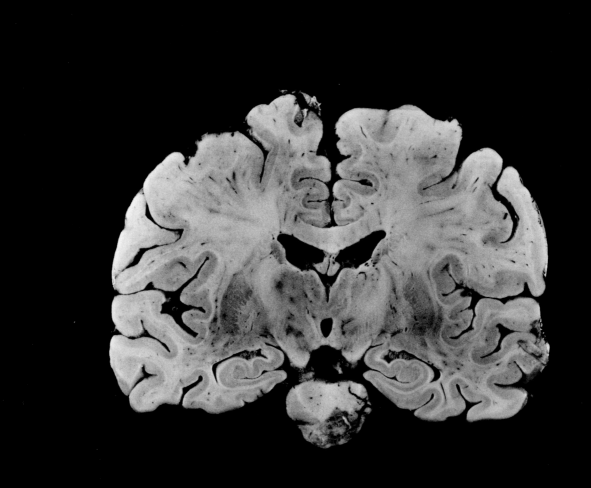

80° section, No. 13, uppersurface.

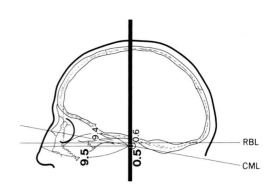

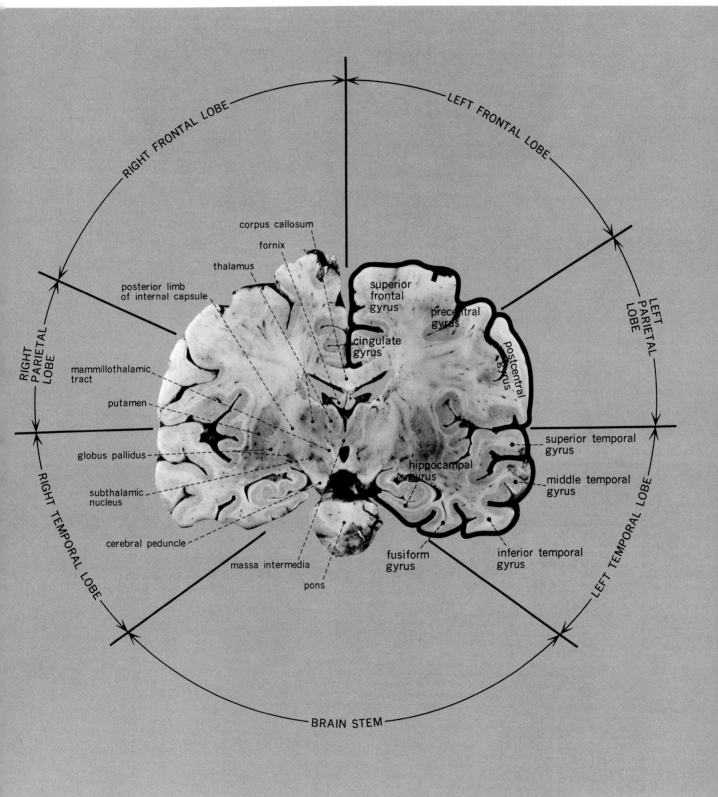

RIGHT FRONTAL LOBE

LEFT FRONTAL LOBE

corpus callosum

fornix

thalamus

posterior limb
of internal capsule

superior
frontal
gyrus

precentral
gyrus

cingulate
gyrus

postcentral
gyrus

RIGHT
PARIETAL
LOBE

LEFT
PARIETAL
LOBE

mammillothalamic
tract

putamen

globus pallidus

superior temporal
gyrus

middle temporal
gyrus

hippocampal
gyrus

subthalamic
nucleus

cerebral peduncle

RIGHT TEMPORAL LOBE

LEFT TEMPORAL LOBE

massa intermedia

fusiform
gyrus

inferior temporal
gyrus

pons

BRAIN STEM

RBL

CML

9.5 9.4 0.5 0.6

80° section, No. 13, uppersurface indicating prominent structures, lobes and gyri.

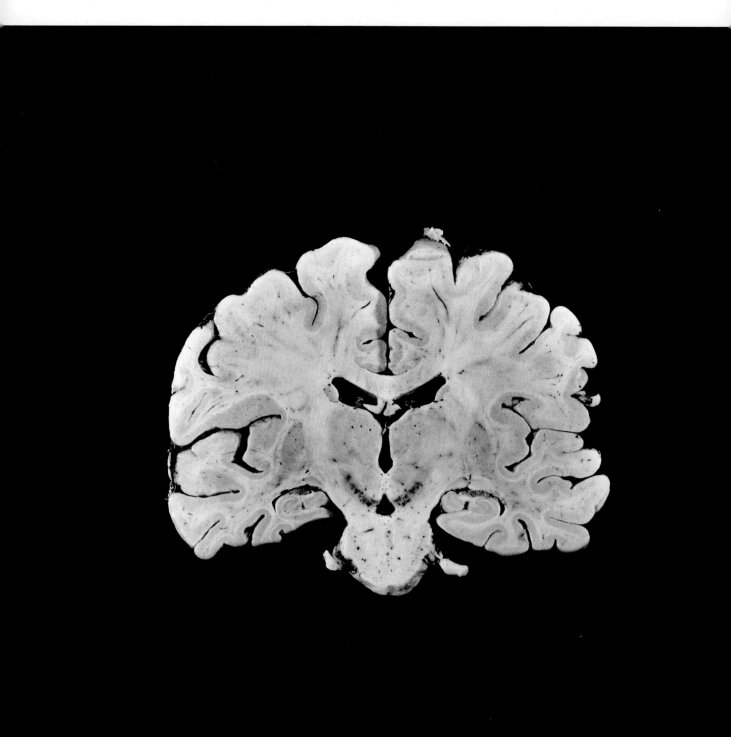

80° section, No. 14, uppersurface.

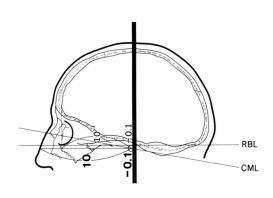

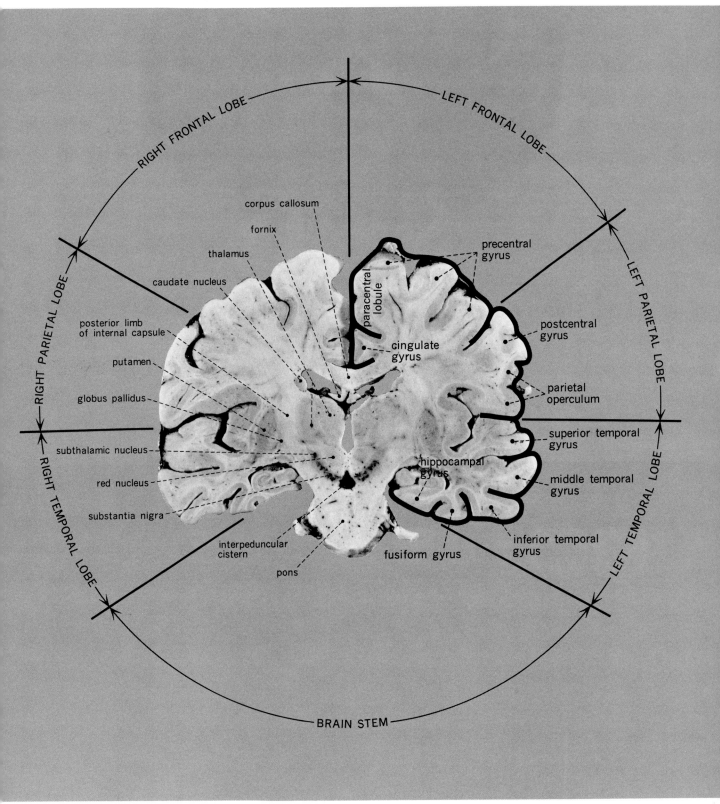

80° section, No. 14, uppersurface indicating prominent structures, lobes and gyri.

80°- 15

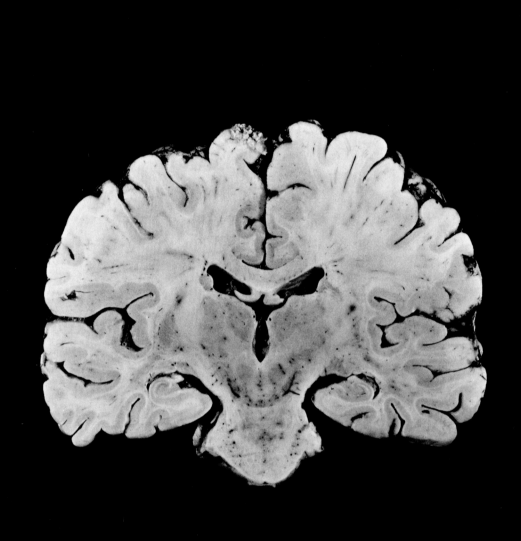

80° section, No. 15, uppersurface.

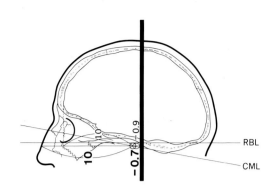

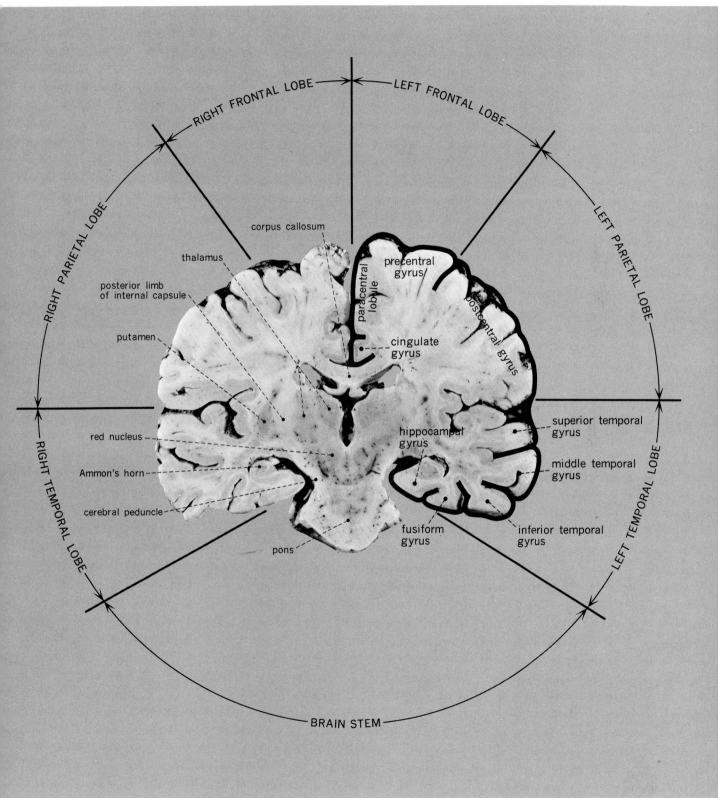

RIGHT FRONTAL LOBE — LEFT FRONTAL LOBE

RIGHT PARIETAL LOBE

LEFT PARIETAL LOBE

corpus callosum

thalamus

precentral gyrus

paracentral lobule

postcentral gyrus

posterior limb of internal capsule

putamen

cingulate gyrus

hippocampal gyrus

superior temporal gyrus

red nucleus

middle temporal gyrus

Ammon's horn

cerebral peduncle

RIGHT TEMPORAL LOBE

fusiform gyrus

inferior temporal gyrus

LEFT TEMPORAL LOBE

pons

BRAIN STEM

80° section, No. 15, uppersurface indicating prominent structures, lobes and gyri.

429

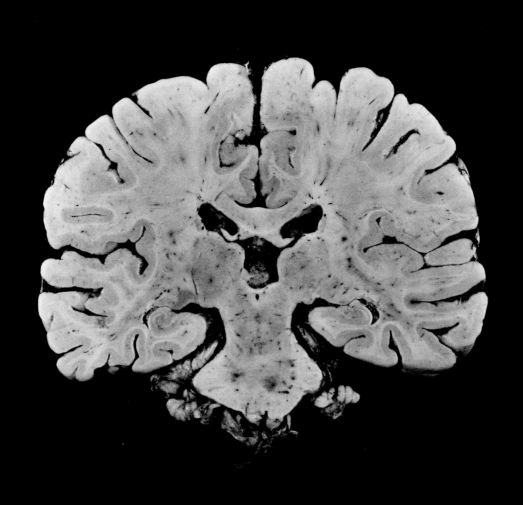

80° section, No. 16, uppersurface.

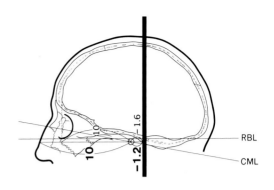

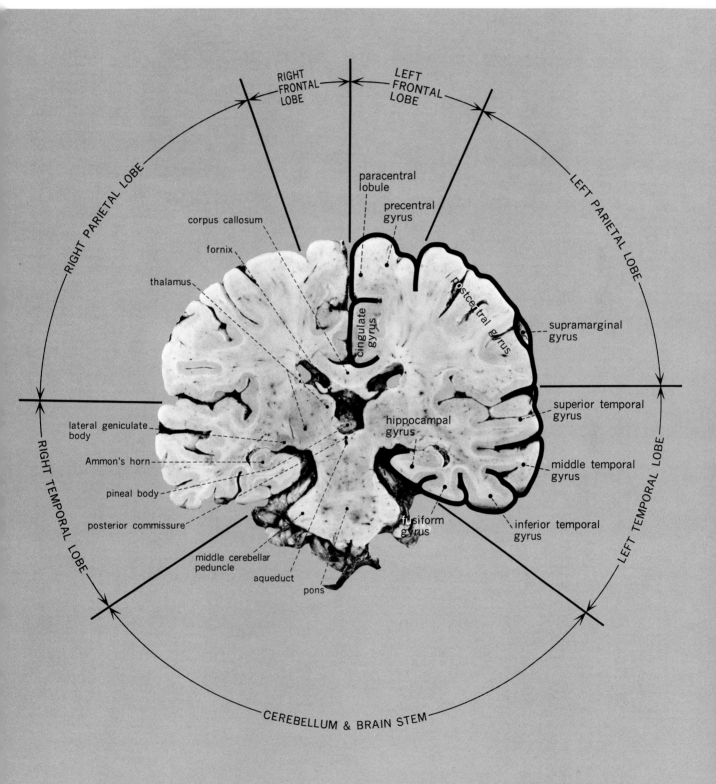

RIGHT FRONTAL LOBE

LEFT FRONTAL LOBE

RIGHT PARIETAL LOBE

LEFT PARIETAL LOBE

paracentral lobule

precentral gyrus

corpus callosum

fornix

postcentral gyrus

thalamus

cingulate gyrus

supramarginal gyrus

superior temporal gyrus

hippocampal gyrus

lateral geniculate body

middle temporal gyrus

Ammon's horn

pineal body

inferior temporal gyrus

posterior commissure

fusiform gyrus

RIGHT TEMPORAL LOBE

LEFT TEMPORAL LOBE

middle cerebellar peduncle

aqueduct

pons

CEREBELLUM & BRAIN STEM

80° section, No. 16, uppersurface indicating prominent structures, lobes and gyri.

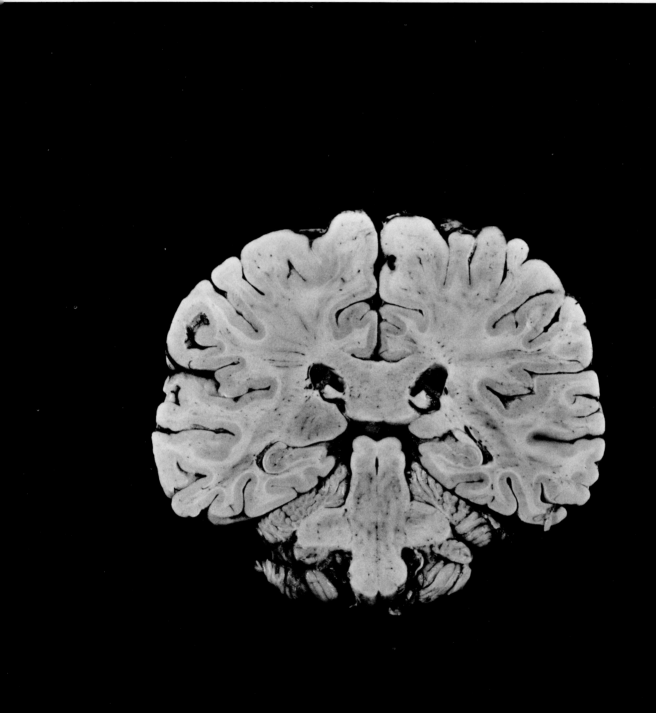

80° section, No. 17, uppersurface.

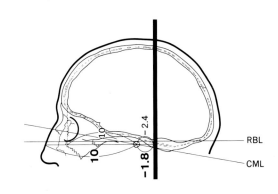

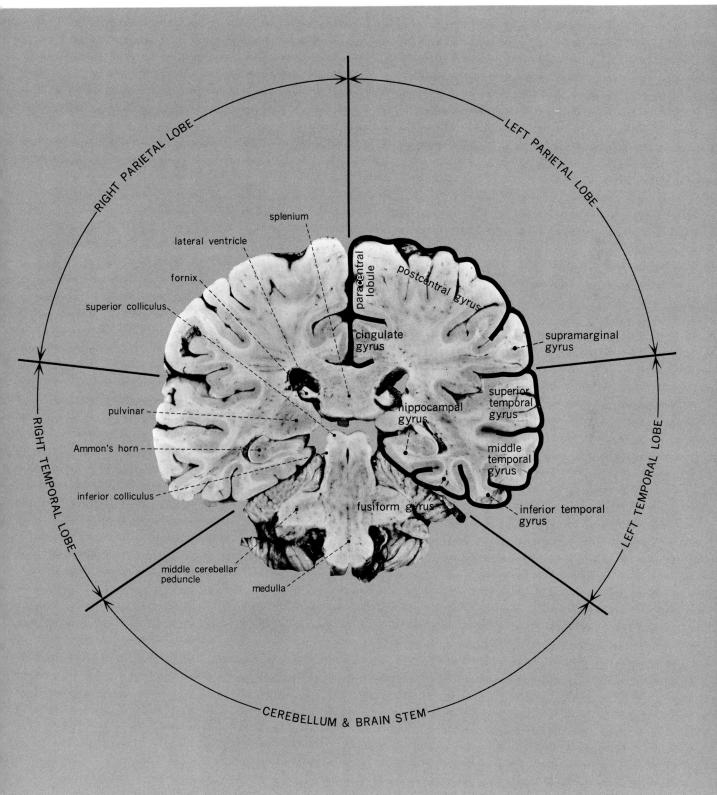

80° section, No. 17, uppersurface indicating prominent structures, lobes and gyri.

433

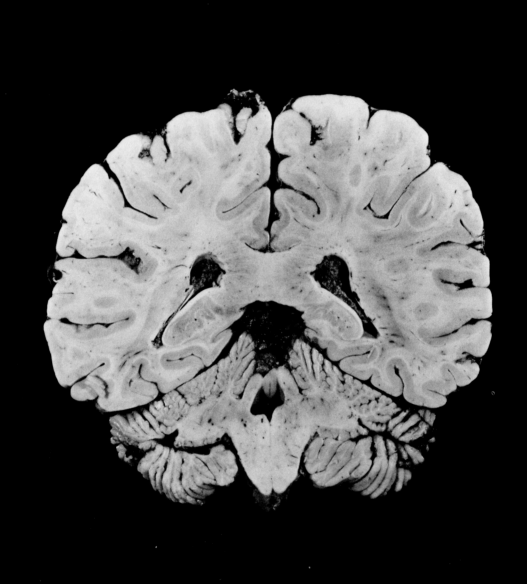

80° section, No. 18, uppersurface.

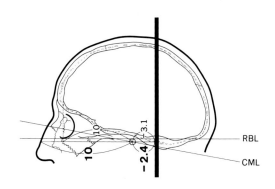

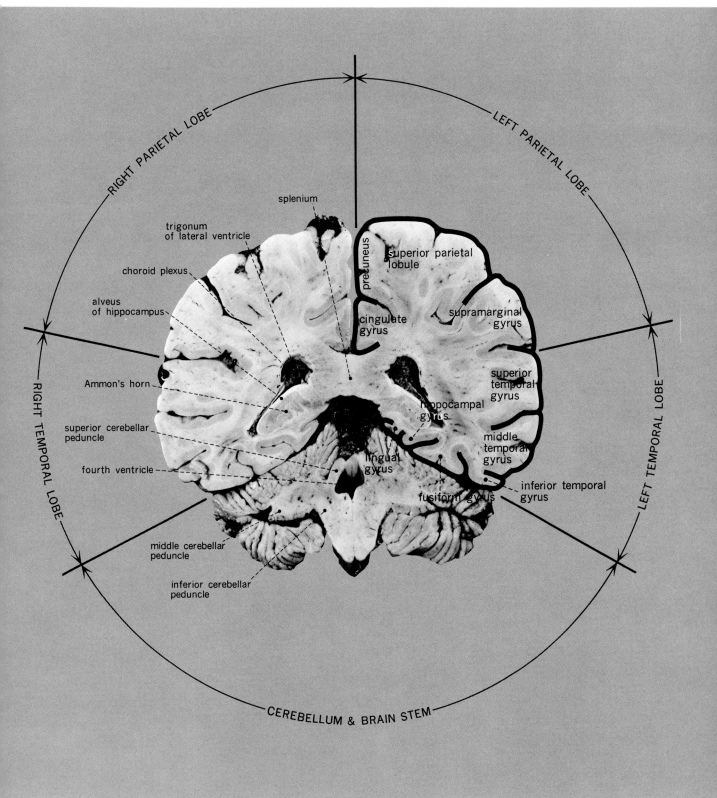

80° section, No. 18, uppersurface indicating prominent structures, lobes and gyri.

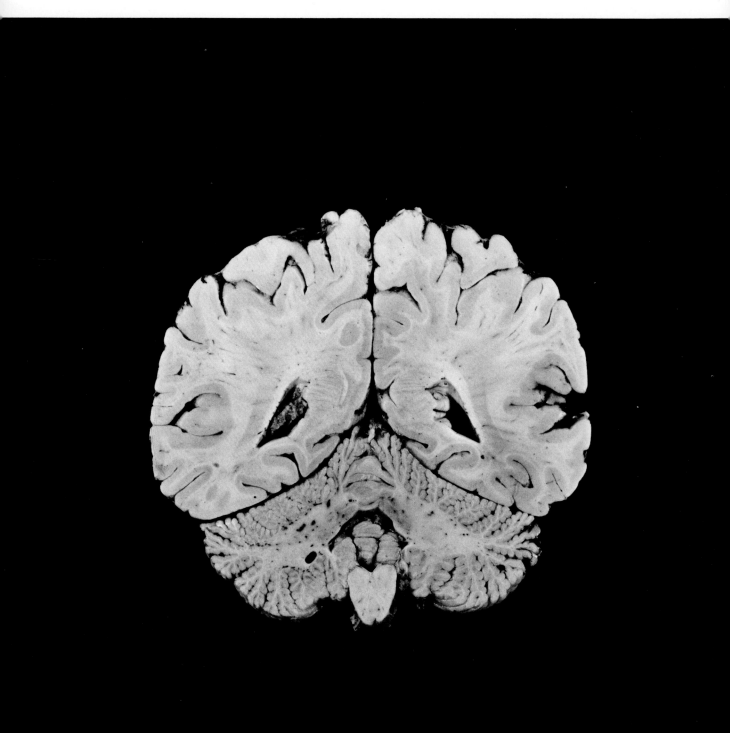

80° section, No. 19, uppersurface.

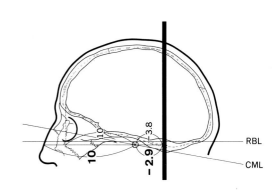

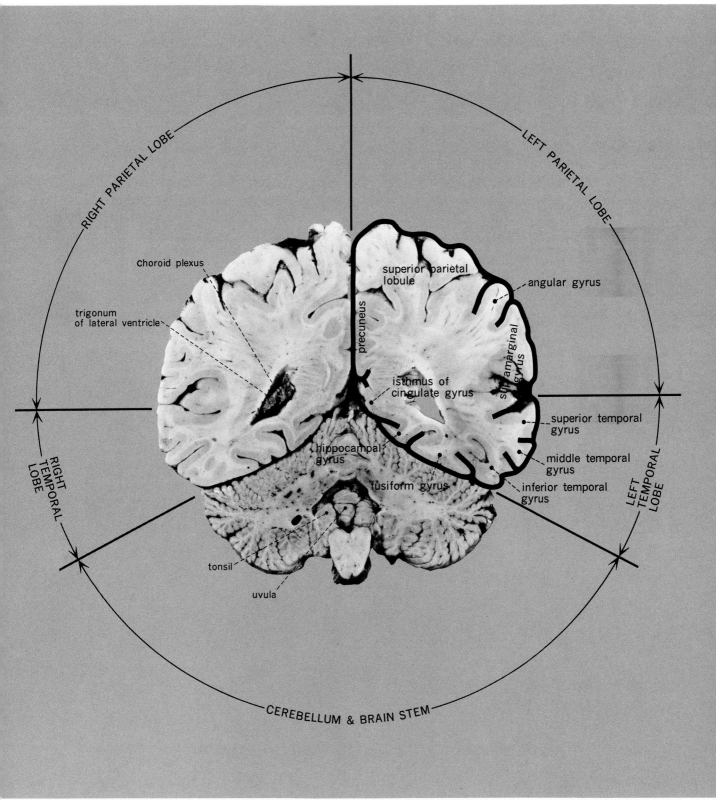

80° section, No. 19, uppersurface indicating prominent structures, lobes and gyri.

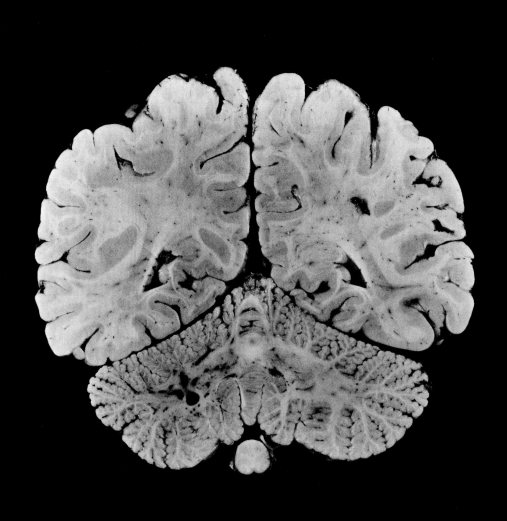

80° section, No. 20, uppersurface.

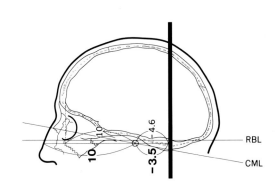

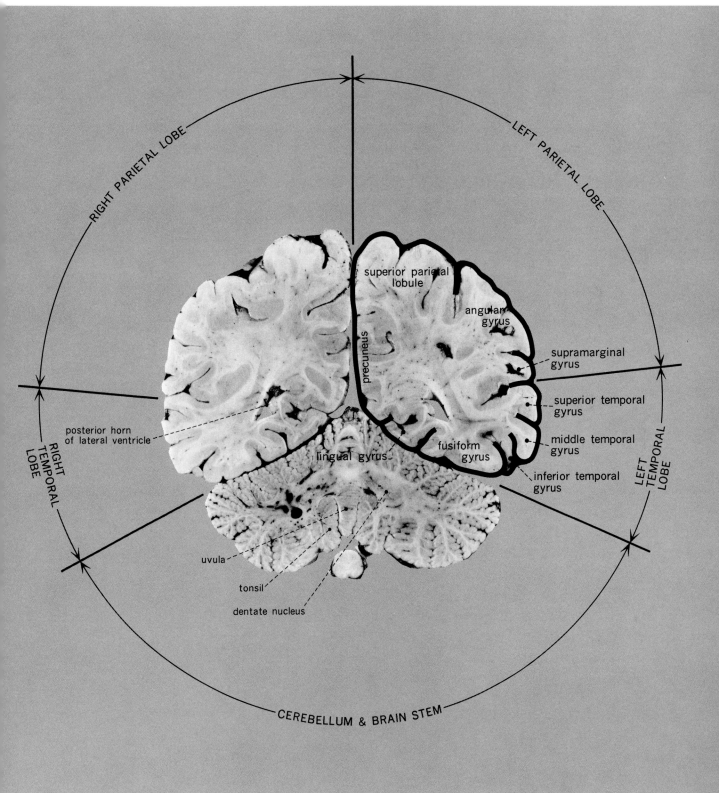

superior parietal lobule

angular gyrus

precuneus

supramarginal gyrus

superior temporal gyrus

middle temporal gyrus

fusiform gyrus

inferior temporal gyrus

posterior horn of lateral ventricle

lingual gyrus

RIGHT TEMPORAL LOBE

LEFT TEMPORAL LOBE

RIGHT PARIETAL LOBE

LEFT PARIETAL LOBE

CEREBELLUM & BRAIN STEM

uvula

tonsil

dentate nucleus

80° section, No. 20, uppersurface indicating prominent structures, lobes and gyri.

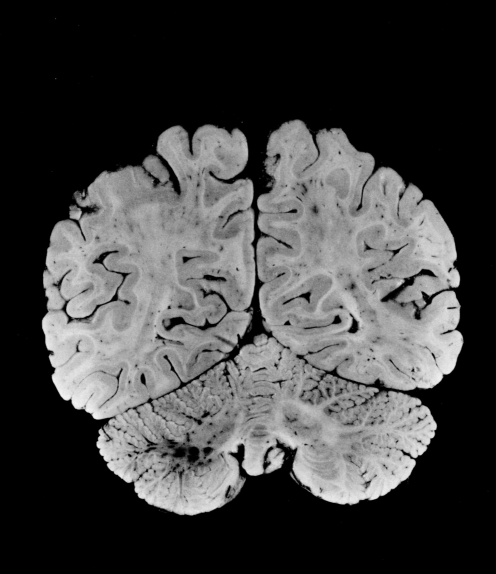

80° section, No. 21, uppersurface.

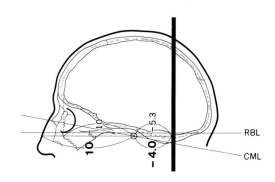

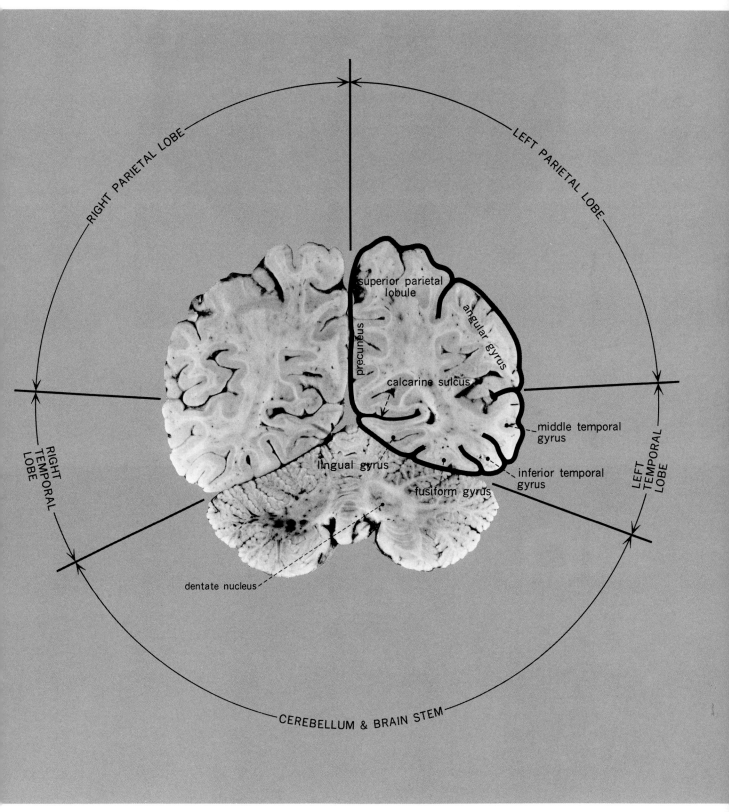

80° section, No. 21, uppersurface indicating prominent structures, lobes and gyri.

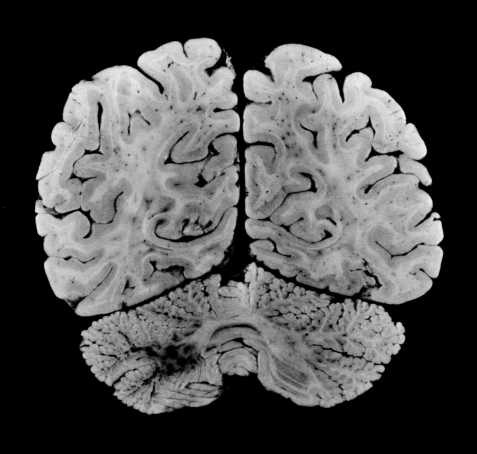

80° section, No. 22, uppersurface.

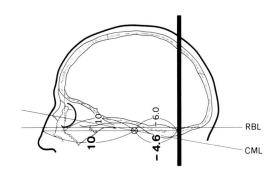

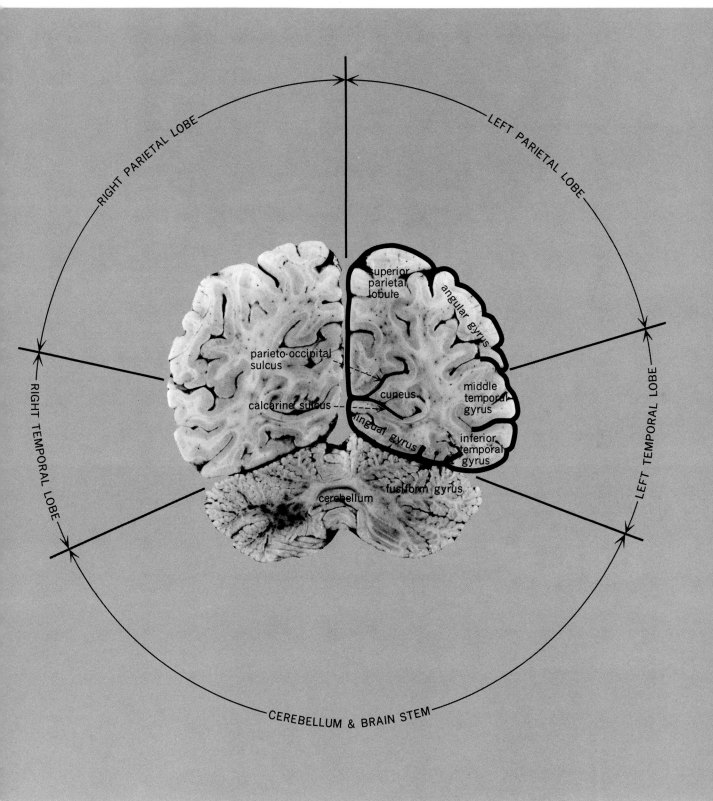

RIGHT PARIETAL LOBE

LEFT PARIETAL LOBE

RIGHT TEMPORAL LOBE

LEFT TEMPORAL LOBE

superior parietal lobule

angular gyrus

parieto-occipital sulcus

cuneus

middle temporal gyrus

calcarine sulcus

lingual gyrus

inferior temporal gyrus

fusiform gyrus

cerebellum

CEREBELLUM & BRAIN STEM

80° section, No. 22, uppersurface indicating prominent lobes and gyri.

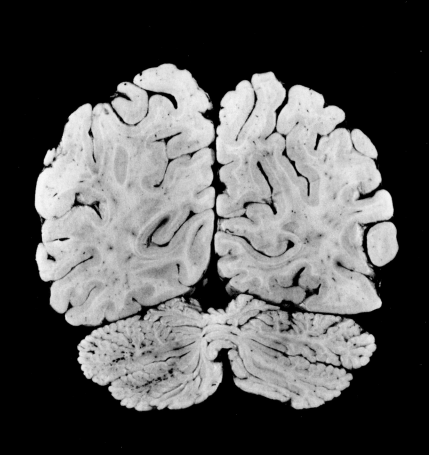

80° section, No. 23, uppersurface.

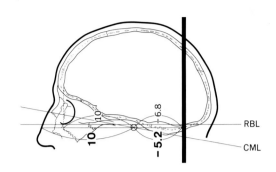

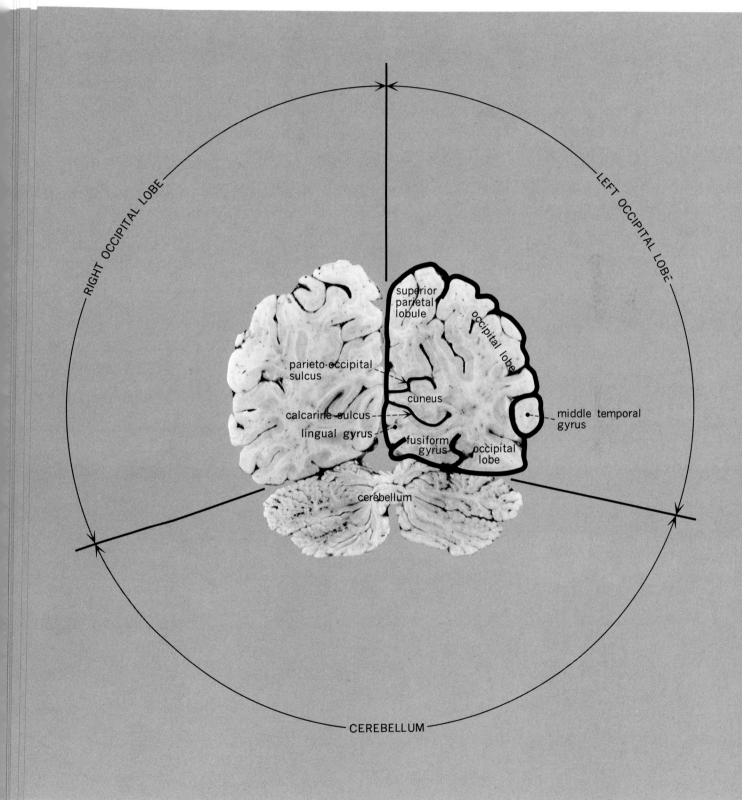

RIGHT OCCIPITAL LOBE

LEFT OCCIPITAL LOBE

superior parietal lobule

occipital lobe

parieto-occipital sulcus

cuneus

calcarine sulcus

lingual gyrus

middle temporal gyrus

fusiform gyrus

occipital lobe

cerebellum

CEREBELLUM

80° section, No. 23, uppersurface indicating prominent lobes and gyri.

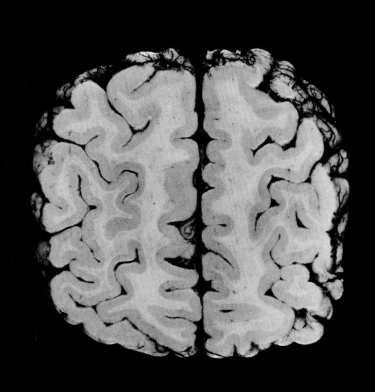

110° section, No. 3, uppersurface.

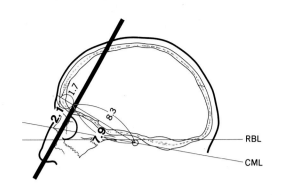

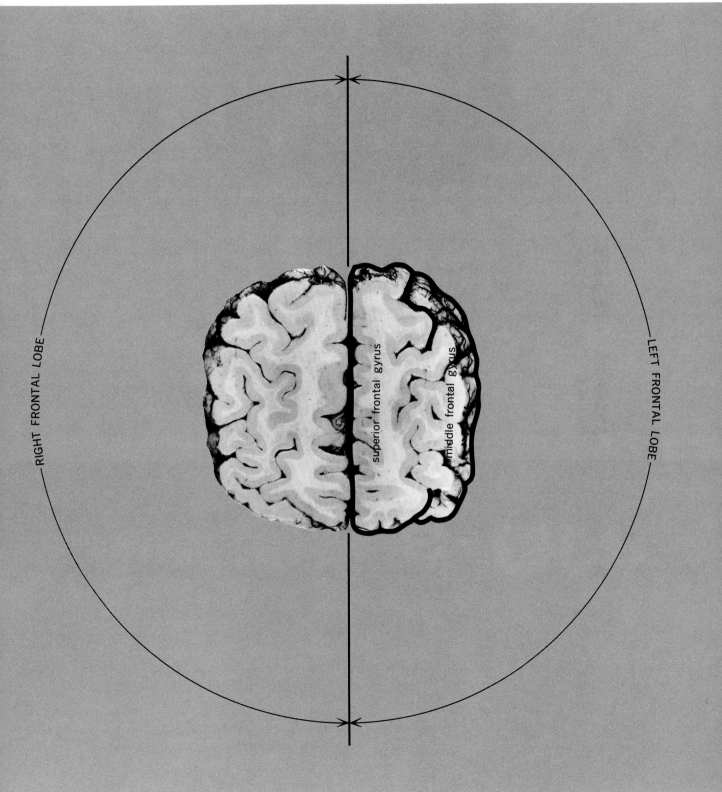

110° section, No. 3, uppersurface indicating prominent lobes and gyri.

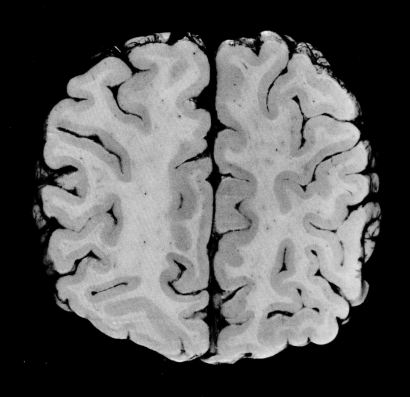

110° section, No. 4, uppersurface.

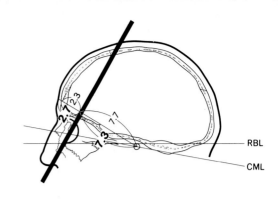

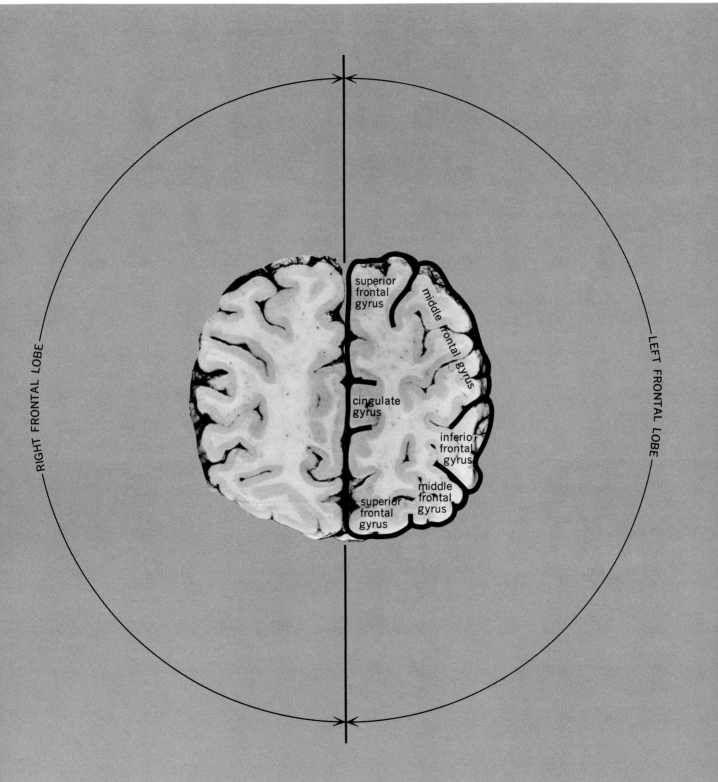

RIGHT FRONTAL LOBE

LEFT FRONTAL LOBE

superior frontal gyrus

middle frontal gyrus

cingulate gyrus

inferior frontal gyrus

middle frontal gyrus

superior frontal gyrus

110° section, No. 4, uppersurface indicating prominent lobes and gyri.

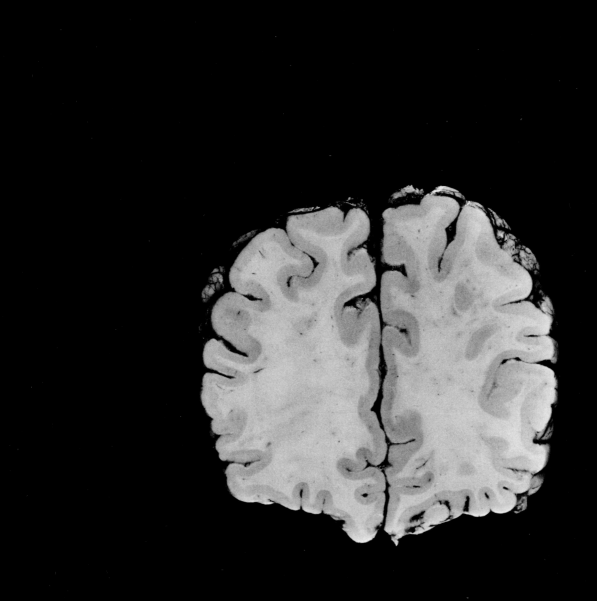

110° section, No. 5, uppersurface.

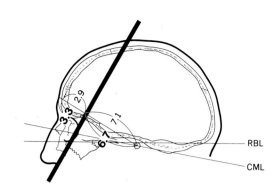

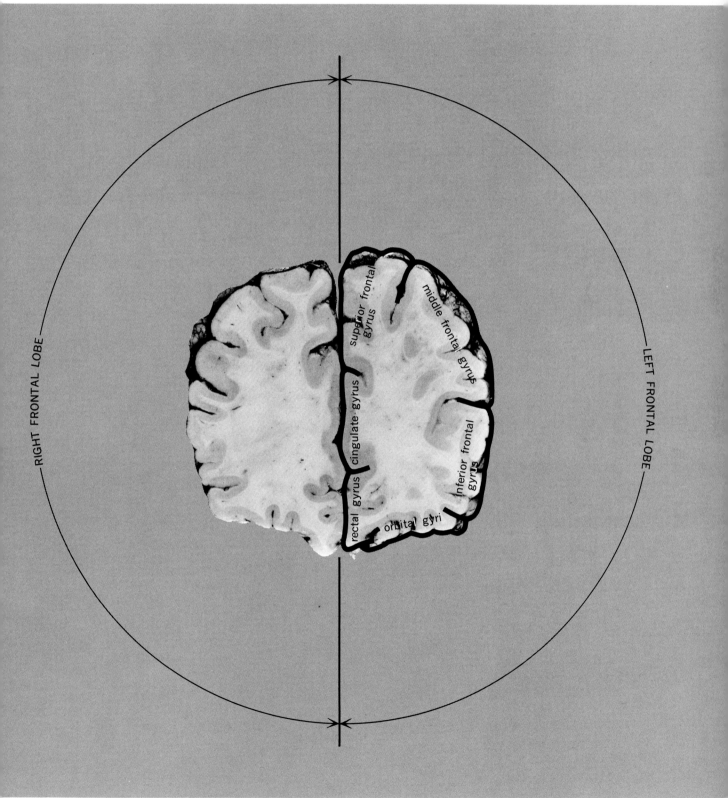

110° section, No. 5, uppersurface indicating prominent lobes and gyri.

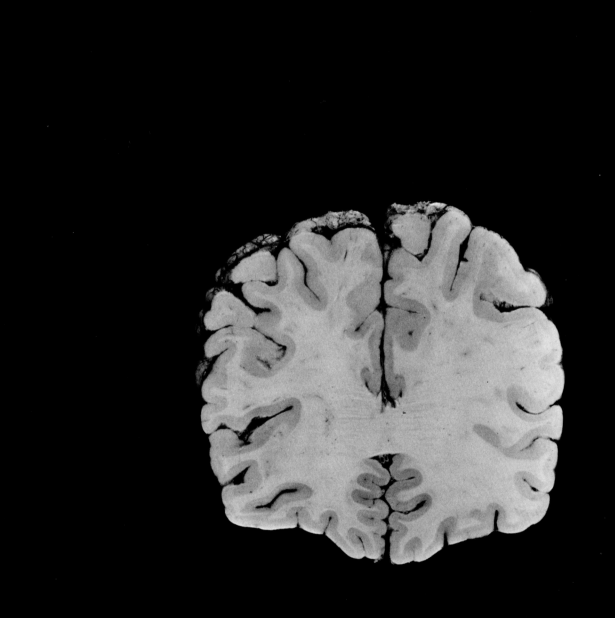

110° section, No. 6, uppersurface.

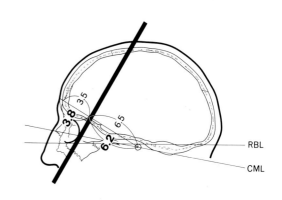

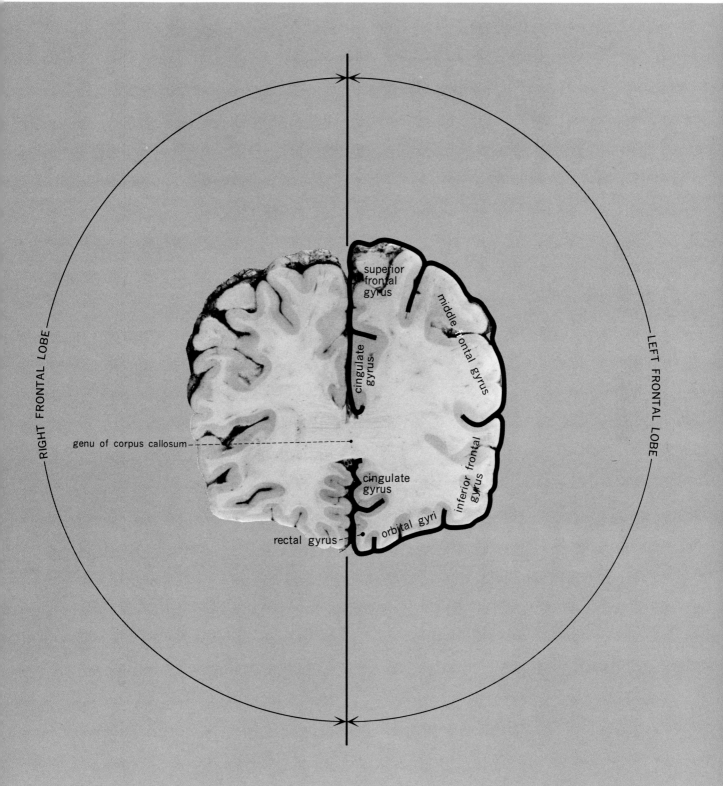

RIGHT FRONTAL LOBE

LEFT FRONTAL LOBE

superior frontal gyrus

middle frontal gyrus

cingulate gyrus

genu of corpus callosum

cingulate gyrus

inferior frontal gyrus

orbital gyri

rectal gyrus

110° section, No. 6, uppersurface indicating prominent structures, lobes and gyri.

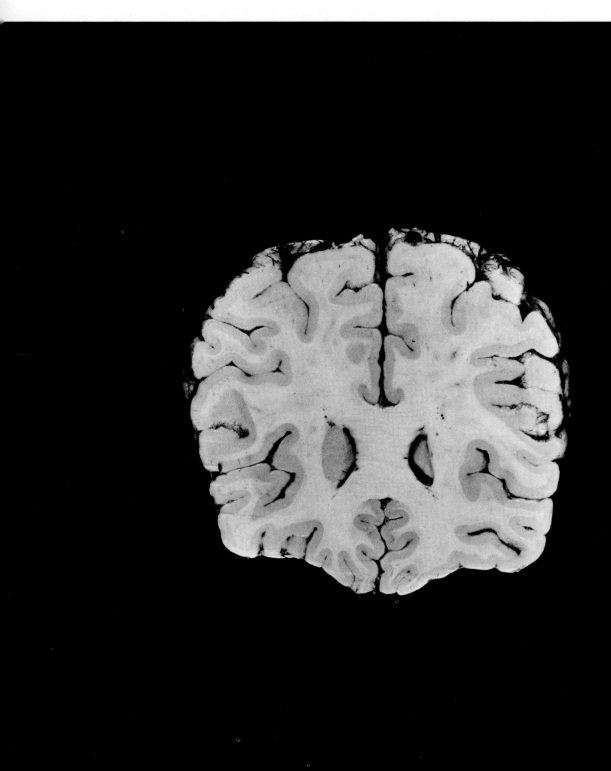

110° section, No. 7, uppersurface.

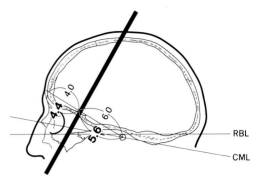

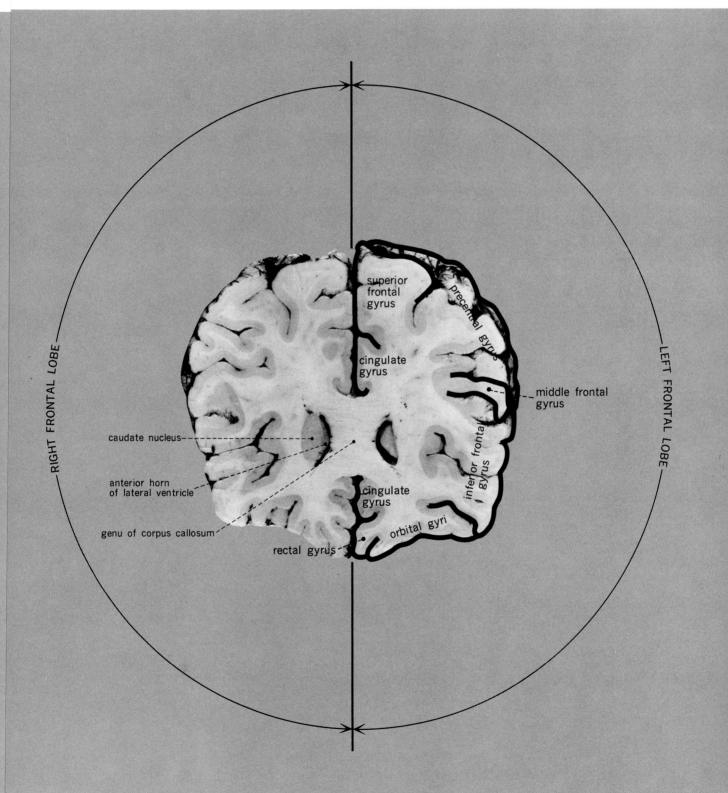

110° section, No. 7, uppersurface indicating prominent structures, lobes and gyri.

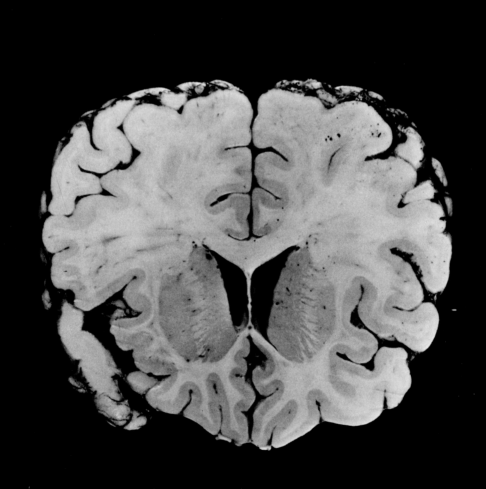

110° section, No. 9, uppersurface.

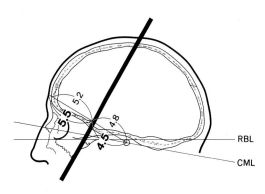

RBL

CML

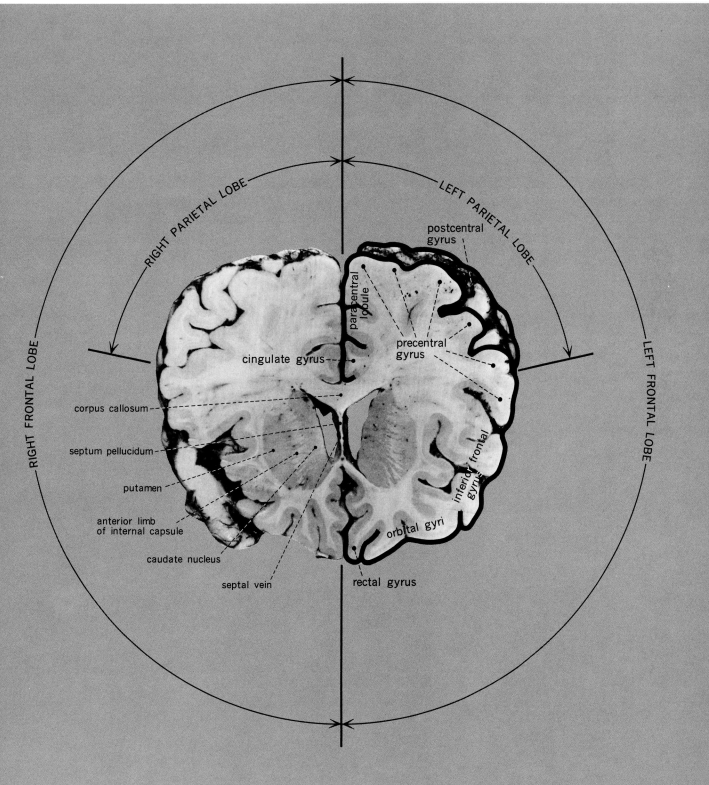

110° section, No. 9, uppersurface indicating prominent structures, lobes and gyri.

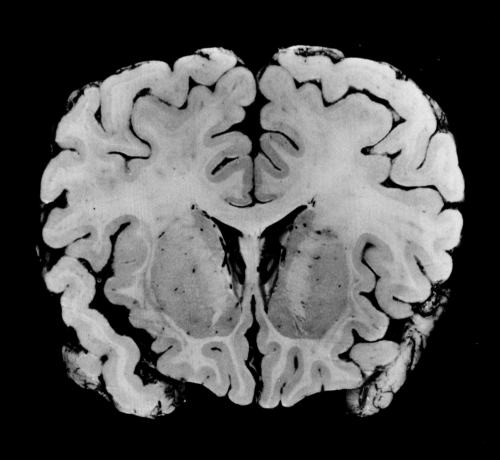

110° section, No. 10, uppersurface.

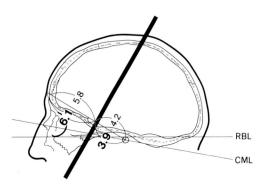

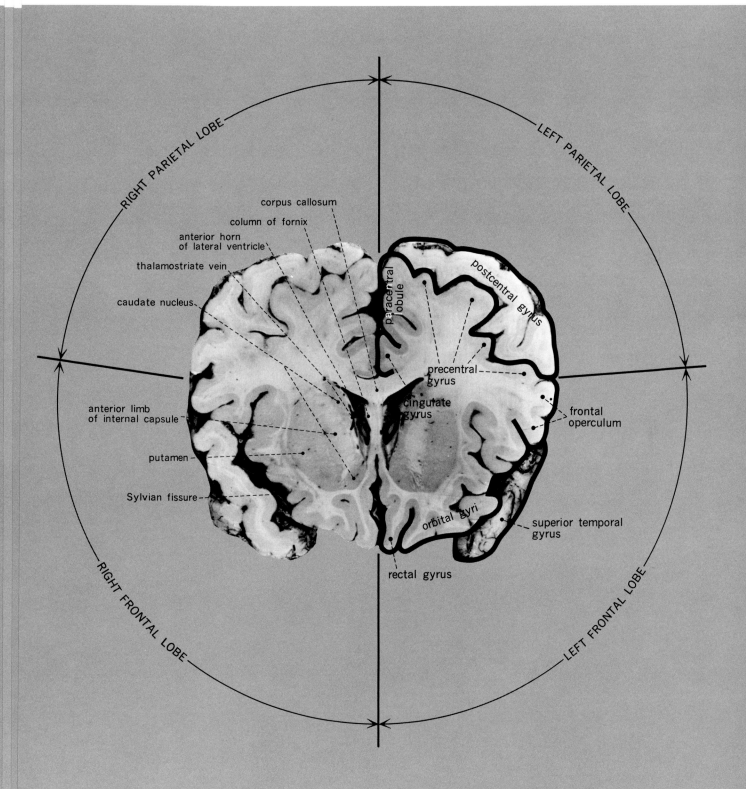

corpus callosum

column of fornix

anterior horn
of lateral ventricle

thalamostriate vein

caudate nucleus

RIGHT PARIETAL LOBE

LEFT PARIETAL LOBE

paracentral lobule

postcentral gyrus

precentral gyrus

cingulate gyrus

anterior limb
of internal capsule

frontal operculum

putamen

Sylvian fissure

orbital gyri

superior temporal gyrus

rectal gyrus

RIGHT FRONTAL LOBE

LEFT FRONTAL LOBE

RBL

CML

110° section, No. 10, uppersurface indicating prominent structures, lobes and gyri.

471

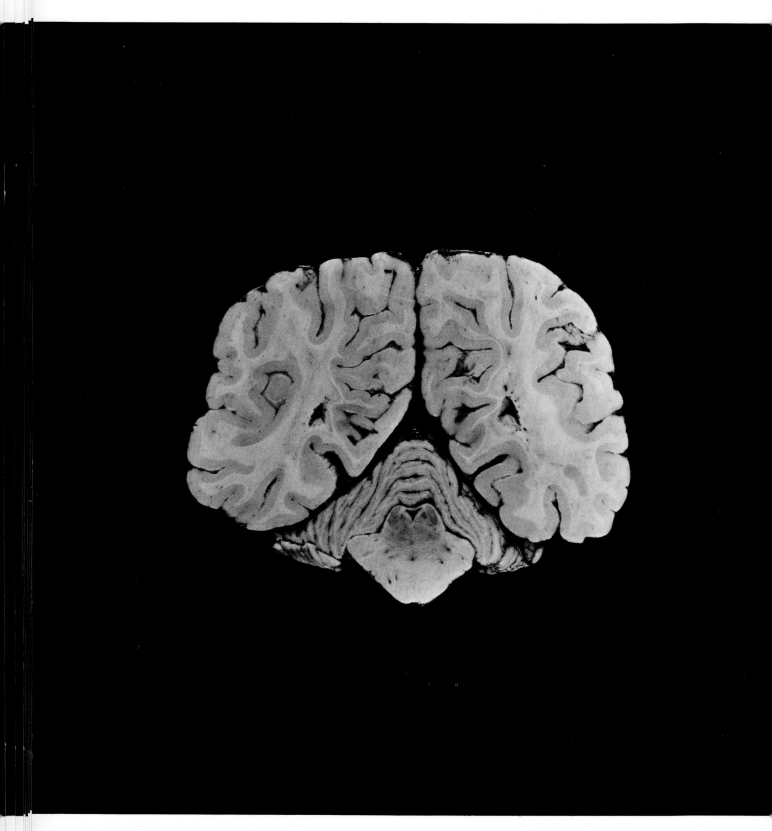

110° section, No. 18, uppersurface.

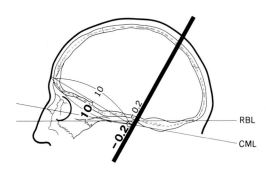

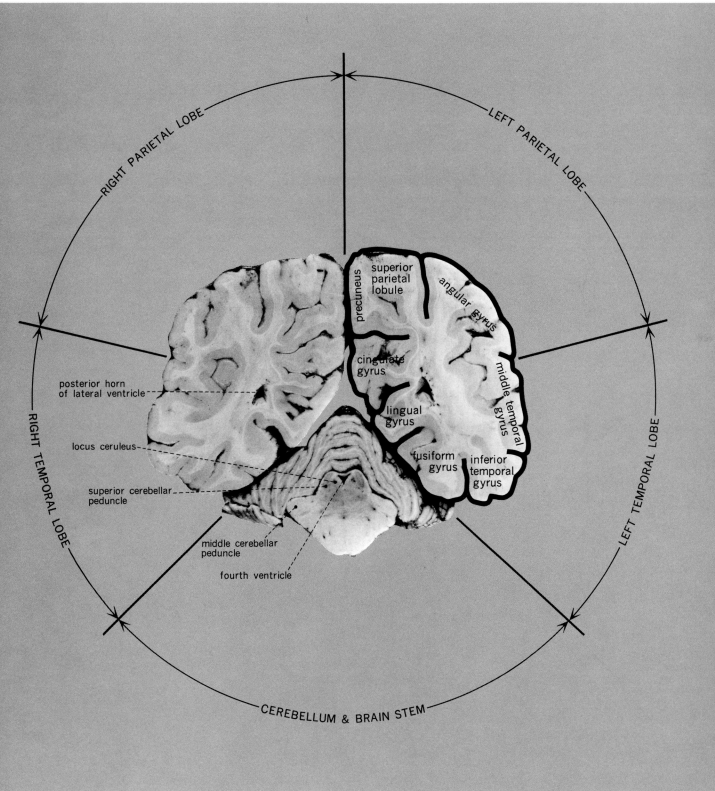

110° section, No. 18, uppersurface indicating prominent structures, lobes and gyri.

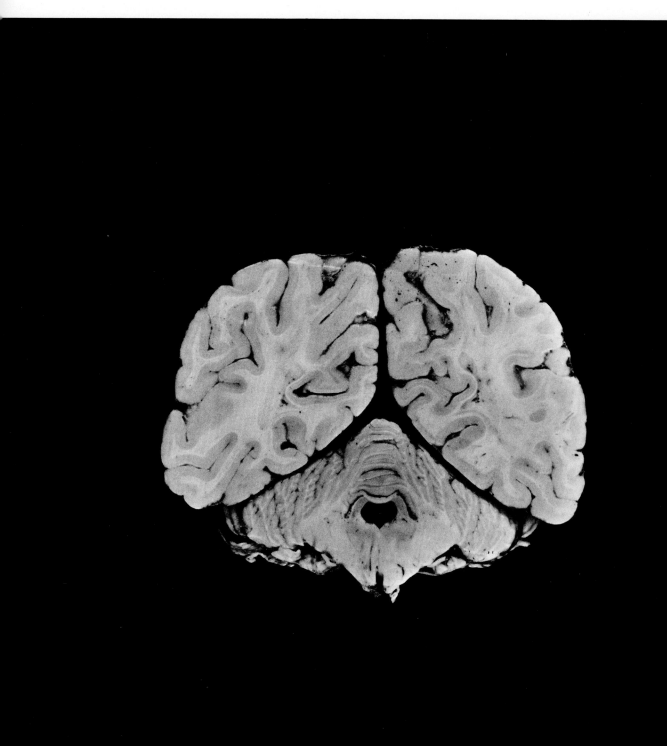

110° section, No. 19, uppersurface.

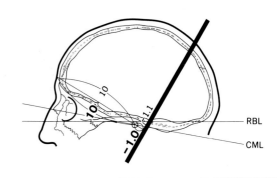

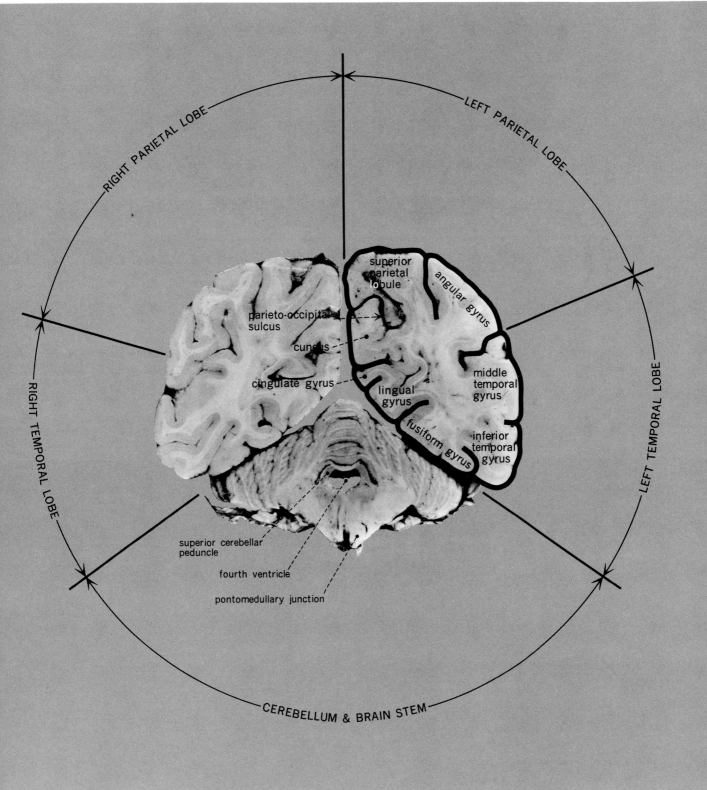

110° section, No. 19, uppersurface indicating prominent structures, lobes and gyri.

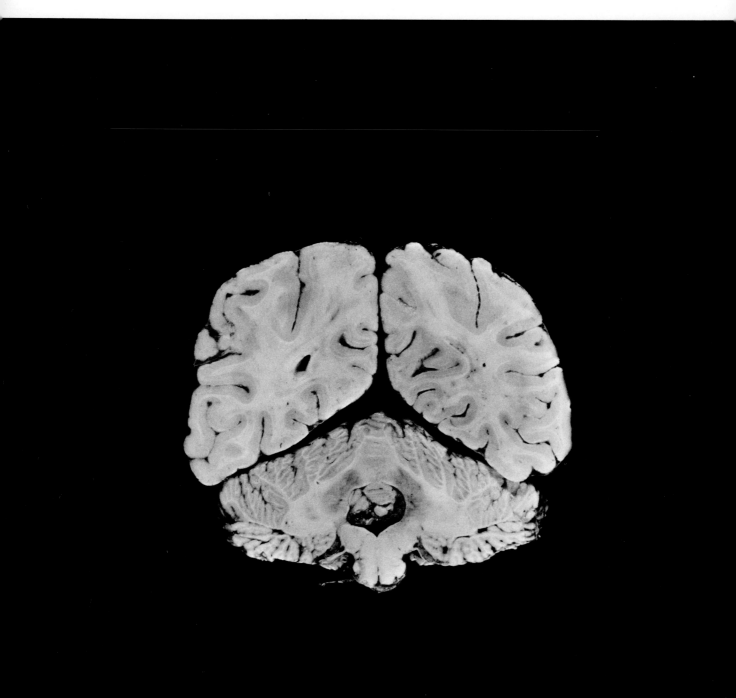

110° section, No. 20, uppersurface.

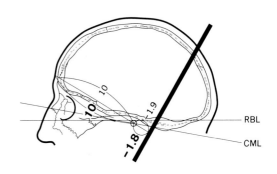

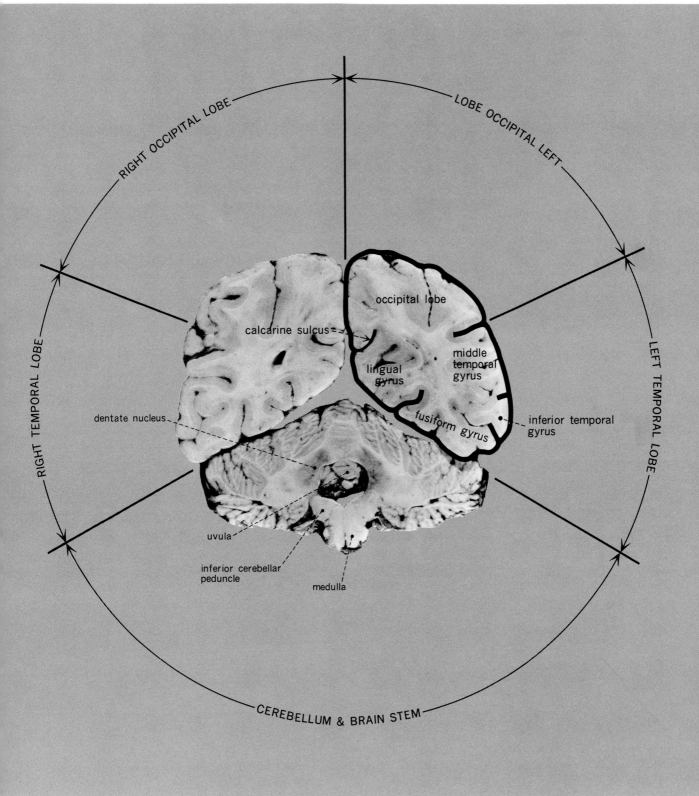

110° section, No. 20, uppersurface indicating prominent structures, lobes and gyri.

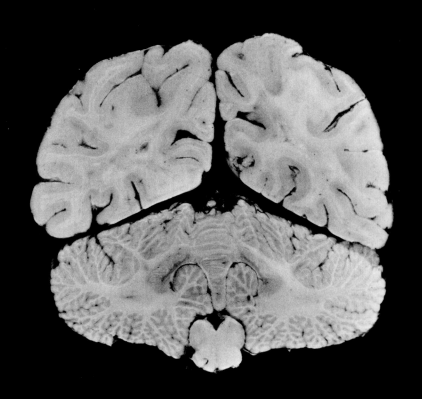

110° section, No. 21, uppersurface.

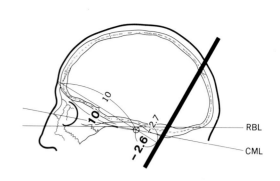

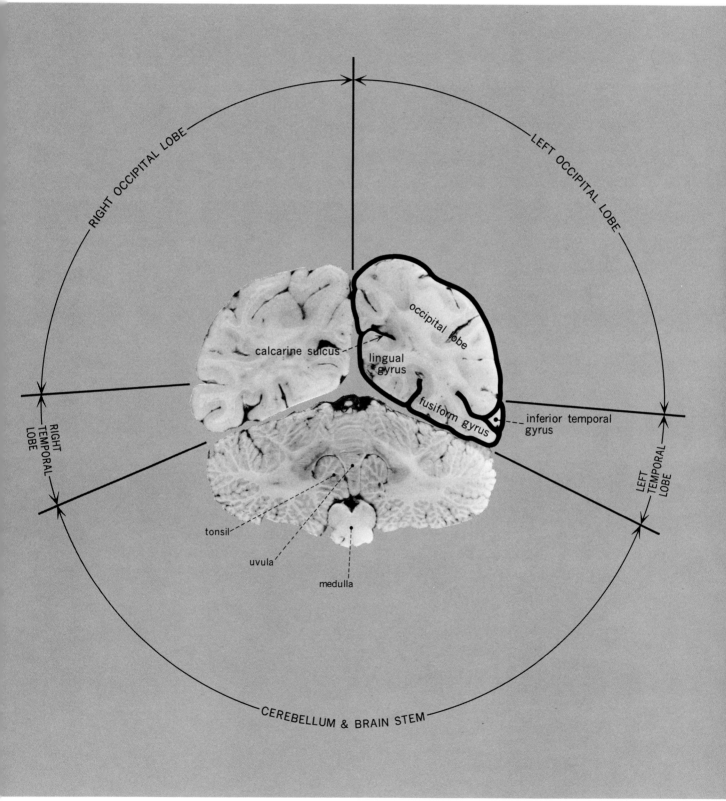

110° section, No. 21, uppersurface indicating prominent structures, lobes and gyri.

110°-22

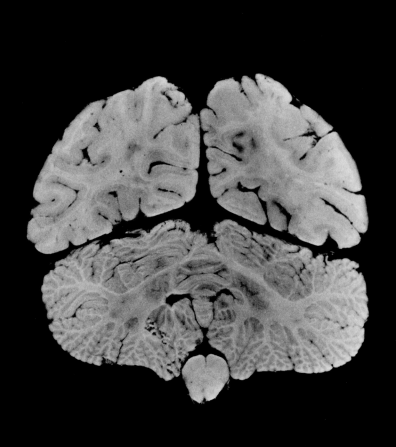

110° section, No. 22, uppersurface.

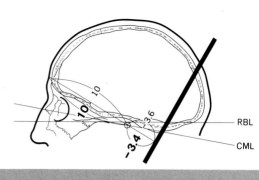

RBL

CML

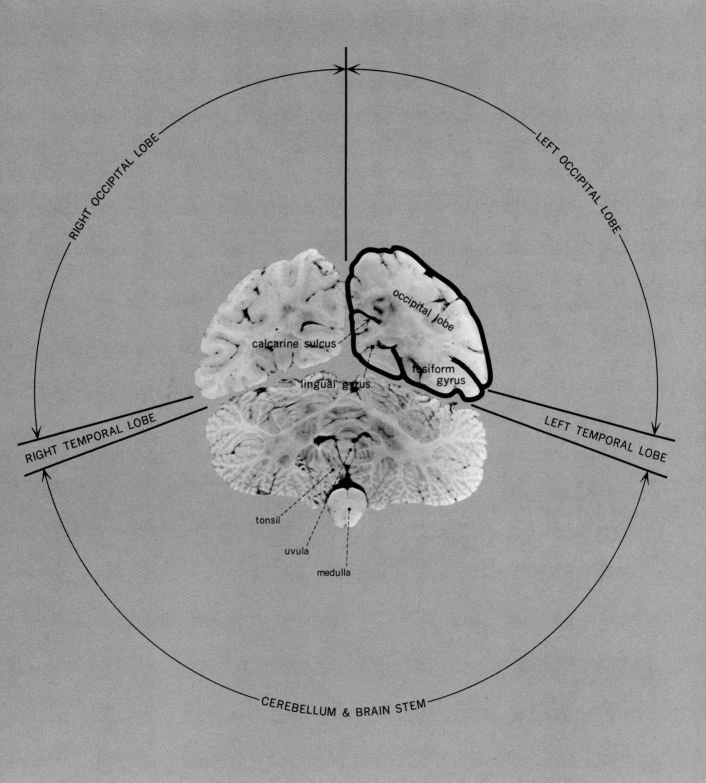

RIGHT OCCIPITAL LOBE

LEFT OCCIPITAL LOBE

occipital lobe

calcarine sulcus

lingual gyrus

fusiform gyrus

RIGHT TEMPORAL LOBE

LEFT TEMPORAL LOBE

tonsil

uvula

medulla

CEREBELLUM & BRAIN STEM

110° section, No. 22, uppersurface indicating prominent structures, lobes and gyri.

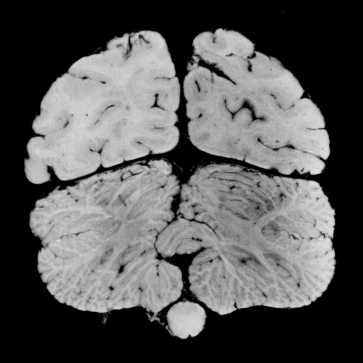

110° section, No. 23, uppersurface.

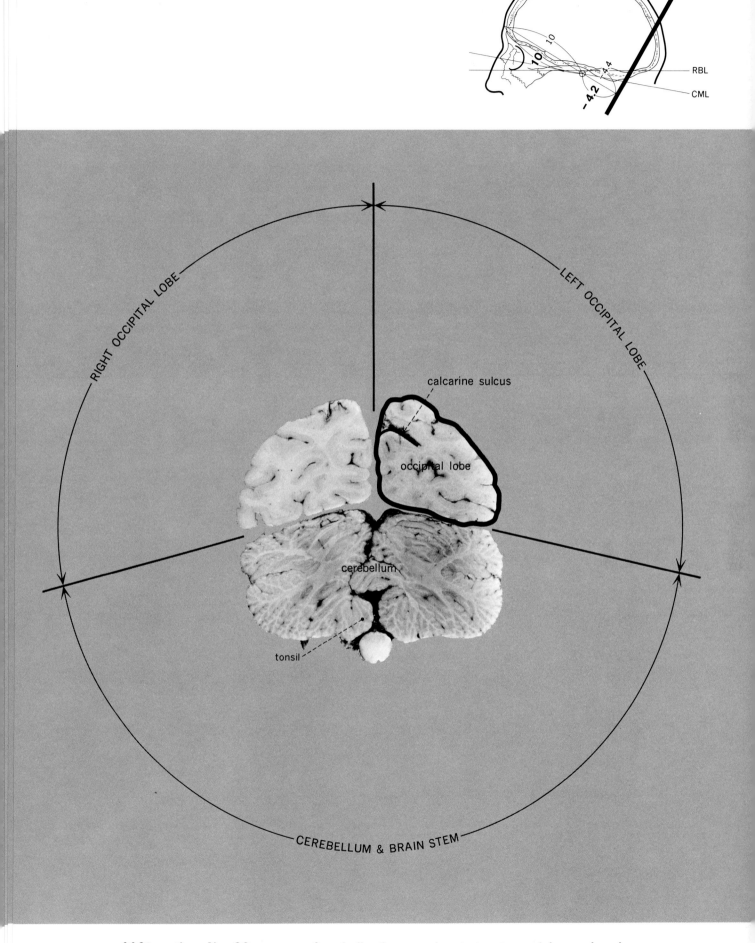

RBL

CML

calcarine sulcus

occipital lobe

RIGHT OCCIPITAL LOBE

LEFT OCCIPITAL LOBE

cerebellum

tonsil

CEREBELLUM & BRAIN STEM

110° section, No. 23, uppersurface indicating prominent structures, lobes and gyri.

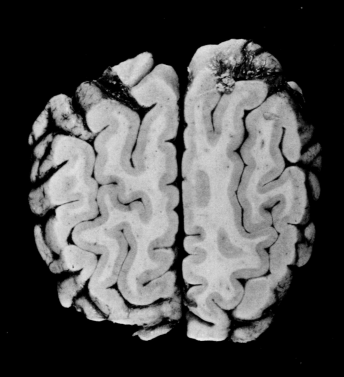

140° section, No. 2, uppersurface.

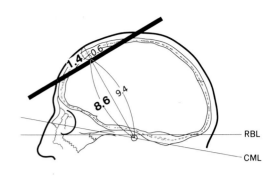

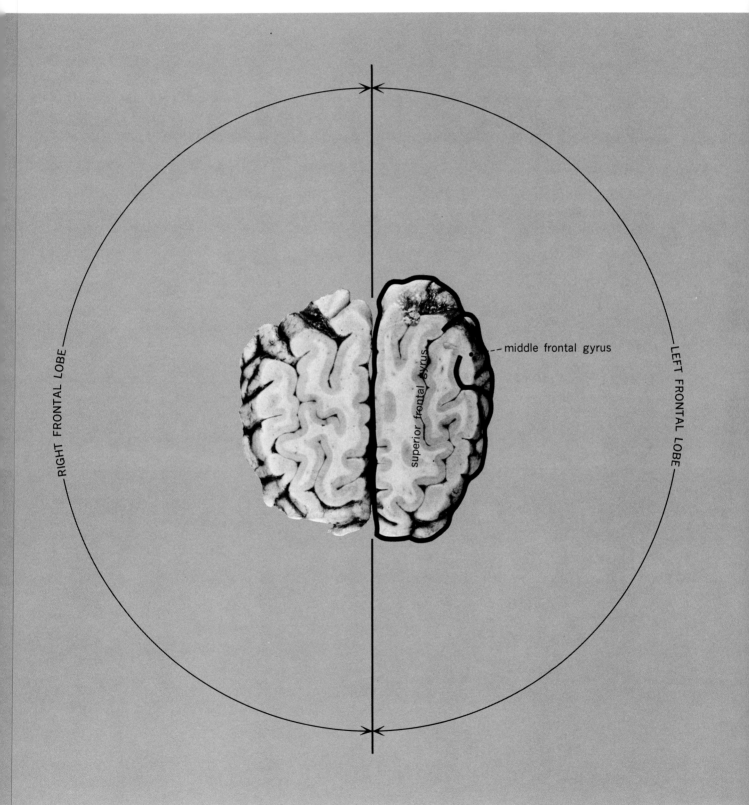

middle frontal gyrus

superior frontal gyrus

RIGHT FRONTAL LOBE

LEFT FRONTAL LOBE

140° section, No. 2, uppersurface indicating prominent lobes and gyri.

140°-4

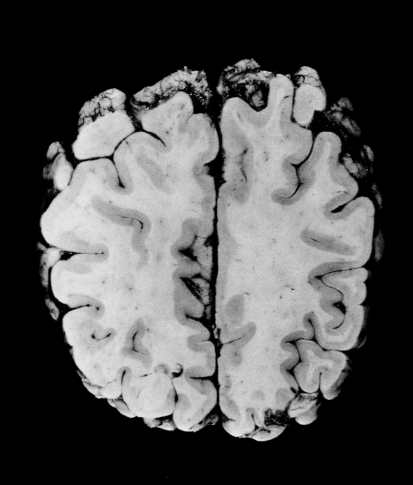

140° section, No. 4, uppersurface.

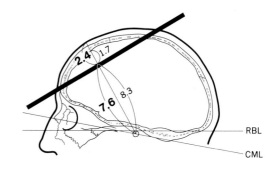

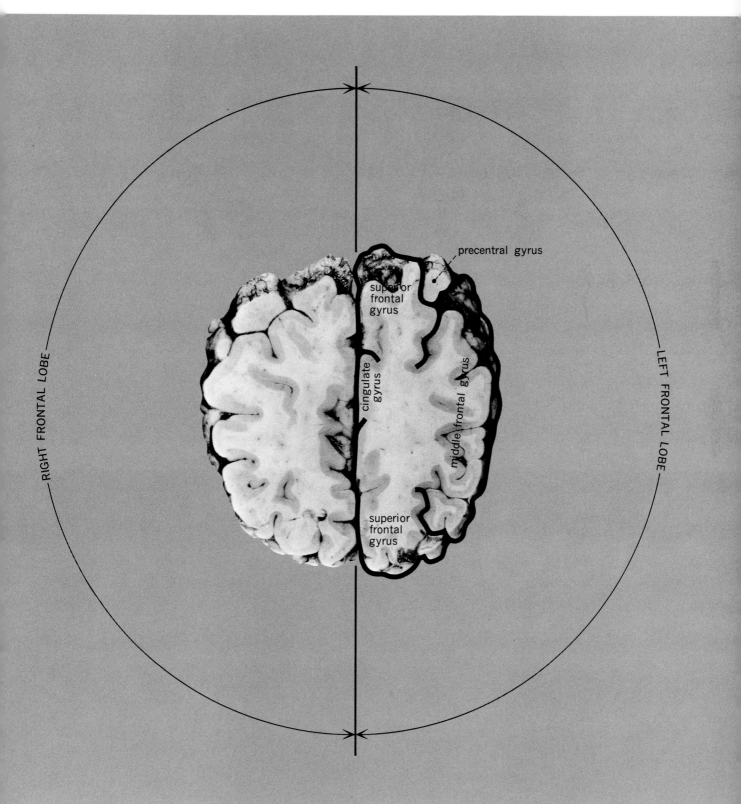

140° section, No. 4, uppersurface indicating prominent lobes and gyri.

140°-5

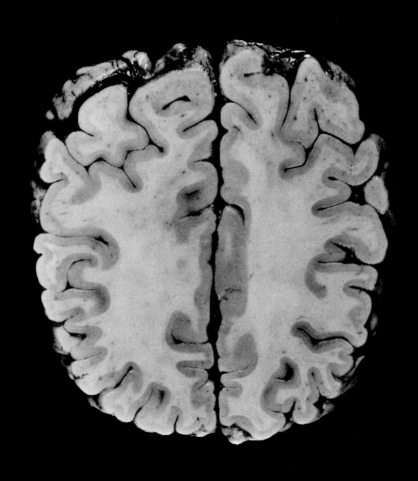

140° section, No. 5, uppersurface.

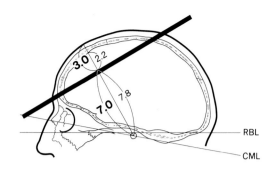

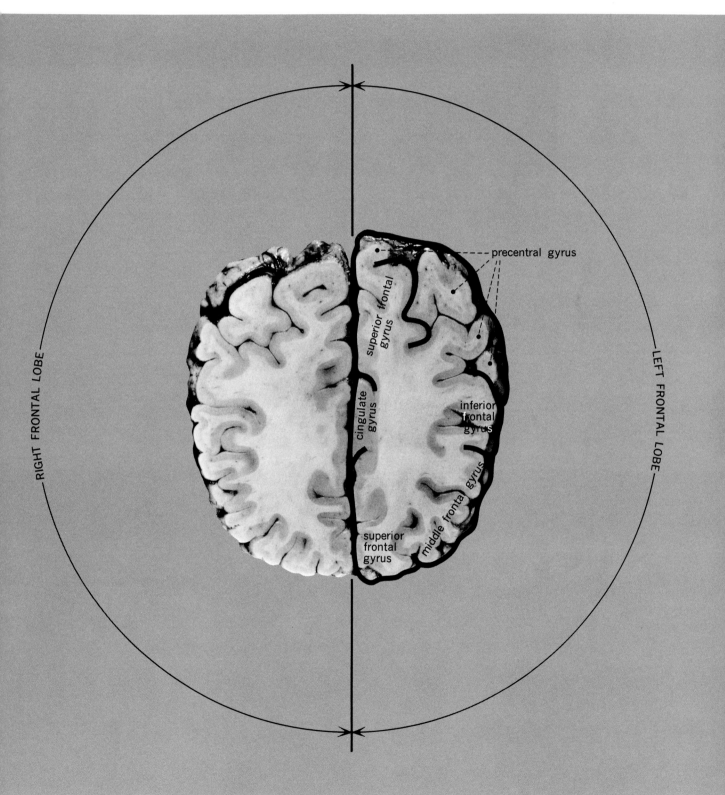

RIGHT FRONTAL LOBE

LEFT FRONTAL LOBE

precentral gyrus

superior frontal gyrus

cingulate gyrus

inferior frontal gyrus

middle frontal gyrus

superior frontal gyrus

140° section, No. 5, uppersurface indicating prominent lobes and gyri.

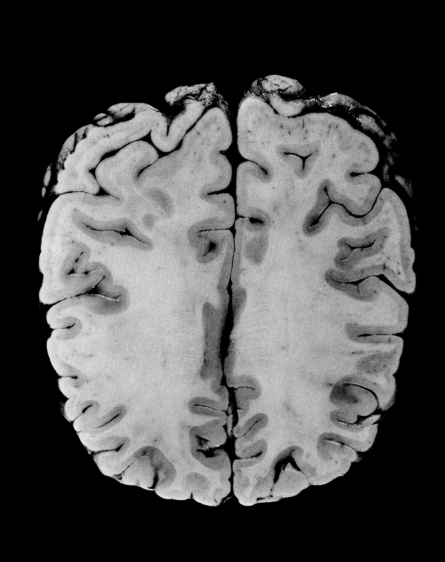

140° section, No. 6, uppersurface.

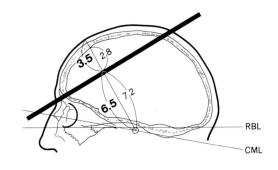

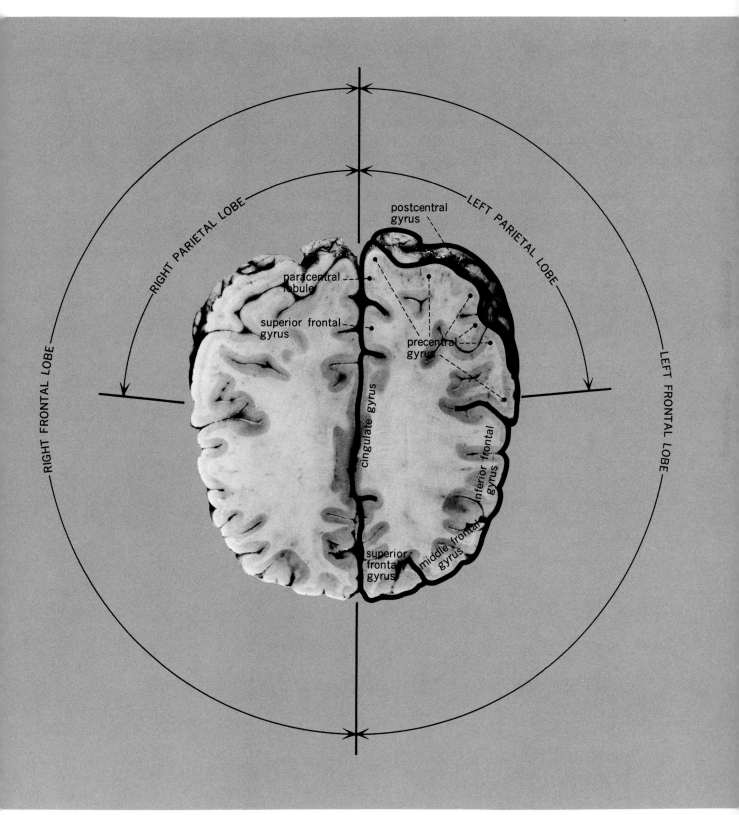

140° section, No. 6, uppersurface indicating prominent lobes and gyri.

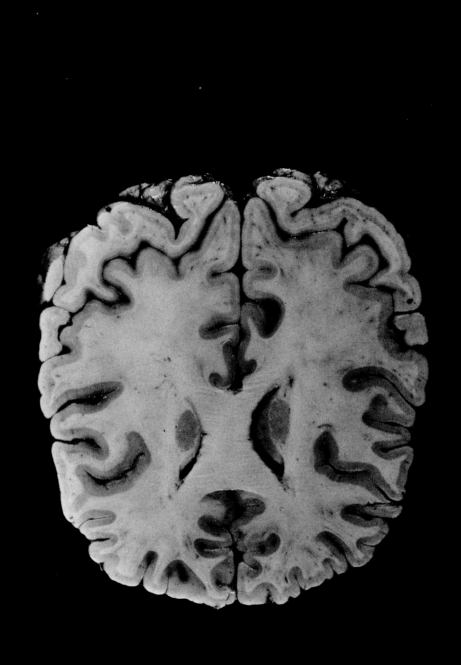

140° section, No. 7, uppersurface.

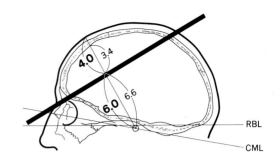

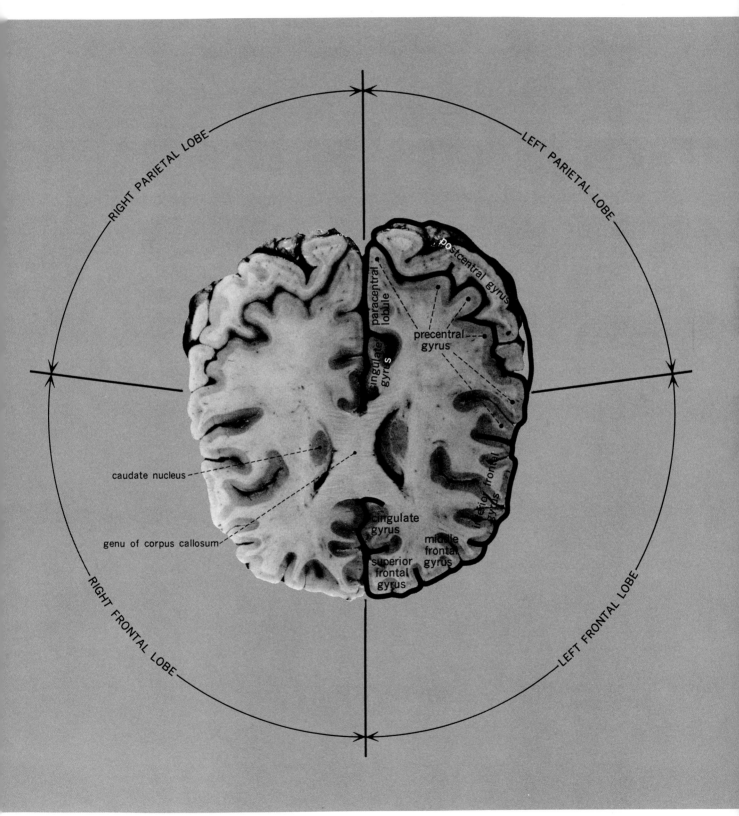

140° section, No. 7, uppersurface indicating prominent structures, lobes and gyri.

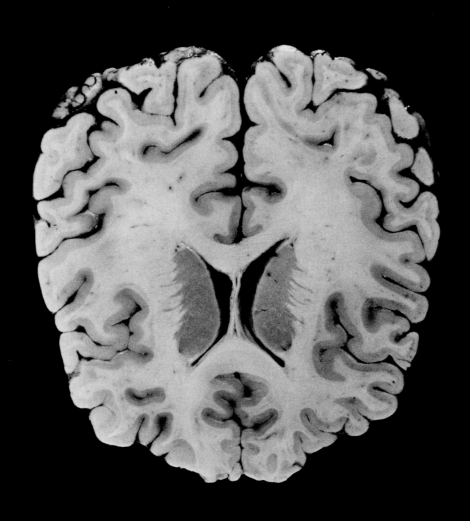

140° section, No. 8, uppersurface.

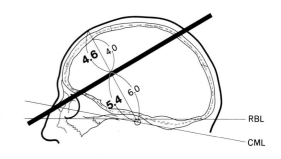

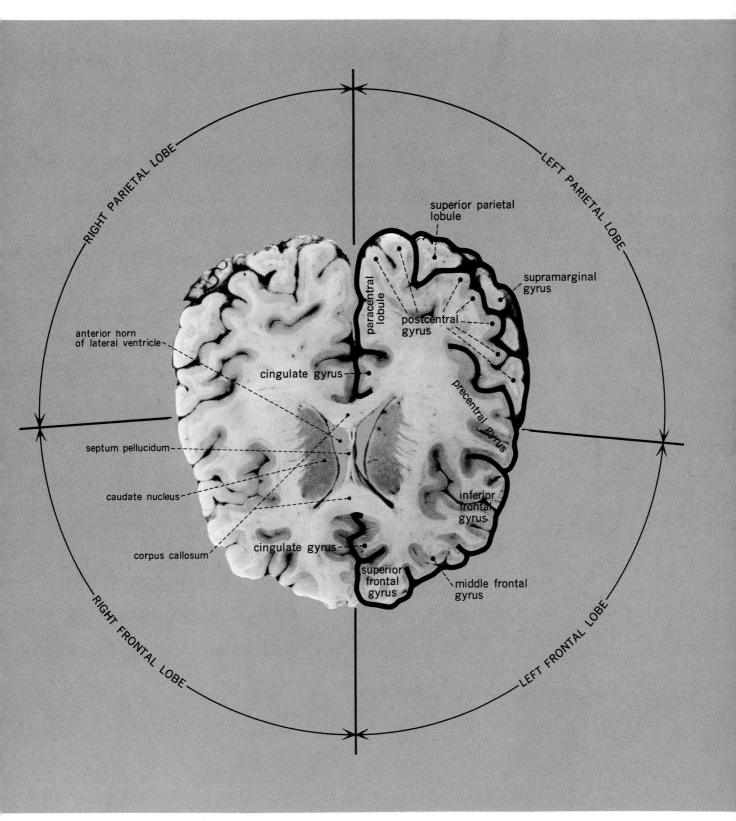

superior parietal
lobule

supramarginal
gyrus

paracentral
lobule

postcentral
gyrus

precentral gyrus

RIGHT PARIETAL LOBE

LEFT PARIETAL LOBE

anterior horn
of lateral ventricle

cingulate gyrus

septum pellucidum

caudate nucleus

inferior
frontal
gyrus

corpus callosum

cingulate gyrus

superior
frontal
gyrus

middle frontal
gyrus

RIGHT FRONTAL LOBE

LEFT FRONTAL LOBE

140° section, No. 8, uppersurface indicating prominent structures, lobes and gyri.

517

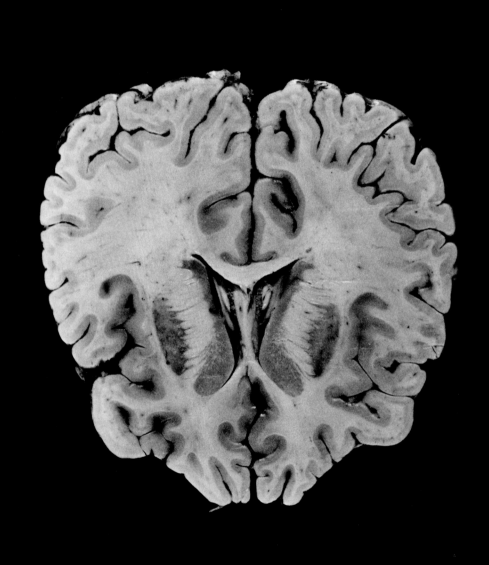

140° section, No. 9, uppersurface.

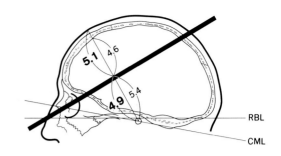

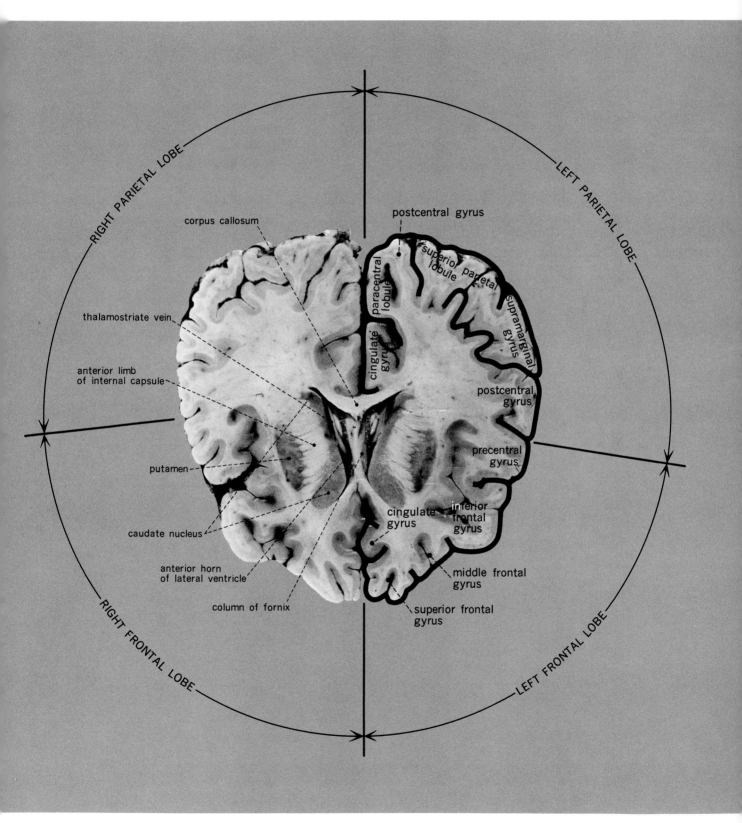

RBL
CML

140° section, No. 9, uppersurface indicating prominent structures, lobes and gyri.

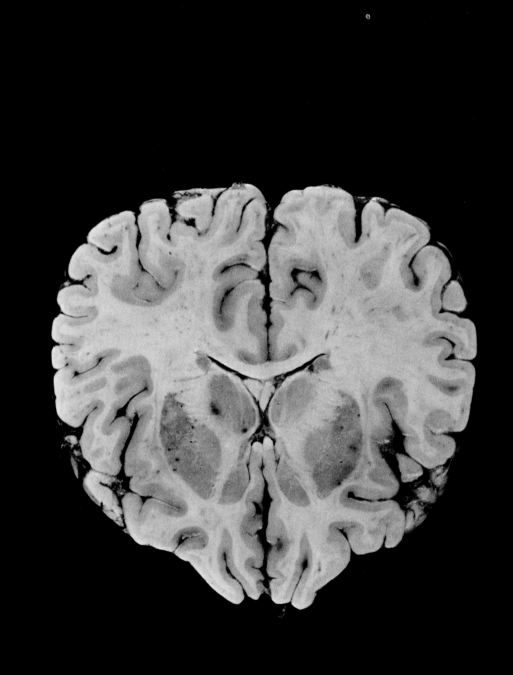

140° section, No. 10, uppersurface.

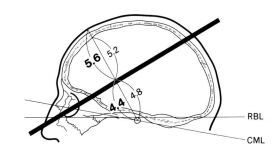

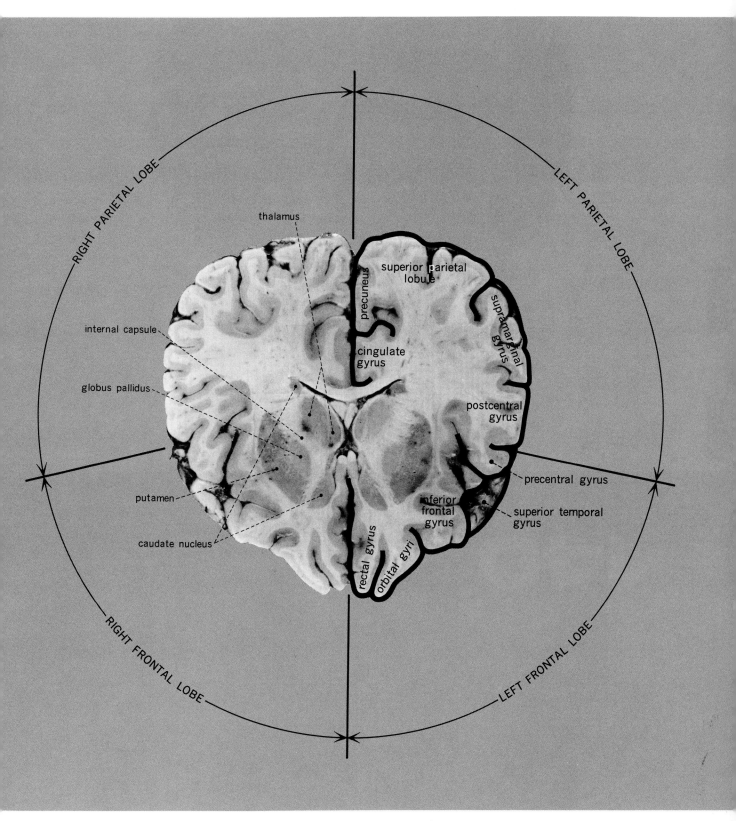

140° section, No. 10, uppersurface indicating prominent structures, lobes and gyri.

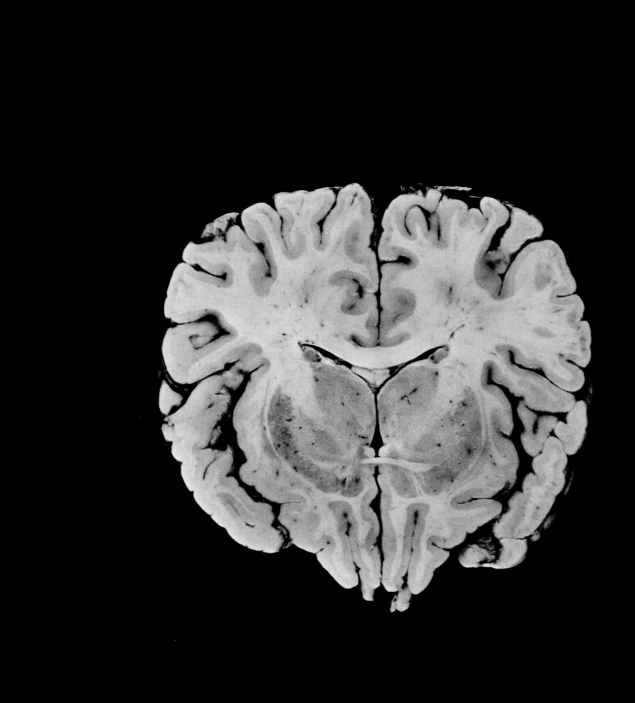

140° section, No. 11, uppersurface.

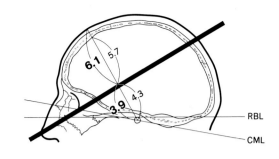

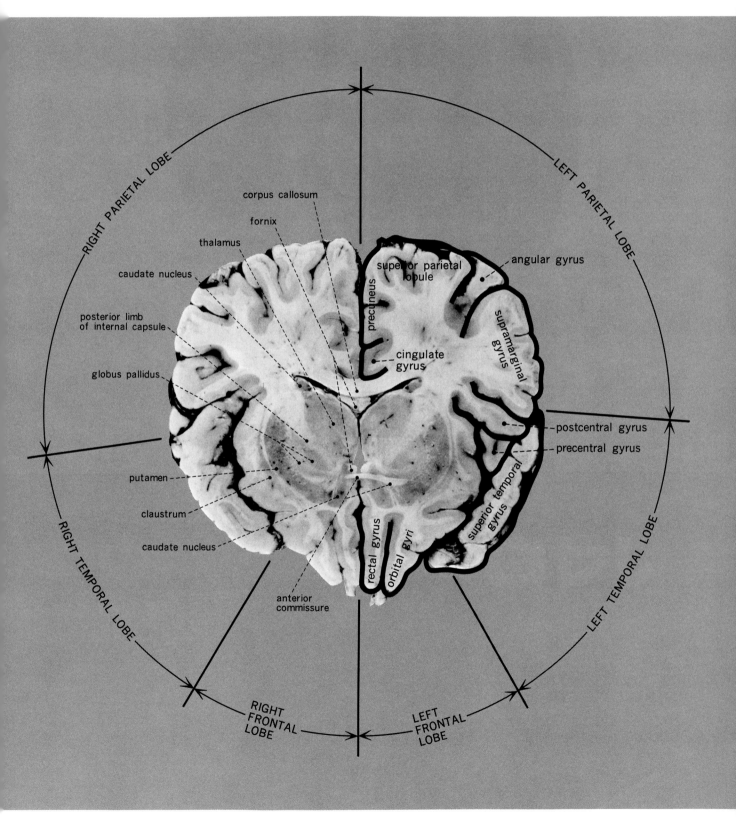

140° section, No. 11, uppersurface indicating prominent structures, lobes and gyri.

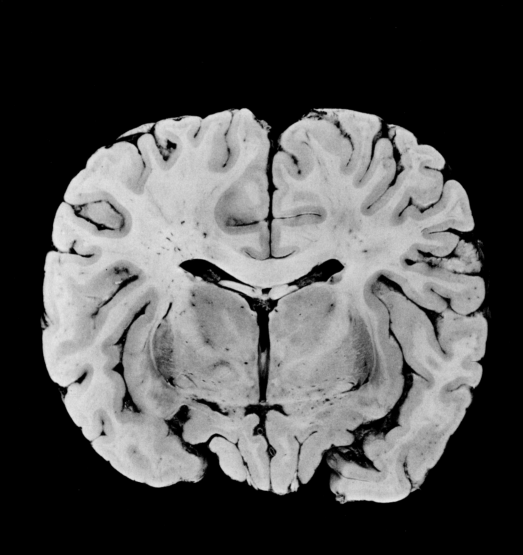

140° section, No. 12, uppersurface.

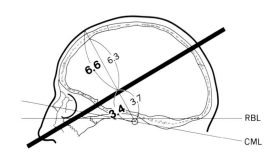

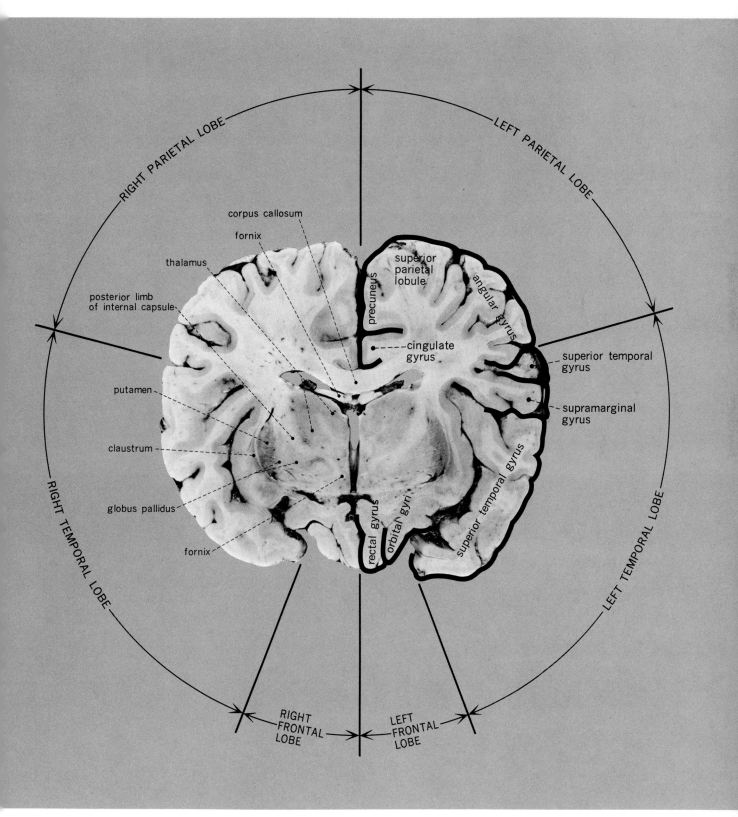

140° section, No. 12, uppersurface indicating prominent structures, lobes and gyri.

525

140°-13

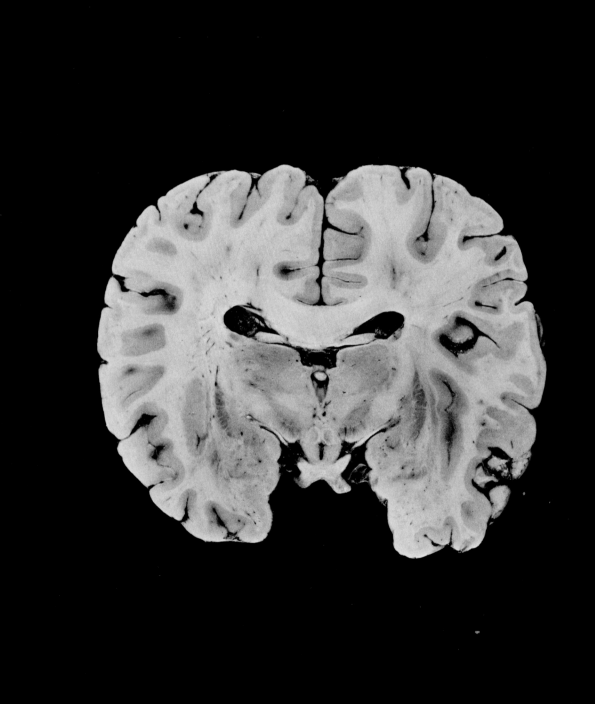

140° section, No. 13, uppersurface.

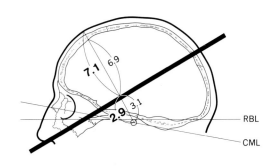

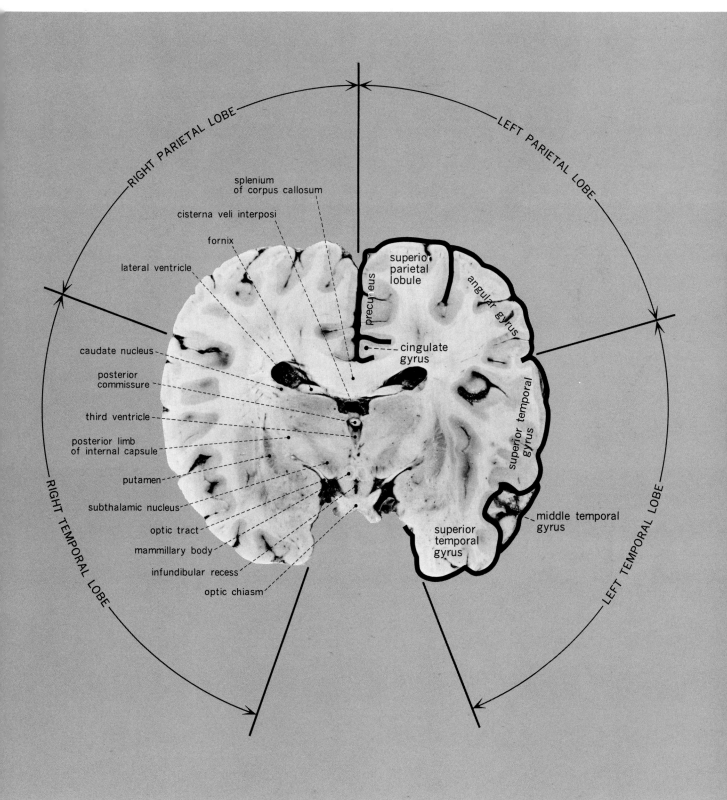

RIGHT PARIETAL LOBE

LEFT PARIETAL LOBE

splenium
of corpus callosum

cisterna veli interposi

fornix

lateral ventricle

superior
parietal
lobule

angular gyrus

precuneus

cingulate
gyrus

caudate nucleus

posterior
commissure

third ventricle

posterior limb
of internal capsule

putamen

subthalamic nucleus

optic tract

mammillary body

infundibular recess

optic chiasm

superior temporal gyrus

middle temporal
gyrus

superior
temporal
gyrus

RIGHT TEMPORAL LOBE

LEFT TEMPORAL LOBE

140° section, No. 13, uppersurface indicating prominent structures, lobes and gyri.

140°- 14

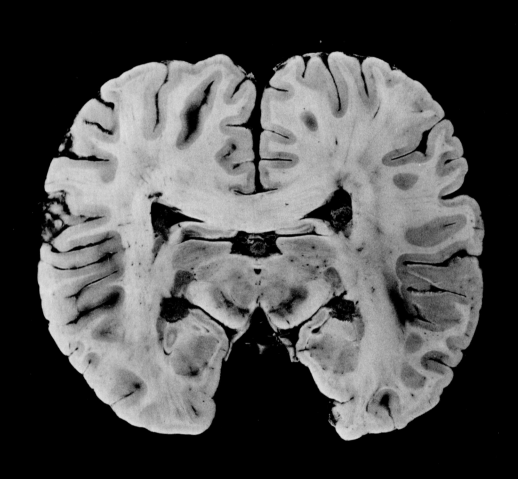

140° section, No. 14, uppersurface.

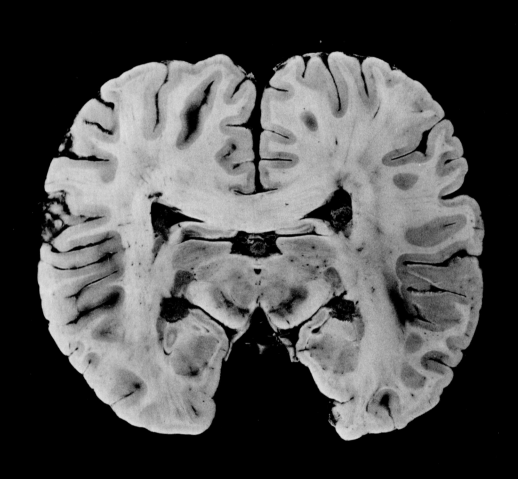

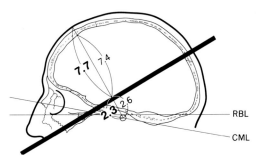

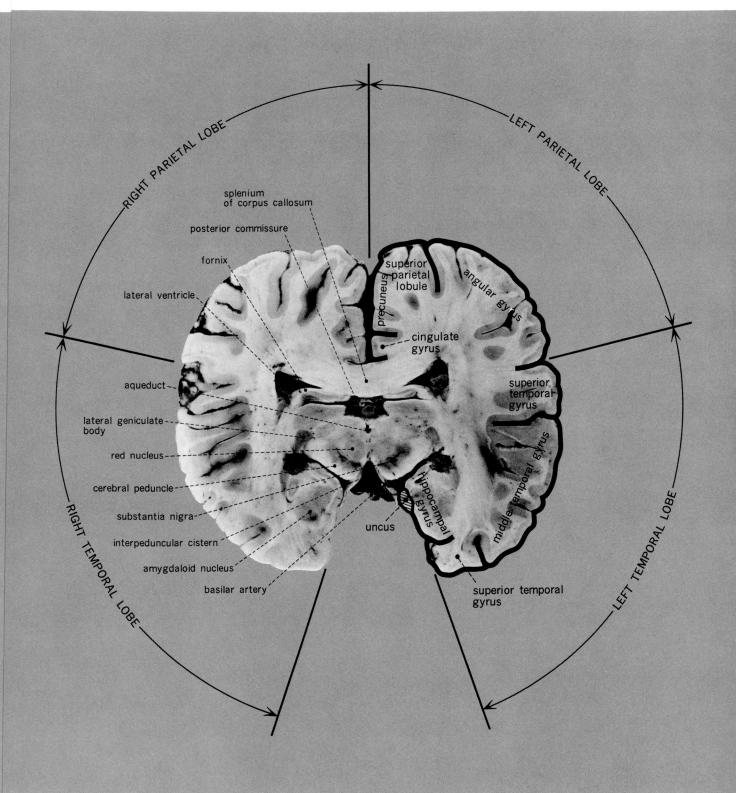

splenium
of corpus callosum

posterior commissure

fornix

lateral ventricle

aqueduct

lateral geniculate
body

red nucleus

cerebral peduncle

substantia nigra

interpeduncular cistern

amygdaloid nucleus

basilar artery

RIGHT PARIETAL LOBE

LEFT PARIETAL LOBE

RIGHT TEMPORAL LOBE

LEFT TEMPORAL LOBE

precuneus

superior
parietal
lobule

angular gyrus

cingulate
gyrus

superior
temporal
gyrus

middle temporal gyrus

hippocampal gyrus

uncus

superior temporal
gyrus

RBL

CML

140° section, No. 14, uppersurface indicating prominent structures, lobes and gyri.

529

140°- 16

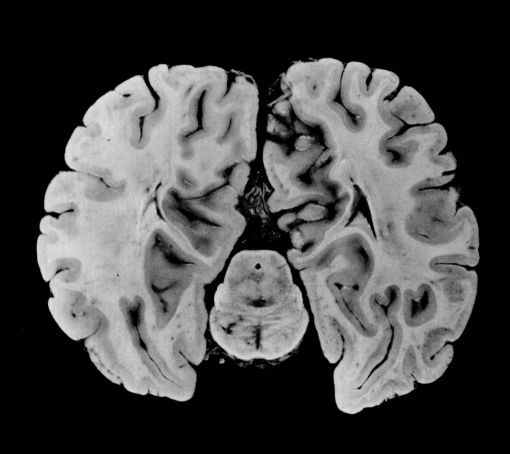

140° section, No. 16, uppersurface.

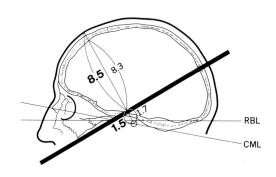

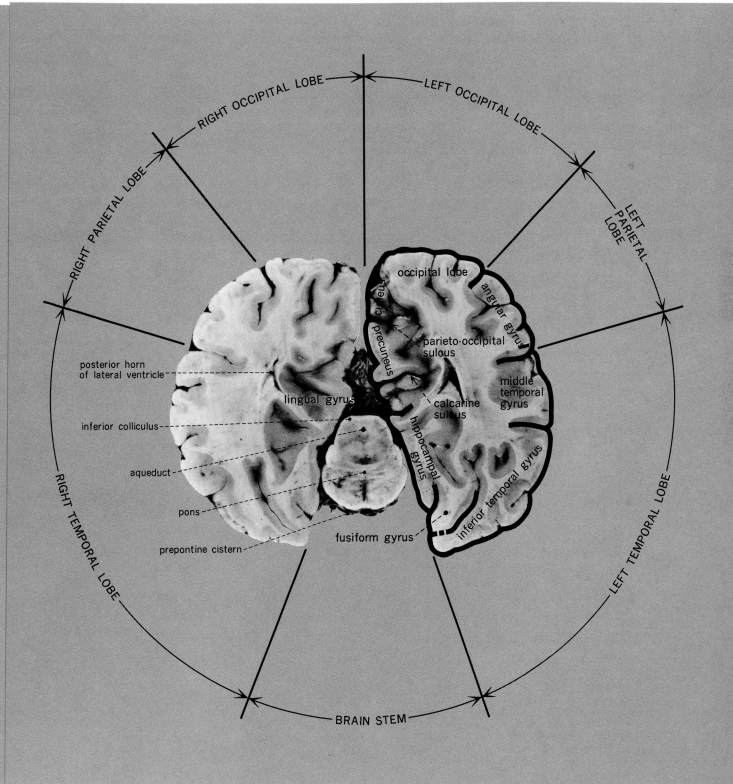

140° section, No. 16, uppersurface indicating prominent structures, lobes and gyri.

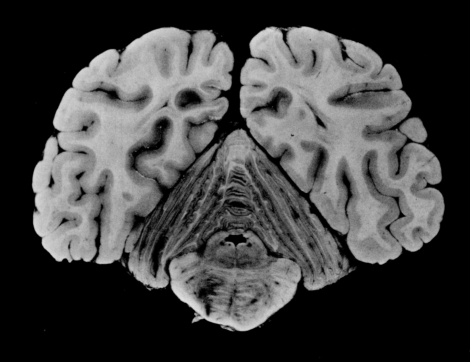

140° section, No. 18, uppersurface.

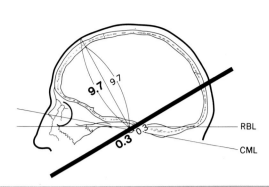

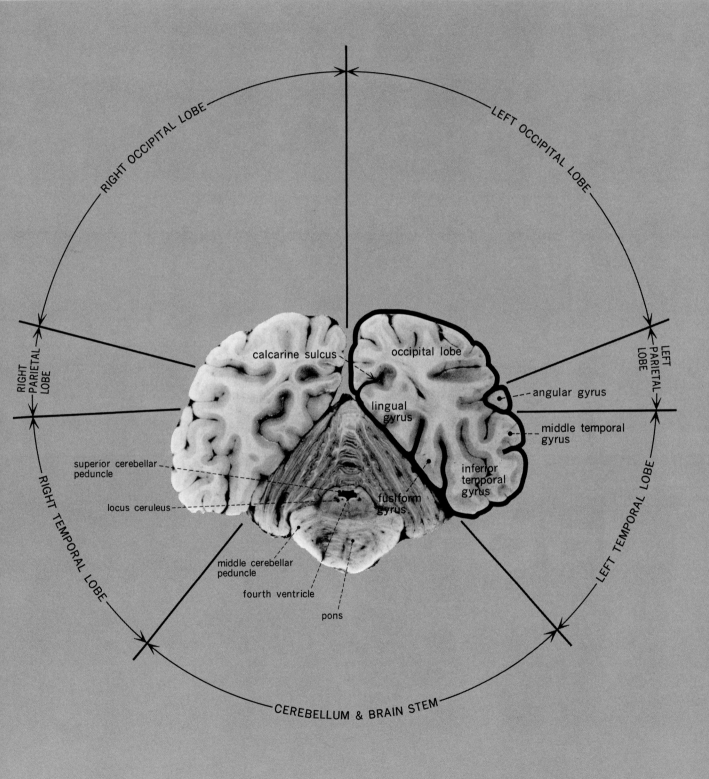

calcarine sulcus

occipital lobe

lingual
gyrus

angular gyrus

middle temporal
gyrus

inferior
temporal
gyrus

RIGHT OCCIPITAL LOBE

LEFT OCCIPITAL LOBE

RIGHT PARIETAL LOBE

LEFT PARIETAL LOBE

superior cerebellar
peduncle

locus ceruleus

fusiform
gyrus

RIGHT TEMPORAL LOBE

LEFT TEMPORAL LOBE

middle cerebellar
peduncle

fourth ventricle

pons

CEREBELLUM & BRAIN STEM

140° section, No. 18, uppersurface indicating prominent structures, lobes and gyri.

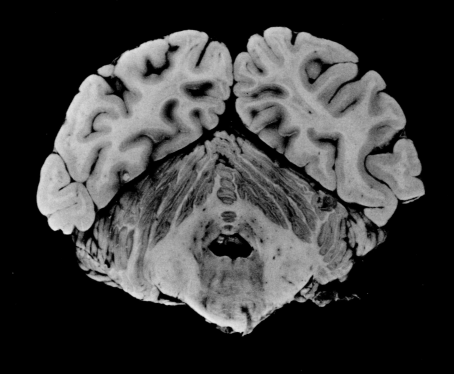

140° section, No. 19, uppersurface.

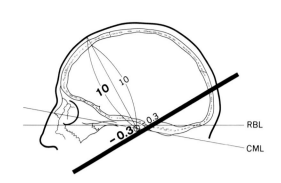

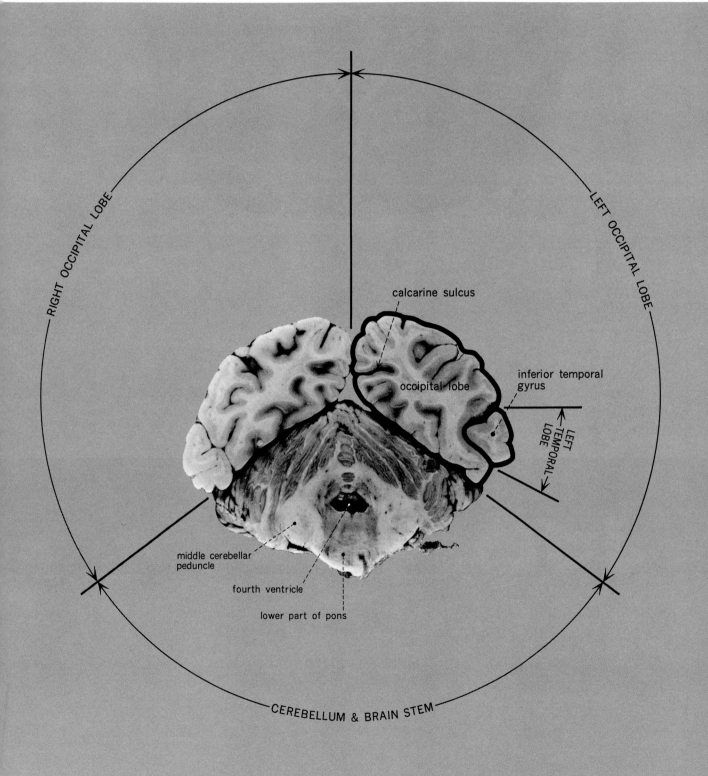

140° section, No. 19, uppersurface indicating prominent structures, lobes and gyri.

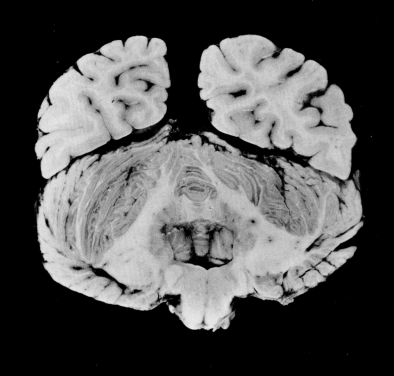

140° section, No. 20, uppersurface.

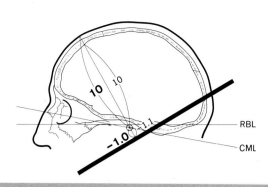

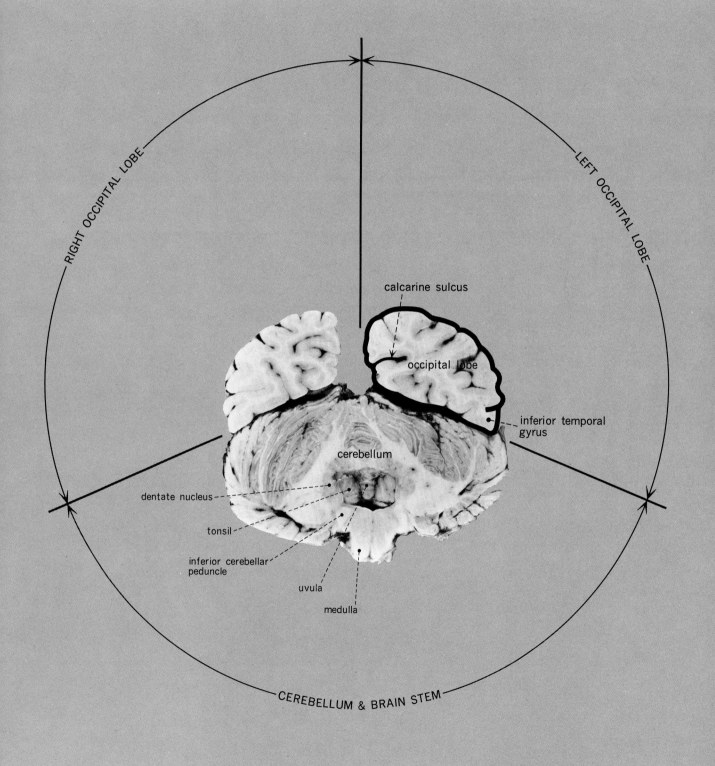

calcarine sulcus

occipital lobe

inferior temporal gyrus

cerebellum

dentate nucleus

tonsil

inferior cerebellar peduncle

uvula

medulla

RIGHT OCCIPITAL LOBE

LEFT OCCIPITAL LOBE

CEREBELLUM & BRAIN STEM

140° section, No. 20, uppersurface indicating prominent structures, lobes and gyri.

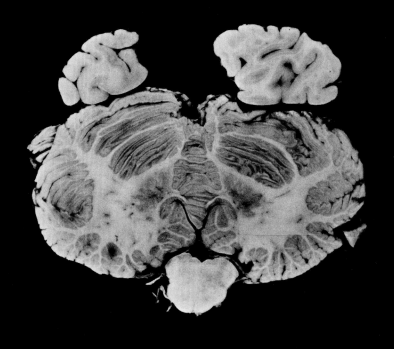

140° section, No. 21, uppersurface.

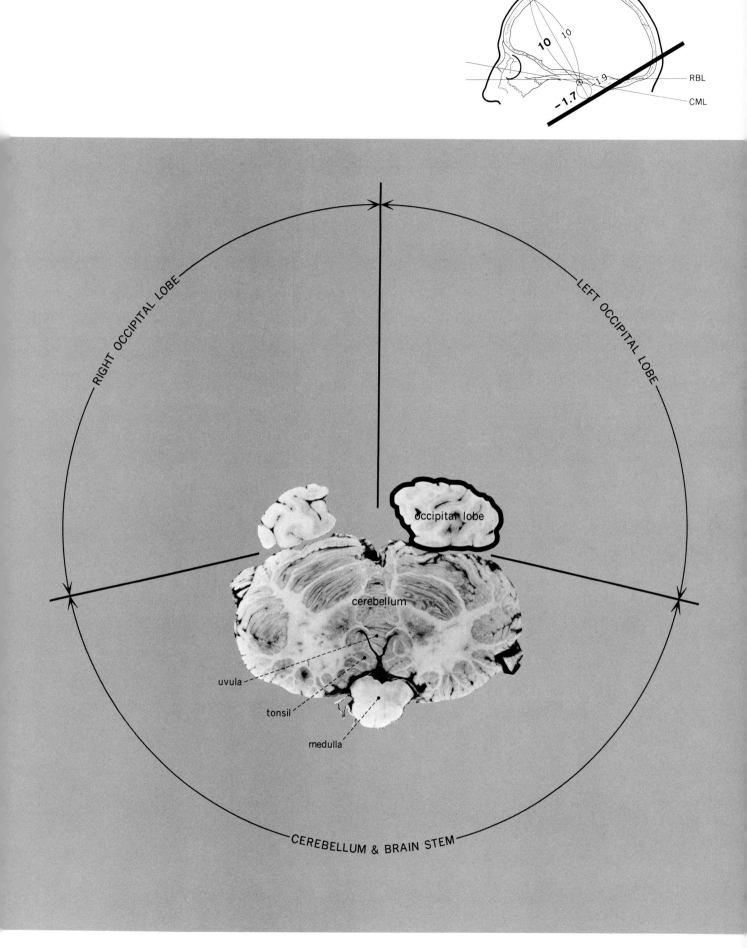

RBL

CML

10 10

-1.7 1.9

RIGHT OCCIPITAL LOBE

LEFT OCCIPITAL LOBE

occipital lobe

cerebellum

uvula

tonsil

medulla

CEREBELLUM & BRAIN STEM

140° section, No. 21, uppersurface indicating prominent structures, lobes and gyri.

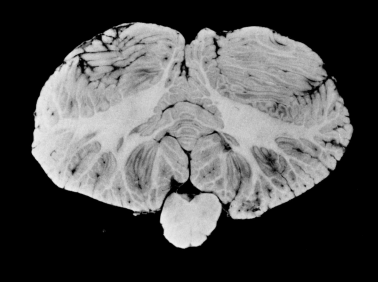

140° section, No. 22, uppersurface.

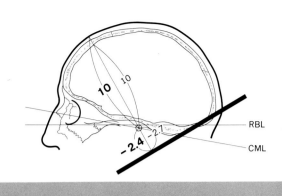

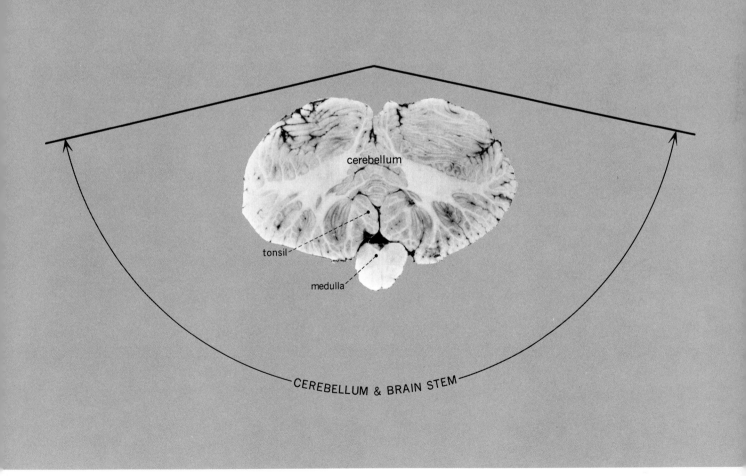

cerebellum

tonsil

medulla

CEREBELLUM & BRAIN STEM

140° section, No. 22, uppersurface indicating prominent structures, lobes and gyri.

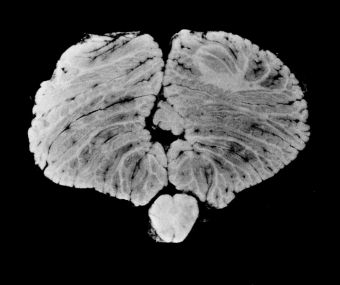

140° section, No. 23, uppersurface.

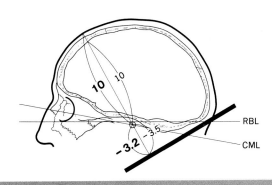

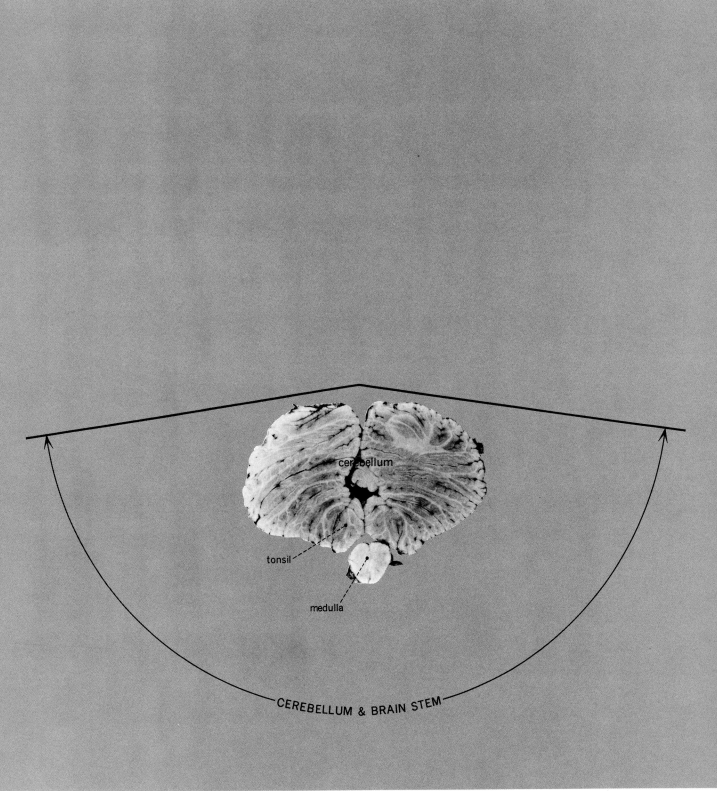

140° section, No. 23, uppersurface indicating prominent structures, lobes and gyri.

References

Adams, D.F., Hessel, S.J., Judy, P.F., et al. : Computed tomography of the normal and infarcted myocardium. Am. J. Roentgenol., *126* : 786-791, 1976.

Aidinis, S.J., Zimmerman, R.A., Shapiro, H.M., et al. : Anesthesia for brain computer tomography. Anesthesiology, *44* : 420-425, 1976.

Alderson, P.O., Mikhael, M., Coleman, R.E., et al. : Optimal utilization of computerized cranial tomography and radionuclide brain imaging. Neurol., *26*: 803-807, 1976.

Alfidi, R.J. : Computerized tomography of the gallbladder and biliary tract Semin. Roentgenol., *11* : 143, 1976.

Alfidi, R, J., Haaga, J., Meaney, T.F., et al. : Computed tomography of the thorax and abdomen. A preliminary report. Radiology, *117* : 257-264, 1975.

Alfidi, R.J. and Haaga, J.R. : Computed tomography of the body. A new horizon. Postgrad. Med., *60* : 133-136, 1976.

Alfidi, R.J., Haaga, J.R., Havrilla, T.R., et al.´ : Computed tomography of the liver. Am. J.Roentgenol., *127* : 69-74, 1976.

Alfidi, R.J. and Laval-Jeantet, M. : AG 60.99; A promising contrast agent for computed tomography of the liver and spleen. Radiology, *121* : 491, 1976.

Alfidi, R.J. and MacIntyre, W.J. : Computed tomography standardization. Radiology, *119* : 743-744, 1976.

Alfidi, R.J., MacIntyre, M.J. and Haaga, J.R. : The effects of biological motion on CT resolution. Am. J.Roentgenol., *127* : 11-15, 1976.

Alfidi, R.J., MacIntyre, W.J., Meaney, T.F., et al.: Experimental studies to determine application of CAT scanning to the human body. Am. J. Roentgenol. Radium Ther. Nucl. Med., *124* : 199-207, 1975.

Alfidi, R.J., Rodriguez-Antunez, A. and Meaney, T.F. : On CATs and Territorial Imperative. Radiology, *120* : 453, 1976.

Ambrose, J. : Computerized transverse axial scanning (tomography). Part 2. Clinical application. Br.J. Radiol., *46* : 1023-1047, 1973.

Ambrose, J. : Computerized transverse axial scanning of the brain. Proc. Roy. Soc. Med., *66* : 833-834, 1973.

Ambrose, J. : Computerized x-ray scanning of the brain. J. Neurosurg., *40* : 679-695, 1974.

Ambrose, J. and Hounsfield, G. : Computerized transverse axial tomography. Br.J. Radiol., *46* : 148-149, 1973.

Ambrose, J.A.E., Lloyd, G.A.S. and Wright, J.E. : A preliminary evaluation of fine matrix computerized axial tomography (Emiscan) in the diagnosis of orbital space-occupying lesions. Br.J. Radiol., *47* : 747-751, 1974.

Ambrose, J., Gooding, M.R., Griver, J., et al. : A quantitative study of the EMI values obtained for normal brain cerebral infarction and certain tumours. Br. J. Radiol., *49* : 827-830, 1976.

Ambrose, J., Gooding, M.R. and Richardson, A.E. : Sodium iothalamate as an aid to diagnosis of intracranial lesions by computerized transverse axial scanning. Lancet, *2* : 669-674, 1975.

Axelbaum, S.P., Schellinger, D., Gomes, M.N., et al. : Computed tomographic evaluation of aortic aneurysms. Am. J. Roentgenol. *127* : 75-78, 1976.

Baily, N.A., Keller, R.A., Jakowatz, C.V., et al. : The capability of fluoroscopic systems for the production of computerized axial tomograms. Invest. Radiol., *11* : 434-439, 1976.

Bajraktari, X., Bergström, M., Brismar, K., et al. : Diagnosis of intrasellar cisternal herniation (empty sella) by computed assisted tomography. Computed Tomography, *1* : 105-116, 1977.

Baker, H.L., Jr. : The impact of computed tomography on neuroradiologic practice. Radiology, *116* : 637-640, 1975.

Baker, H.L., Jr. : Computed tomography and neuroradiology; a fortunate primary union. Am. J. Roentgenol., *127* : 101-110, 1976.

Baker, H.L., Jr., Campbell, J.K., Houser, O.W., et al. : Computer assisted tomography of the head; An early evaluation. Mayo Clin. Proc., *49* : 17-27, 1974.

Baker, H.L., Jr., Campbell, J.K., Houser, O.W., et al. : Early experience with the EMI scanner for study of the brain. Radiology, *116* : 327-333, 1975.

References

Baker, H.L., Hauser, O.W., Campbell, J.K., et al. : Computerized tomography of the head. JAMA, *233* : 1304-1308, 1975.

Baker, H.L., Jr. and Houser, O.W. : Computed tomography in the diagnosis of posterior fossa lesions. Radiol. Clin. North Am., *14* : 129-147, 1976.

Baker, H.L., Jr., Kearns, T.P., Campbell, J.K., et al. : Computerized transaxial tomography in neuro-ophthalmology. Trans. Am. Ophthalmol. Soc., *72* : 49-64, 1974.

Baker, H.L., Jr., Kearns, T.P., Campbell, J.K., et al. : Computerized transaxial tomography in neuro-ophthalmology. Am. J. Ophthalmol., *78* : 285-294, 1974.

Banna, M. : Interpretation of the computerized tomographic scan. Can.J.Neurol. Sci., *3* : 123-132, 1976.

Banna, M. : Basic introduction to computerized tomography. J. Can. Assoc. Radiol., *27* : 143-148, 1976.

Banna, M., Molot, M.J., Kapur, P.L., et al. : Computer tomography of the brain in Hamilton. Can. Med. Assoc. J., *113* : 303-307, 1975.

Barrett, H,H., Gordon, S.K. and Hershel, R.S. : Statistical limitations in transaxial tomography. Comput. Biol. Med., *6* : 307-323, 1976.

Barron, S.T., Jacobs, L. and Kinkel, W.R. : Changes in size of normal lateral ventricles during aging determined by computerized tomography. Neurol., *26* : 1011-1013, 1976.

Battino, D., Luzzatti, C. and Spinnler, H. : Unforeseen clinicoanatomical correlation in the brain detected by computerized tomography, Med. J., *1* : 759-760, 1976.

Becker, M.H., McCarthy, J.G., Chase, N., et al. : Computerized axial tomography of craniofacial malformations. A preliminary report. Am. J. Dis. Child, *130* : 17-20, 1976.

Berger, P.E., Harwood-Nash, D.C. and Fitz, C.R. : Computerized tomography; abnormal intracerebral collections of blood in children. Neuroradiology, *11* : 29-33, 1976.

Berger, P.E., Kirks, D.R., Gilday, D.L., et al. : Computed tomography in infants and children; Intracranial neoplasms. Am. J.Roentgenol., *127* : 129-137, 1976.

Bergström, M., Ericson, K., Levander, B., et al. : Variation with time of the attenuation values of intracranial hematomas. Computed Tomography, *1* : 57-63, 1977.

Bergström, M. and Greitz, T. : Stereotaxic computed tomography. Am. J.Roentgenol., *127* : 167-170, 1976.

Bergström, M., Riding, M. and Greitz, T. : The limitations of definition of blood vessels with computer intravenous angiography. Neuroradiology, *11* : 35-40, 1976.

Bergström, M. and Sundman, R. : Analysis of regions of interest in EMI scans. Br. J. Radiol., *49* : 549-550, 1976.

Bergström, M. and Sundman, R. : Picture processing in computed tomography. Am. J. Roentgenol., *127* : 17-21, 1976.

Bergvall, U. : Temporal course of contrast medium enhancement in differential diagnosis of intracranial lesions with computer tomography. In : Advances in cerebral angiography (edited by Salamon, G.), Springer, Berlin, 1975, p.346-348.

Bergvall, U. Greitz, T. and Steiner, C. : Computer tomography in post-mortem examination of the brain and other specimens. Acta Radiol., Suppl. (Stockh.), *346* : 39-44, 1975.

Bjorgen, J.E. and Gold, L.H.A. : Computed tomographic appearance of methotrexateinduced necrotizing leukoencephalopathy. Radiology, *122* : 377-378, 1977.

Bligh, A.S., Frazer, A.K., Graham, J.G., et al. : Computer-assisted tomography of the brain. Lancet, *2* : 1260, 1974.

Boltshauser, E. and Isler, W. : Computerized axial tomography in spongy degeneration. Lancet, *1* : 1123, 1976.

Bogdanoff, B.M., Stafford, C.R., Green, L., et al. : Computerized transaxial tomography in the evaluation of patients with focal epilepsy. Neurol., *25* : 1013-1017, 1975.

Bosch, E.P., Cancilla, P.A. and Cornell, S.H. : Computerized tomography in progressive multifocal leukoencephalopathy. Arch. Neurol., *33* : 216, 1976.

Bracewell, R.N. : Correction for collimeter width (restration) in reconstructive x-ray tomography. Computed Tomography, *1* : 6-15, 1977.

Bracewell, R.N. and Raddle, A.C. : Inversion of fan-beam scans in radio-astronomy. Astrophys J., *150* : 427-434, 1967.

Braun, I.F., Naidich, T.P., Leeds, N.E., et al. : Dense intracranial epidermoid tumors; Computed tomographic observations. Radiology, *122* : 717-719, 1977.

Brismar, J., Davis, K.R., Dallow, R.L., et al. : Unilateral endocrine exophthalmos; Diagnostic problems in association with computed tomography. Neuroradiology, *12* : 21-23, 1976.

Brismar, J., Robertson, G.H. and Davis, K.R. : Radiation necrosis of the brain; Neuroradiological considerations with computed tomography. Neuroradiology, *12* : 109-113, 1976.

Britton, K.E. and Williams, E.S. : E.M.I. and radioisotope brain imaging. Lancet, *1* : 477-478, 1976.

Britton, K.E. and Williams, E.S. : E.M.I. and radioisotope brain imaging. Lancet, *1* : 904-905, 1976.

Brooks, R.A. and Di Chiro, G. : Theory of image reconstruction in computed tomography. Radiology, *117* : 561-572, 1975.

Brooks, R.A. and Di Chiro, G. : Beam hardening in x-ray reconstructive tomography. Phys. Med. Biol., *21* : 390-398, 1976.

Brooks, R.A. and Di Chiro, G. : Principles of computer assisted tomography (CAT) in radiographic and radioisotopic imaging. Phys. Med. Biol., *21* : 689-732, 1976.

Boulware, F.T., Jr. : Computerized transaxial tomogram; Relationship to other neurodiagnostic procedures. Rocky Mt. Med. J., *72* : 435-438, 1975.

Budinger, T.F., Derenzo, S.E., Gullberg, G.T., et al. : Emission computer assisted tomography with single-photon and positron annihilation photon emitters. Computed Tomography, *1* : 131-145, 1977.

Butzer, J.F., Cancilla, P.A. and Cornell, S.H. : Computerized axial tomography of intracerebral hematoma; A clinical and neuropathological study. Arch. Neurol., *33* : 206-214, 1976.

Campbell, J.K., Baker, H.L. and Laws, E.R., Jr. : Computer assisted axial tomography (EMI scan) in neurologic investigation. Trans. Am. Neurol. Assoc., *99* : 117-120, 1974.

Carella, R.J., Ray, N., Newall, J., et al. : Computerized (axial) tomography in the serial study of cerebral tumors treated by radiation; A preliminary report. Cancer, *37* : 2719-2728, 1976.

Carter, B.L. and Ignatow, S.B. : Neck and mediastinal angiography by computed tomography scan, Radiology, *122* : 515-516, 1977.

Carter, B.L., Kahn, P.C., Wolpert, S.M., et al. : Unusual pelvic masses; A comparison of computed tomographic scanning and ultrasonography. Radiology, *121* : 383-390, 1976.

Chernak, E.S., Rodriguez-Antunez, A., Jelden, G.L., et al. : The use of computed tomography for radiation therapy treatment planning. Radiology, *117* : 613-614, 1975.

Chesler, D.A., Riederer, S.J. and Pelc, N.J. : Noise due to photon counting statistics in computed x-ray tomography. Computed Tomography, *1* : 64-74, 1977.

Chiu, L.C., Fodor, L.B., Cornell, S.H., et al. : Computed tomography and brain scintigraphy in ischemic stroke. Am. J. Roentgenol., *127* : 481-486, 1976.

Cho, Z.H. and Ahn, I.S. : Computer algorithm for the tomographic image reconstruction with x-ray transmission scans. Comut. Biomed. Res., *8* : 8-25, 1975.

Cho, Z.H., Ahn, I., Bohn, C., et al. : Computerized image reconstruction methods with multiple photon/x-ray transmission scanning. Phys. Med. Biol., *19* : 511-522, 1974.

Cho, Z.H., Tsai, C.M. and Wilson, G. : Study of contrast and modulation mechanisms in x-ray/photon transverse axial transmission. Phys. Med. Biol., *20* : 879-889, 1975.

Christle, J.H., Mori, H., Go, R.T., et al. : Computed tomography and radionuclide studies in the diagnosis of intracranial disease. Am. J.Roentgenol. *127* : 171-174, 1976.

Chu, F.C. : Radiological methods of studying the orbit. Computerized Tomography, *1* : 45-50, 1977.

Clark, J.W. : Can radiology retain computed tomography? Radiology, *117* : 739, 1975.

Clarke, R.L., Milne, E.N. and Van Dyk, G. : The use of Compton scattered gamma rays for tomography. Invest. Radiol. *11* : 225-235, 1976.

Claveria, L. E., Du Boulay, G.H. and Moseley, I.F. : Intracranial infections; investigation by computerized axial tomography. Neuroradiology, *12* : 59-71, 1976.

Claveria, L.E., Sutton, D. and Tress, B.M. : The radiological diagnosis of meningiomas, the impact of EMI scanning. Br. J.Radiol. *50* : 15-22. 1976.

Clifford, J.R., Connolly, E.S. and Voorhies, R.M. : Comparison of radionuclide scans with computer-assisted tomography in diagnosis of intracranial disease. Neurol., *26* : 1119-1123, 1976.

Cloe, L.E. : Health planning for computed tomography : perspectives and problems. Am. J. Roentgenol., *127* : 187-190, 1976.

Coin, C.G., Coin, J.W. and Glover, M.B. : Vascular tumors of the choroid plexus; Diagnosis by computed tomography. Computed Tomography, *1* : 146-148, 1977.

Coin, C.G., Wilson, G.H. and Klebanoff, R. : Contrast enhancement by arterial perfusion during computerized tomography. Neuroradiology, *11* : 119-121, 1976.

Collard, M. and Dupont, H. : Indications de la tomodensitométrie cérébrale. Bilan de 2000 observations. J. Radiol. Electrol. Méd. Nucl., *57* : 589-591, 1976.

Collard, M., Dupont, H. and Noël, G. : Ere nouvelle de la neuroradiologie; La tomographie axiale transverse computérisée-T.A.T.C. (EMI-Scanner) et ses indications. J. Radiol. Electrol. Méd. Nucl., *56* : 453-469, 1975.

Constant, P., Renou, A.M., Caille, A.M., et al. : Cerebral metastasis—A study of computerized tomography. Computerized Tomography, *1* : 87-94, 1977.

Cormack, A.M. : Representation of a function of its line integrals, with some radiological applications. J. Appl. Physics, *34* : 27722-2727, 1963.

Cornell, S.H., Christie, J.H., Chiu, C.L., *et al.* : Computerized axial tomography of the cerebral ventricles and subarachnoid spaces. Am. J. Roentgenol. Radium Ther. Nucl. Med., *124* : 186-194, 1975.

Cornel, S.H., Musallam, J.J., Chiu, C.L., et al. : Individualized computer tomography of the skull with the EMI scanner using 160 x 160 matrix. Am. J. Roentgenol., *126* : 779-785, 1976.

Crockard, H.A., Hanlon, K., Ganz, E., et al. : Intracranial pressure gradients in a patient with a thalamic tumor. Surg. Neurol., *5* : 151-155, 1976.

References

Crocker, E.F., Zimmerman, R.A., Phelps, M.E., et al. : The effect of steroids on the extravascular distribution of radiographic contrast material and technetium pertechnetate in brain tumors as determined by computed tomography. Radiology, *119* : 471-474, 1976.

Cronqvist, S., Brismar, J., Kjellin, K., et al. : Computer assisted axial tomography in cerebrovascular lesions. Acta Radiol. [Diag.] (Stockh.), *16* : 135-145, 1975.

Dallow, R.L., Momose, K.J., Weber, A.L., et al. : Comparison of ultrasonography, computerized tomography (EMI scan), and radiographic techniques in evaluation of exophthalmos. Trans. Am. Acad. Ophthlmol. Otolaryngol., *81* : 305-322, 1976.

Danziger, J., Bloch, S. and Podlas, H. : Computer axial tomography of the head. S. Afr. Med. J., *50* 1398-1402, 1976.

Davis, D.O., Marden, D. and Staples, G.S. : A head-holding device for computed tomography, Radiology, *117* : 480, 1975.

Davis, D.O. and Pressman, B.D. : Computerized tomography of the brain; Symposium on the skull and brain (edited by Chase, N.E. & Kricheff, I.I.). Radiol. Clin. North. Am., *12* : 297-313, 1974.

Davis, K.R., Ackerman, R.H., Kistler, J.P., et al. : Computed tomography of cerebral infarction; Hemorrhagic, contrast enhancement, and time of appearance. Computerized Tomography, *1* : 71-86, 1977.

Davis, K.R., New, P.F.J., Ojemann, R.G., et al. : Computed tomographic evaluation of hemorrhage secondary to intracranial aneurysm. Am. J.Roentgenol., *127* : 143-153, 1976.

Davis, K.R., Robertson, G.H., Taveras, J.M., et al. : Diagnosis of epidermoid tumor by computed tomography. Analysis and evaluation of findings. Radiology, *119* : 347-353, 1976.

Davis, K.R., Taveras, J.M., New, P.F.J., et al. : Cerebral infarction. Diagnosis by computerized tomography analysis and evaluation of findings. Am. J. Roentgenol. Radium Ther. Nucl. Med., *124* : 643-660, 1975.

Davis, K.R., Taveras, J.M., Robertson, G.H. : Some limitations of computed tomography in the diagnosis of neurological diseases. Am. J.Roentgenol., *127* : 111-123, 1976.

Deck, M.D.F., Messina, A.V. and Sackett, J.F. : Computed tomography in metastatic disease of the brain. Radiology, *119* : 115-120, 1976.

Delaney, P. and Schellinger, D. : Computerized tomography and benign intracranial hypertension. JAMA *236* : 951-952, 1976.

Di Chiro, G. : Of CAT and other beasts. Am. J. Roentgenol. Radium Ther. Nucl. Med., *122* : 659-661, 1974.

Di Chiro, G., Axelbaum, S.P., Schellinger, D., et al. : Computerized axial tomography in syringomyelia, New Engl. J. Med., *292* : 13-16, 1975.

Di Chiro, G., Hammock, M.K. and Bleyer, W.A. : Spinal descent of cerebrospinal fluid in man. Neurol., *26* : 1-8, 1976.

Di Chiro, G. and Schellinger, D. : Computed tomography of spinal cord after lumber intrathecal introduction of Metrizamide (Computer-assisted myelography). Radiology, *120* : 101-103, 1976.

Doppman, J.L., Brennan, M.F., Koehler, J.O., et al. : Computed tomography for parathyroid localization. Computed Tomography, *1* : 30-36, 1977.

Douglas, M.A. : Computerized axial tomography. J.Miss. State Med. Assoc., *17* : 155-160, 1976.

Dryer, B.P. and Rosenbaum, A.E. : Suprasellar masses on computerized tomography with intrathecal metrizamide. Lancet, *2* : 736-737, 1976.

Dublin, A.B., French, B.N. and Rennick, J.M. : Computed tomography in head trauma. Radiology, *122* : 365-370, 1977.

Dublin, A.B., Rennick, J.M. and Sivalingam, S. : Failure of computerized axial tomography to demonstrate a chronic subdural hematoma. Surg. Neurol., *6* : 23-24, 1976.

Du Boulay, G.H. and Marshall, J. : Comparison of E.M.I. and radioisotope imaging in neurological disease. Lancet, *2* : 1294-1297, 1975.

Du Boulay, G.H. and Marshall, J. : E.M.I. and radioisotope brain scanning. Lancet, *1* : 583-584, 1976.

Duda, E.E. and Huttenlocher, P.R. : Computed tomography in adrenoleukodystrophy: Correlation of radiological and histological findings. Radiology, *120* : 349-350, 1976.

Duggan, H.E. : C.T. scanning—a rapidly changing field. J. Can. Assoc. Radiol., *27* : 134, 1976.

Dyment, P.G., Rothner, A.D., Duchesneau, P.M., et al. : Computerized tomography in the detection of intracranial metastasis in children. Pediatrics, *58* : 72-77, 1976.

Edholm. P. : Image construction in transversal computer tomography. Acta Radiol., Suppl. (Stockh.), *346* : 21-38, 1975.

Edholm, P. : Datortomografi en revolutionerande ny röntgen metod. Lakartidningen, *73* : 2408-2412, 1976.

Elke, M., Hunig, R., Wiggli, U., et al. : Die computerisierte Tomographie des Schädels; Eine neue Dimension der Röntgendiagnostik. Roentgenpraxis, *29* : 1-11, 1976.

Enzman, D., Donaldson, S.S., Marshall, W.H., et al. : Computed tomography in orbital pseudotumor (Idiopathic orbital inflammation). Radiology, *120* : 597-601, 1976.

Enzmann, D. and Gates, G.F. : "Watershed" infarction in sickle cell disease. Radiology, *118* : 337-339, 1976.

552

Enzmann, D.R., Hayward, R.W., Norman, D., et al. : Cranial computed tomographic scan appearance of Sturge-Weber disease; Unusual presentation. Radiology, *122* : 721-724, 1977.

Enzmann, D., Marshall, W.H., Jr., Rosenthal, A.R., et al. : Computed tomography in Graves' ophthalmopathy. Radiology, *118* : 615-620, 1976.

Enzman, D.R., Norman, D., Mani, J., et al. : Computed tomography of granulomatous basal arachnoiditis. Radiology, *120* : 341-344, 1976.

Eriksson, L. and Cho, Z.H. : Efficiency optimization analysis for dynamic function studies with 3-D transaxial positron cameras. Comput. Biol. Med., *6* : 361-372, 1976.

Evens, R.G. : New frontier for radiology; Computed tomography. 40th Annual Preston M. Hickey Memorial Lecture. Am. J. Roentgenol., *126* : 1117-1129, 1976.

Evens, R.G. and Jost, G.R. : Economic analysis of computed tomography units. Am. J. Roentgenol., *127* : 191-198, 1976.

Eycleshymer, A.C. and Schoemaker, D.M. : A cross-section anatomy. Appleton-Century-Crofts, New York, 1970.

Eyler, W.R. and Figley, M.M. : Computed tomography display. Radiology, *119* : 487-488, 1976.

Fawcitt, R.A. and Isherwood, I. : Radiodiagnosis of intracranial pearly tumours with particular reference to the value of computer tomography. Neuroradiology, *11* : 235-242, 1976.

Feindel, W. : Head and body scanning by computer tomography. Can. Med. Assoc. J., *113* : 273-274, 1975.

Fields, S.W., Bell., R. M., Campbell, J.K., et al. : Computed tomography in the management of cerebrovascular disease. Stroke, *6* : 105-107, 1975.

Figley, M.M. and Eyler, W.R. : Orientation of CT images. Am. J.Roentgenol., *127* : 199, 1976.

Fischgold, H. : L'EMI-scanner. J. Radiol. Electrol. Méd. Nucl., *54* : 1-5, 1973.

Fox, J.H. and Huckman, M.S. : Computerized tomography. A recent advance in evaluating senile dementia. Geriatrics, *30* : 97-100, 1975.

Fox, J.H., Topel, J.L. and Huckman, M.S. : The use of computerized tomography in senile dementia. J. Neurol. Neurosurg. Psychiatry, *38* : 948-953, 1975.

Freedman, G.S. : C.T. in CT. for CATS in Conn. or computerized axial tomography in Connecticut. Conn. Med., *40* : 763-769, 1977.

Gado, M.H., Coleman, R.E., Merlis, A.L., et al. : Comparison of computerized tomography and radionuclide imaging in "stroke". Stroke, *7* : 109-113, 1976.

Gado, M.H., Coleman, R.E., Lee, K.S., et al. : Correlation between computerized transaxial tomography and radionuclide cisternography in dementia. Neurol., *26* : 555-560, 1976.

Gado, M.H. and Phelps, M.E. : The peripheral zone of increased density in cranial computed tomography. Radiology, *117* : 71-74, 1975.

Gado, M.H., Phelps, M.E. and Coleman, R.E. : An extravascular component of contrast enhancement in cranial computed tomography; Part 1. The tissue-blood ratio of contrast enhancement. Radiology, *117* : 589-593, 1975.

Gado, M.H., Phelps, M.E. and Coleman, R.E. : An extravascular component of contrast enhancement in cranial computed tomography; Part 2. Contrast enhancement and the blood-tissue barrier. Radiology, *117* : 595-597, 1975.

Gastaut, H. : Conclusion; Computerized transeverse axial tomography in epilepsy. Epilepsia, *17* : 337-338, 1976.

Gastaut, H. and Gastaut, J.L. : Computerized transverse axial tomography in epilepsy. Epilepsia, *17* : 325-336, 1976.

Gastaut, H., Gastaut, J.L. and Pinsard, N. : Diagnostic de la maladie de Bourneville par la tomographic cérébrale commandée par ordinateur. Nouv. Presse Méd., *5* : 864, 1976.

Gastaut, H., Gastaut, J.L. and Régis, H. : Etude des épilepsies par la tomographie axiale transverse de l'encéphale commandée par ordinateur. Nouv. Presse Méd., *5* : 481-486, 1976.

Gastaut, J.L., Rayband, C. and Régis, H. : Preliminary study of the application of computerized axial tomography in the etiologic diagnosis of epilepsy. In : Advances in cerebral angiography (edited by Salamon, G.), Springer, Berlin, 1975, p.358-360.

Gastaut, H., Salamon, G., Régis, H., et al. : Place de la tomographie axiale avec ordinateur en neuroradiologie. Premiers résultats. Nouv. Presse Méd., *5* : 1239-1243, 1976.

Gawler, J. : EMI scanning in relation to other investigations of the brain. Br. J.Radiol., *48* : 606-607, 1975.

Gawler, J., Bull, J.W., Du Boulay, G.H., et al. : Computer-assisted tomography (EMI scanner). Its place in investigation of suspected intracranial tumors. Lancet, *2* : 419-423, 1974.

Gawler, J., Bull, J.W.D., Du Boulay, G, H., et al. : Computerized axial tomography. The normal EMI scan. J. Neurol. Neurosurg. Psychiatry, *38* : 935-947, 1975.

Gawler, J., Du Boulay, G.H., Bull, J.W.D., et al. : Computerized tomography (the EMI scanner); A comparison with pneumoencephalography and ventriculography. J. Neurol. Neurosurg. Psychiatry, *39* : 203-211, 1976.

References

Gawler, J., Du Boulay, G.H., Bull, J.W., et al. : A comparison of computer assisted tomography (EMI scanner) with conventional neuroradiologic methods in the investigation of patients clinically suspected of intracranial tumor. J.Can. Assoc. Radiol., *27* : 157-159, 1976.

Gawler, J., Sanders, M.D., Bull, J.W., et al. : Orbital scanning Br. J. Ophthalmol., *58* : 571-587, 1974.

Gawler, J., Sanders, M.D., Bull, J.W.D, et al. : Computer-assisted tomography in orbiatl disease. Br. J. Ophthalmol., *58* : 571-587, 1974.

Gendell, H., Maroon, J. and Wisotzkey, H. : Epidermoid of the fourth ventricle; Discovery by computerized tomography. Surg. Neurol., *5* : 37-39, 1976.

Gerger, P.E., Harwood-Nash, D.C. and Fitz, C.R. : Computerized tomography; Abnormal intracerebral collections of blood in children. Neuroradiology, *11* : 29-33, 1976.

Glenn, W.V., Jr., Johnston, R.J., Morton, P.E., et al. : Image generation and display techniques for CT scan data; Thin transverse and reconstructed coronal and sagittal planes. Invest. Radiol., *10* : 403-416, 1975.

Glenn, W.V., Jr., Johnston, R.J. and Morton, P.E. : Further investigation and initial clinical use of advanced CT display capability. Invest. Radiol. *10* : 479-489, 1975.

Goddé-Jolly, D., Massin, M., Haut, J., et al. : Apport de la tomographie axiale transverse avec calculateur intégré au diagnostic ophtalmologique et neuro-ophtalmologique. Bull. Soc. Ophtalmol. Fr., *75* : 851-856, 1976.

Goitein, M. : Three-dimensional density reconstruction from a series of two-dimensional projections. Nucl. Inst. Meth., *101* : 509-518, 1972.

Gomes, M.N. : ACTA scanning in the diagnosis of abdominal aortic aneurysms. Computerized Tomography, *1* : 51-61, 1977.

Gomez, M.R., Mellinger, J.F. and Reese, D.F. : The use of computerized transaxial tomography in the diagnosis of tuberous sclerosis. Mayo Clin. Proc., *50* : 553-556, 1975.

Gomez. M.R. and Reese, D.F. : Computed tomography of the head in infants and children. Pediatr. Clin. North Am., *23* : 473-498, 1976.

Goodenough, D.J., Weaver, K.E. and Davis, D.O. : Potential artifacts associated with the scanning pattern of the EMI scanner. Radiology, *117* : 615-620, 1975.

Gordon, R., Bender, R. and Herman, G. : Algebraic reconstruction techniques (ART) for three-dimensional electron microscopy and X-ray photography. J. Theor. Biol., *29* : 471-481, 1970.

Gramlak, R. and Waag, R.C. : Cardiac reconstruction imaging in relation to other ultrasound systems and computed tomography. Am. J.Roentgenol., *127* : 91-99, 1976.

Gray, W.R. Jr., Parkey, R.W., Buja, L.M., et al. : Computed tomography; In vitro evaluation of mycardial infarction. Radiology, *122* : 511-513, 1977.

Gregg, E.C. : Tomography with monoenergetic photons. AAPM Quart. Bull., *7* : 96-97, 1973.

Gregorius, F.K. and Batzdorf, U. : Diagnosis of intrathalamic cyst by computerized tomographic scan. Surg. Neurol., *6* : 191-193, 1976.

Gregorius, F.K., Crandall, P.H. and Baloh, R.W. : Positional vertigo with cerebellar astrocytoma. Surg. Neurol., *6* : 283-286, 1976.

Greitz, T. : I year's experience with computer tomography. Acta Radiol., Suppl. (Stockh.), *346* : 7-13, 1975.

Greitz, T. : Computer tomography for diagnosis of intracranial tumours compared with other neuroradiologic procedures. Acta Radiol., Suppl. (Stockh.), *346* : 14-20, 1975.

Greitz, T. : Svenska erfarenheter av datortomografi. Lakartidningen, *73* : 2403-2407, 2412, 1976.

Greitz, T. : Trends in the development of reconstruction tomography in neuroradiology. Am. J. Roentgenol., *127* : 125-127, 1976.

Greitz, T. and Hindmarsh, T. : Computer assisted tomography of intracranial and CSF circulation using a water-soluble contrast medium. Acta Radiol. [Diag.] (Stockh.), *15* : 497-507, 1974.

Grepe, A. and Norén, G. : Computer cisternography of extracerebral tomours using lumbar injection of water-soluble contrast medium. Acta Radiol., Suppl. (Stockh.), *346* : 51-62, 1975.

Grepe, A., Areitz, T. and Norén, G. : Computer cisternography of extracerebral tumors using lumbar injection of water-soluble contrast medium. Acta Radio., Suppl. (Stockh.), *346* : 45-50, 1975.

Griffith, H. and Thomson, J.L.C. : Computer-assisted tomography of the brain. Lancet, *2* : 1205-1206, 1974.

Griver, J., Ambrose, J. and Perry, B.J. : A graphic display system for use with a computer-assisted tomographic scanner. Br. J.Radiol., *49* : 547-549, 1976.

Gromme, Th., Lanksch, W., Kazner, E., et al. : Zur Diagnose des chronischen subduralen Hämatoms im Computer-Tomogramm. Neurochirurgia, *19* : 95-103, 1976.

Gross, G. and McCullough, E.C. : Exposure values around an x-ray scanning transaxial tomograph (EMI scanner). Med. Phys., *2* : 282, 1975.

Gross, G.P. and McCullough, E.C. : Radiation protection requirements for a whole-body CT scanner. Radiology, *122* : 825-827, 1977.

Grossman, Z.D., Wistow, B.W., Wallinga, H.A., et al. : Recognition of vertebral abnormalities in computed tomography of the chest and abdomen. Radiology, *121* : 369-373, 1976.

Grove, A.S., Jr., New., P.F.J. and Momose, K.J. : Computerized tomographic (CT) scanning for orbital evaluation. Trans. Am. Acad. Ophthalmol. Otolaryngol., *79* : 137-149, 1975.

Grumme, T., Meese, W. and Lange, S. : Kraniale Computertomographie (EMI-Scan). Wert und Einsazmoglichkeit. Dtsch. Med. Wochenschr., *101* : 765-769, 1976.

Guner, M., Shaw, M.D.M., Turner, J.W., et al. : Computed tomography in the diagnosis of colloid cyst. Surg. Neurol., *6* : 345-348, 1976.

Guy, H.J., Gaines, R.A., Hill, P.M., et al. : Computerized, noninvasive tests of lung function; A flexible approach using mass spectrometry. Am. Rev. Respir. Dis., *113* : 737-744, 1976.

Gvozdanovic, V., Nutrizio, V., Papa, J. et al. : Computerized tomography in the diagnostics of acousticus neuroma. Acta Med. Iugosl., *30* : 355–356, 1976.

Gyldensted, C. : Computer tomography of the cerebrum in multiple sclerosis. Neuroradiology, *12* : 33-42, 1976.

Gyldensted, C. : Computer tomography of the brain in multiple sclerosis—A radiological study of 110 patients with special reference of demonstration of cerebral plaques. Acta Neurol. Scand., *53* : 386-389, 1976.

Gyldensted., C., Lester, J. and Thomsen, J. : Computer tomography in the diagnosis of cerebellopontine angle tumours. Neuroradiology, *11* : 191-197, 1976.

Haaga, J.R. and Alfidi, R.J. : Precise biopsy localization by computed tomography. Radiology, *118* : 603-607, 1976.

Haaga, J.R., Alfidi, R.J. and Cooperman, A.M. : Definitive treatment of a large pyogenic liver abscess with CT guidance. Cleve. Clin. Q., *43* : 85-88, 1976.

Haaga, J.R., Alfidi, R.J., Zelch, M.G., et al. : Computed tomography of the pancreas. Radiology, *120* : 589-595, 1976.

Hacker, H. : Tomometry—Experience of 1,200 CT-scans with the Siretom. Br. J.Radiol., *48* : 607, 1975.

Hahn, F.J.Y. and Rim, K. : Frontal ventricular dimensions on normal computed tomography. Am. J. Roentgenol., *126* : 593-596, 1976.

Hahn, F.J.Y., Rim, K. and Schapiro, R.L. : The normal range and position of the pineal gland on computed tomography. Radiology, *119* : 599-600, 1976.

Hahn, F.J.Y. and Schapiro, R.L. : The excessively small ventricle on computed axial tomography of the brain. Neuroradiology, *12* : 137-139, 1976.

Hammerschlag, S.B., Wolpert, S.M. and Carter, B.L. : Computed coronal tomography. Radiology, *120* : 219-220, 1976.

Hammerschlag, S.B., Wolpert, S.M. and Carter, B.L. : Computed tomography of the skull base. Computed Tomography, *1* : 75-80, 1977.

Hammerschlag, S.B., Wolpert, S.M. and Carter, B.L. : Computed tomography of the spinal canal. Radioology, *121* : 361-367, 1976.

Hanson, J., Levander, B. and Liliequist, B. : Size of the intracerebral ventricles as measured with computer tomography, encephalography and echoventriculograhy. Acta Radiol., Suppl. (Stockh.), *346* : 98-106, 1975.

Harwood-Nash, D.C. and Breckbill, D.L. : Computed tomography in children; a new diagnostic technique. J. Pediatr., *89* : 343-357, 1976.

Harwood-Nash, D.C. and Fitz, C.R. : Neuroradiology in infants and children. C.V.Mosby Co., St. Luis, 1976.

Harwood-Nash, D.C., Fitz, C.R. and Reilly, B.J. : Cranial computed tomography in infants and children. Can. Med. Assoc. J., *113* : 546-549, 1975.

Hassani, N., Khomeini, R. and Bard, R. : Principles of computerized tomography. J. Natl. Med. Assoc., *68* : 110-112, 1976.

Hatam, A., Bergvall, U., Lewander, R., et al. : Contrast medium enhancement with time in computer tomography; Differential diagnosis of intracranial lesions. Acta Radiol., Suppl. (Stockh.), *346* : 63-81, 1975.

Hayward, R. D. : Intracranial arteriovenous malformations; observations after experience with computerized tomography. J. Neurol. Neurosurg. Psychiatry, *39* : 1027-1033, 1976.

Hayward, R.D. and O'Railly, G.V. : Intracerebral hemorrhage; Accuracy of computerized transverse axial scanning in predicting the underlying aetiology. Lancet, *1* : 1-4, 1976.

Hayward, R.W. and Zatz, L.M. : A thin-section collimater for the EMI scanner. Radiology, *117* : 475-478, 1975.

Herman, G.T., Lakshminarayanan, A.V. and Naparstek, A. : Convolution reconstruction techniques for divergent beams. Comput. Biol. Med., *6* : 259-271, 1976.

Herman, G.T. and Lent, A. : Iterative reconstruction algorithms. Comput. Biol. Med., *6* : 273-294, 1976.

References

Herman, G.T. and Liu, H.K. : Display of three-dimensional information in computed tomography. Computed Tomography, *1* : 155-160, 1977.

Hilal, S.K., Trokel, S.L. and Coleman, D.J. : High resolution computerized tomography and B-scan ultrasonography of the orbits. Trans. Am. Acad. Ophthalmol. Otolaryngol., *81* : OP 607-617, 1976.

Hill, K.R. and Joyner, R.W. : Computerized x-ray tomography. Sci. Prog., *62* : 237-262, 1975.

Hill, K.R. and Joyner, R.W. : The EMI-scanner. Radiography, *40* : 147-157, 1974.

Hindmarsh, T. : Elmination of water-soluble contrast media form the subarachnoid space—Invetsigation with computer tomography. Acta Radiol., Suppl. (Stockh.), *346* : 45-49, 1975.

Hindmarsh, T. and Greitz, T. : Computer cisternography in the diagnosis of communicating hydrocephalus. Acta Radiol., Suppl. (Stockh.), *346* : 91-97, 1975.

Hockley, A.D., Hoffman, H.J. and Hendrick, E.B. : Occipital mesenchymal tumors of infancy. Report of three cases. J.Neurosurg., *46* : 239-244, 1977.

Hoffman, E.J. and Phelps, M.E. : An analysis of some of the physical aspects of positron transaxial tomography. Comput. Biol. Med., *6* : 345-360, 1976.

Holm, H.H. : Ultralydscanning eller computerized axial tomography. Ugeskr. Laeger., *138* : 2625-2640, 1976.

Holtz, D.M. : Computerized transverse axial tomography in brain disease : a new challenge for technologists. Radiol. Technol., *46* : 139-147, 1974.

Hounsfield, G.N. : Computerized transverse axial scanning (tomography). Part 1. Description of system. Br. J. Radiol., *46* : 1016-1022, 1973.

Hounsfield, G.N. : Historical notes on computerized axial tomography. J. Can. Assoc. Radiol., *27* : 135-142, 1976.

Hounsfield. G.N. : Picture quality of computed tomography. Am. J.Roentgenol., *127* : 3-9, 1976.

Houser, O.W., Baker, H.L.Jr., Campbell, J.K. et al. : Recent advances in neuroradiology. Some aspects of computerized transaxial tomography of the head. Minn. Med., *58* : 122-128, 1975.

Houser, O.W., Smith, J.B., Gomez, M.R., et al. : Evaluation of intracranial disorders in children by computerized transaxial tomography. A preliminary report. Neurol., *25* : 607-613, 1975.

Huang, H. K. and Ledley, R.S. : Three-dimensional image reconstruction from in vivo consecutive transverse axial sections. Comput. Biol. Med., *5* : 165-170, 1975.

Huang, H.K. and Wu, S.C. : The evaluation of mass densities of the human body in vivo from CT scans. Comput. Biol. Med., *6* : 337-343, 1976.

Hubschmann, O., Kasoff, S., Doniger, D., et al. : Cavernous haemangioma in the pineal region. Surg. Neurol., *6* : 349-351, 1976.

Huckaman, M.S. : Clinical experience with the intravenous infusion of iodinated contrast material as an adjunct to computed tomography. Surg. Neurol., *4* : 297-318, 1975.

Huckman, M.S. : Computerized tomography in relation to the diagnosis of gliomas. Recent Results Cancer Res., *51* : 79-87, 1975.

Huckman, M.S. and Ackerman, L.V. : Use of automated measurement of mean density as an adjunct to computed tomography. Computed Tomography, *1* :37-42, 1977.

Huckman, M.S., Fox, J.S., Ramsey, R.G., et al. : Computed tomography in the diagnosis of pseudotumor cerebri. Radiology, *119* : 593-597, 1976.

Huckman, M.S., Fox, J. and Topel, J. : The validity of criteria for the evaluation of cerebral atrophy by computed tomography. Radiology, *116* : 85-92, 1975.

Humphreys, R.P., Hockley, A.D., Freedman, M.H., et al. : Management of intracerebral hemorrhage in idiopathic thrombocytopenic purpura; Report of four cases. J. Neurosurg., *45* : 700-704, 1976.

Hungerford, G.D., Du Boulay, G.H. and Zilkha, K.J. : Computerized axial tomography in patients with severe migraine; a preliminary report. J.Neurol. Neurosurg. Psychiatry, *39*: 990-994, 1976.

Idstrom, L.G. : New images in radiology. Jerman Memorial Lecture. Radiol. Tehnol., *47* : 357-363, 1976.

Jacobs, L. and Kinkel, W. : Computerized axial transeverse tomography in the diagnosis of orbital tumors. Trans. Am. Acad. Ophthalmol. Otolaryngol., *81* : 323-333, 1976.

Jacobs, L. and Kinkel, W. : Computerized axial transverse tomography in normal pressure hydrocephalus. Neurol., *26* : 501-507, 1976.

Jacobs, L., Kinkel, W.R. and Heffner, R.R., Jr. : Autopsy correlation of computerized tomography; Experience with 6,000 CT scans. Neurol., *26* : 1111-1118, 1976.

Jacobs, J.C., Maroum, F.B. and Mangan, M.A. : Computer tomography and diagnosis of CNS lesions. Can. Med. Assoc., *113* : 922, 1975.

Jacobsen, H.H., Jensen, J. and Kragsholm, M. : CT scanning og ultralyd. Ugeskr. Laegr., *138* : 2664-2665, 1976.

Jacobsen, H.H., Kragsholm, M. and Holm, H.H. : The economy of the EMI-Scanner. Neuroradiology, *11* : 183-184, 1976.

Jelden, G.L., Chernak, E.S., Rodriguez-Antunez, A., et al. : Further progress in CT scanning and computerized radiation therapy treatment planning. Am. J. Roentgenol., *127* : 179-185, 1976.

Jennett, B., Galbraith, S., Teasdale, G.M., et al. : E.M.I. scan and head injuries. Lancet, *1* : 1026, 1976.

Jerva, M.J. and Randolph, R. : Non-invasive diagnosis of brain tumors. Pros. Inst. Med. Chic., *30* : 280-281, 1975.

Johns, H. : New methods of imaging in diagnostic radiology. Sylvanus Thompson Memorial Lecture given on October 9, 1975 at the Royal Institution, Albe marle street, London, W.1. Br. J. Radiol., *49* : 745-764, 1976.

Joubert, M.J. : Computerized axial tomography. S. Afr. Med. J., *50* : 1103-1109, 1976.

Judy, P.F. : The line spread function and modulation transfer function of a computed tomographic scanner. Med. Phys., *3* : 233-236, 1976.

Karis, R. and Horenstein, S. : Localisation of speech parameters by brain scan. Neurol., *26* : 226-230, 1976.

Kazner, E. : Effects of computerized axial tomography on the treatment of cerebral abscess. Neuroradiology, *12* : 57-58, 1976.

Kazner, E. : Neue Aspekte in der Diagnostik von Gehirnerkrankungen—die kraniale Computer-Tomographie. Med. Monatsschr., *30* : 97-99, 1976.

Kazner, E., Lanksch, W. and Steinhoff, H. : Cranial computerized tomography in the diagnosis of brain disorders in infants and children. Neuropaediatrie, *7* : 136-174, 1976.

Kazner, E., Lanksch, W., Steinhoff, H., et al. : Die axiale Computer-Tomographie des Gehirnschädels—Anwendungsmöglichkeiten und klinische Ergebnisse. Fortschr. Neurol. Psychiatr., *43* : 487-574, 1975.

Kendall, B.E. and Claveria, L.E. : The use of computerized axial tomography (CAT) for the diagnosis and management of intracranial angiomas. Neuroradiology, *12* : 141-160, 1976.

Kendall, B.E., Lee, B.C.P. and Claveria, E. : Computerized tomography and angiography in subarachnoid haemorrhage. Br. J.Radiol., *49* : 483-501, 1976.

Kinkel, W.R. and Jacobs, L. : Computerized axial transverse tomography in cerebrovascular disease. Neurol., *26* : 924-930, 1976.

Kistler, J.P., Hochberg, F.H., Brooks, B.R., et al. : Computerized axial tomography. Clinicopathologic correlation. Neuol., *25* : 201-209, 1975.

Kjellin, K.G. and Söderström, C.E. : Cerebral haemorrhages with atypical patterns; A study of cerebral haematomas using CSF spectrophotometry and computerized transverse axial tomography (EMI scanning). J. Neurol., Sci., *25* : 211-226, 1975.

Kjellin, K.G., Söderström, C.E. and Cronqvist, S. : Cerebrospinal fluid spectrophotometry and computerized transverse axial tomography (EMI-scanning) in cerebrovascular diseases. Comparative study between two actual diagnostic methods in cerebrovascular disorders. Eur. Neuol., *13* : 315-331, 1975.

Klawans, H.L., Lupton, M. and Simon, L. : Calcification of the basal ganglia as a cause of levodopa-resistant parkinsonism. Neurol., *26* : 221-225, 1976.

Klein, D.M. : Simultaneous subdural effusion and hydrocephalus in infancy. Surg. Neurol., *6* : 363-368, 1976.

Kleman, B. : Datof-tomografin och hjärtat. Lakartinningen, *73* : 3642-3643, 1976.

Kobrine, A.I., Timmins, E., Rajjoub, R.K., et al. : Demonstration of massive traumatic brain swelling within 20 minutes after injury. J. Neurosurg., *46* : 256-258, 1977.

Kormano, M. and Dean, P.B. : Extravascular contrast material; The major component of contrast enhancement. Radiology, *121* : 379-382, 1976.

Kramer, R.A., Janetos, C.P. and Peristein, G. : An approach to contrast enhancement in computed tomography of the brain. Radiology, *116* : 641-647, 1975.

Kreel, L. : Computerized tomography using the EMI general purpose scanner. Br. J.Radiol., *50* : 2-14, 1977.

Kreel, L. : Computerized transverse axial tomography with tissue density measurements. Computed Tomography, *1* : 1-5, 1977.

Kreel, L. : The EMI Whole Body Scanner in the demonstration of lymph node enlargement. Clin. Radiol., *27* : 421-429, 1976.

Kreel, L. : Computerized axial tomography. Nurs. Times, *72*, Suppl. : 17-20, 1976.

Kreel, L. and Osborn, S. : Transverse axial tomography of the spinal column; a comparison of anatomical specimens with EMI scan appearances. Radiography, *42* : 73-80, 1976.

Kricheff, I.I., Lin, J.P. and Chase, N.E. : Computer assisted tomography in intracerebral hematomas and head trauma. *In* : Advances in cerebral angiography (edited by Salamon, G.). Springer, Berlin, 1975, p. 353-357.

Kuhl, D.E. and Edwards, R.Q. : Reorganizing transverse section scan data as a rectilinear matrix using digital processing. J. Nucl. Med., *7* : 332, 1966.

Kuhl, D.E. and Edwards, R.Q. : Reorganizing data from transverse section scans of the brain using digital processing. Radiology, *91* : 975-983, 1968.

Kuhns, L.R., Zeddies, T. and Martin, A.J. : Technical note; A simple method for reproducing polaroid images as transparencies. Computed Tomography, *1* : 161-162, 1977.

References

Ladurner, G., Zilkha, E., Iliff, L.D., et al. : Measurement of regional cerebral blood volume by computerized axial tomography. J.Neurol. Neurosurg. Psychiatry, *39* : 152-158, 1976.

Lampert, V.L., Zelch, J.V. and Cohen, D.N. : Computed tomography of the orbits. Radiology, *113* : 351-354, 1974.

Ledley, R.S. : Innovation and creativeness in scientific research : My experiences in developing computerized axial tomography. Comput. Biol. Med., *4* : 133-136, 1974.

Ledley, R.S. : Introduction to computerized tomography. Comput. Biol. Med., *6* : 239-246, 1976.

Ledley, R.S. : A forthcoming cross-sectional atlas correlating CT scans with anatomical structures. Computerized Tomography, *1* : 125-130, 1977.

Ledley, R.S., Di Chiro, G., Luessenhop, A.J., et al. : Computerized transaxial x-ray tomography of the human body. Science, *186* : 207-212, 1974.

Ledley, R.S., Wilson, J.B., Golab, T., et al. : The ACTA-scanner. The whole body computerized transaxial tomography. Comput. Biol. Med., *4* : 145-155, 1974.

Leibrock, L., Epstein, M.H. and Rybock, J.D. : Cerebral tuberculoma localized by EMI scan. Surg. Neurol., *5* : 305-306, 1976.

Leone, C.R., Jr. and Wilson, F.C. : Computerized axial tomography of the orbit. Ophthalmic Surg., *7* : 34-44, 1976.

Levander, B., Stattin, S. and Svendsen, P. : Computer tomography of traumatic intra-and extracerebral lesions. Acta Radiol., Suppl. (Stockh.), *346* : 107-118, 1975.

Lightfoote, W.E. and Pressman, B.D. : Increased intracranial pressure. Evaluation by computerized tomography. Am. J. Roentgenol. Radium Ther. Nucl. Med., *124* : 195-198, 1975.

Lin, J. P. : Computed tomography of the head in adults. Postgrad. Med., *59* : 113-119, 1976.

Little, J.R. and MacCarthy, C.S. : Tension pneumocephalus after insertion of ventriculo-peritoneal shunt for aqueductal stenosis. J. Neurosurg., *44* : 383-385, 1976.

Lloyd, G.A. and Wright, J.E. : Computer assisted tomography. Br. Med. J., *3* : 114-115, 1974.

Lott, T., El Gammal, T., Dasilva, R., et al. : Evaluation of brain and epidural abscesses by computed tomography. Radiology, *122* : 371-376, 1977.

Lowry, L.D., Keane, W., Bilaniuk, L., et al. : C.A.T. scans. Trans. Pa. Acad. Ophthalmol. Otolaryngol., *29* : 177-178, 1976.

MacGregor, B.J.L., Gawler, J. and South, J.R. : Intracranial epithelial cyst. J.Neurosurg., *44* : 109-115, 1976.

MacIntyre, W.J., Alfidi, R.J., Haaga, J., et al. : Comparative modulation transfer functions of the EMI and Delta scanners. Radiology, *120* : 189-191, 1976.

Macovski, A., Alvarez, R.E., Chan, J.L.H., et al. : Energy dependent reconstruction in x-ray computerized tomography. Comput. Biol. Med., *6* : 325-336, 1976.

Maraist, D.V. and Siville, P.J. : Cystadenoma of the pancreas demonstrated by computed tomography with the ACTA scanner—A case report. Computerized Tomography, *1* : 121-124, 1977.

Mark, V.H. : Computer-assisted tomography. JAMA, *234* : 1169-1170, 1975.

Marshall, C.H. : Principles of computed tomography. Postgrad. Med., *59* : 105-109, 1976.

Martin, G.I. : Computer-assisted tomography and tuberous sclerosis. Lancet, *1* : 147, 1976.

Martin, G.I., Kaiserman, D., Liegler, D., et al. : Computer-assisted cranial tomography in early diagnosis of tuberous sclerosis. JAMA, *235* : 2323-2324, 1976.

Matsui, T. : ACTA scanner; part 1 (in Japanese). Brain & Nerve, *27* : 1046-1051, 1975.

Matsui, T. : ACTA scanner; Part 2 (in Japanese). Brain & Nerve, *27* : 1142-1147, 1975.

Matsui, T. : ACTA scanner; Part 3 (in Japanese). Brain & Nerve, *27* : 1242-1247, 1975.

Matsui, T. : The introduction of CT scanner. Thirty-fourth Annual Meeting of The Japan Neurosurgical Society, Oct. 22-24, 1975, Nagoya,

Matsui, T. : CT scanner; Principle and types of CT scanner (in Japanese). Neurological Medicine, *4* : 449-461, 1976.

Matsui, T. : CT scanner; Its widespread use in the United States and current problems (in Japanese). Neurological Medicine, *4* : 571-572, 1976.

Matsui, T : Present status of CT scanner (in Japanese). Japan Medical Journal, *2738* : 43-45, 1976.

Matsui, T. : The new CT scanner; Anatomical studies of CT scan. Thirty-fifth Annual Meeting of The Japan Neurosurgical Society, Oct. 20-22, 1976, Maebashi.

Matsui, T. : Anatomical correlation of CT scan in infants and children. Nervous System in children, *2* : 151-160, 1977.

Matsui, T. : CT scanner; Analysis of its present status and future (in Japanese). Neurological Medicine, *7* : 166-177, 1977.

Matsui, T : Pathological studies of brain tumors in relation to the CT. First Annual Meeting of Japan CT Society, Jan. 21-22, 1978, Tokyo.

Matsui, T. and Hirano, A. : New technique of CT scan; Multiple angle examinations (the sponcershiop of Taveras, J.M. and New, P.F.J.). March 19-24, 1978, Maiami Beach, Florida.

Matsui, T., Imai, T., Qsugi, T. : Recent publications and scientific meetings on CT scan; A brief review of the world literature (in Japanese). Neurological Medicine, *5* : 31-39, 1976.

Matsui, T., Imai, T., Osugi, T., et al. : Studies of brain sections in relation to computed tomography. International Symposium on Computer Assisted Tomography in Nontumoral Diseases of the Brain; Spinal cord and Eye (The sponcership of Di Chiro, G. and Brooks, R. A.), Oct. 11-15, 1976, Bethesda, Maryland.

Matsui, T., Kawamoto, K., Iwata, M. et al. : Anatomical and pathological study of the brain by CT scanner-1. Anatomical study of normal brain. Computerized Tomography, *1* : 3-43, 1977.

Matsui, T., Kawamoto, K., Hojo, S., et al. : Multiple angle examination with CT scan. Thirty-sixth Annual Meeting of The Japanese Neurosurgical Society, Oct. 27-29, 1977, Osaka.

Matsui, T., Kawamoto, K., Iwata, M., et al. : Anatomical and pathological study of the brain by CT scanner, —2. multiple angle examinations. Computerized Tomography, in print.

Matsui, T. and Ledley, R.S. : A new technique of the CT scanner; Computed Tomography. International Symposium and Course(The sponcership of Taveras, J.M. and New, P.F.J.), April 3-8, 1977, Miami Beach, Florida.

Matsui, T., Luessenhop, A.J. and Axelbaum, S.P. : Development of ACTA scanner and its clinical experience (in Japanese). Jap.j.Clin.Radiol. *21* : 163-168, 1976.

Matsui, T., Luessenhop, A.J. and Ledley, R.S. : Three-window-technique of the CT scanner. Thirty-sixth Annual Meeting of The Japan Neurosurgical Society, Oct. 27-29, 1977, Osaka.

Matsui, T. and Osugi, T. : Anatomical studies of CT scan. Thirty-fifth Annual Meeting of The Japan Neurosurgical Society, Oct. 20-22, 1976, Maebashi.

Matsui, T., Osugi, T., Kawamoto, K., et al. : Anatomical studies of brain sections in relation to the CT scan. Sixth International Congress of Neurological Surgery, June 19-25, 1977, São Paulo, Brazil.

Matsui, T. and Tsutsumi, U. : The new angle of CT examinations. First Annual Meeting of Japan CT Society, Japan. 21-22, 1978, Tokyo.

Mazziotta, J.C. and Suh, J.H. : The value of computed tomography in the radiotherapeutic management of juxtasellar tumors. Computerized Tomography, *1* : 111-119, 1977.

McCort, J.J. : Amebic hepatic abscess; demonstration by total body opacification and tomography. West J. Med., *124* : 426-428, 1976.

McCullough, E.C. : Photon attenuation in computed tomography. Med. Phys. *2* : 307-320, 1975.

McCullough, E.C., Baker, H.L., Jr., Houser, O.W., et al. : An evaluation of the quantitative and radiation features of a scanning x-ray transverse axial tomograph; The EMI scanner. Radiology, *111* : 709-715, 1974.

McCullough, E.C. and Coulam, C.M. : Phyical and dosimetric aspects of diagnostic geometrical and computerassisted tomographic procedures. Radiol. Clin. North Am., *14* : 3-14, 1976.

McCullough, E.C., Payne, J.T., Baker, H.L., Jr. et al. : Performance evaluation and quality assurance of computed tomography scanners, with illustrations from the EMI, ACTA, and Delta scanners. Radiology, *120* : 173-188,1976.

McKusick, K.A., New, P.F.J., Pendergrass, H.P., et al. : Impact of computerized axial tomography upon radionuclide brain scanning in non-neoplastic disease. J. Nucl. Med., *15* : 5-15, 1974.

Menzer, L., Sabin, T. and Mark, W.H. : Computerized axial tomography. Use in the diagnosis of dementia. JAMA, *234* : 754-757, 1975.

Merino-deVillasante, J. and Taveras, J.M. : Computerized tomography (CT) in acute head trauma. Am. J. Roentgenol., *126* : 765-778, 1976.

Mersereau, R.M. : Direct Fourier transform techniques in 3-D image reconstruction. Comput. Biol. Med., *6* : 247-258, 1976.

Messina, A.V. : Computed tomography; Contrast media within subdural hematomas. A preliminary report. Radiology, *119* : 725-726, 1976.

Messina, A.V. : Computerized tomography of the head; a preliminary report on its use in the diagnosis of internal auditory canal and cerebellopontine lesions. Arch. Otolaryngol., *102* : 566-567, 1976.

Messina, A.V. and Chernik, N.L. : Computed tomography; The "resolving" intracerebral hemorrhage. Radiology, *118* : 609-613, 1976.

Messina, A.V., Potts, D.G., Rottenberg, D., et al. : Computed tomography; Demonstration of contrast medium within cystic tumors. Radiology, *120* : 345-347, 1976.

Messina, A.V., Potts, G. and Sackett, J.F. : A system for the accurate correlation of computerized axial tomography with other studies. J.Can. Assoc. Radiol., *27* : 170-177, 1976.

Messina, A.V., Potts, G., Sigel, R.M., et al. : Computed tomography; Evaluation of posterior third ventricle. Radiology, *119* : 581-592, 1976.

Michels, L.G., Bentson, J.R. and Winter, J. : Computed tomography of cerebral venous angiomas. Computed Tomography, *1* : 149-154, 1977.

Miller, E.M., Mani, R.L. and Townsend, J.J. : Cerebellar glioblastoma multiforme in an adult. Surg. Neurol., *5* : 341-343, 1976.

References

Mills, S.R., Doppman, J.L. and Nienhuis, A.W. : Computed tomography in the diagnosis of disorders of excessive iron storage of the liver. Computed Tomography, *1* : 101-104, 1977.

Momose, K.J., New, P.F.J., Grove, A.S., Jr. et al. : The use of computed tomography in ophthalmology. Radiology, *115* : 361-368, 1975.

Monro, P. : E.M.I. and radioisotope brain imaging. Lancet, *1* : 640, 1976.

Monro, P. : E.M.I. and radioisotope brain imaging. Lancet, *1* : 1123-1124, 1976.

Moseley, I.F. and Bull, J.W. : Computerized axial tomography, carotid angiography and orbital phlebography in the diagnosis of space-occupying lesions of the orbit. In : Advances in cerebral angiography (edited by Salamon, G.), Springer, Berlin, 1975, p.361-369.

Mostowycz, L., Ware, R.W. and Dochterman, D. : Computerized transverse axial tomography. J.Ky. Med. Assoc., *74* : 128-134, 1976.

Müller, H.R., Wüthrich, R., Hünig, R., et al. : A graphical reporting system for computerized axial x-ray tomography (Emi-scanning). Eur. Neurol., *11* : 197-207, 1974.

Müller, H.R., Wüthrich, R., Wiggli, U., et al. : The contribution of computerized axial tomography to the diagnosis of cerebellar and pontine hematomas. Stroke, *6* : 467-475, 1975.

Murphy, J.V., D'So'uza, B.J. and Haughton, V.M. : CT scans and tuberous sclerosis. JAMA, *236* : 1115, 1976.

Naidichi, T.P., Epstein, F., Lin, J.P., et al. : Evaluation of pediatric hydrocephalus by computed tomography. Radiology. *119* : 337-345, 1976.

Naidich, T.P. and Kricheff, I.I. : Computed tomography of the head in children. Postgrad. Med., *59* : 123-129, 1976.

Naidich, T.P., Lin, J.P., Leeds, N.E., et al. : Computed tomography in the diagnosis of extra-axial posterior fossa masses. Radiology, *120* : 333-339, 1976.

Naidichi, T.P., Pinto, R.S., Kushner, M.J., et al. : Evaluation of sellar and parasellar masses by computer tomography. Radiology, *120* : 91-99, 1976.

Naidich, T.P., Pudlowski, R.M., Leeds, N.E., et al : The normal contrast-enhanced axial tomogram of the brain. Computed Tomography, *1* : 16-29, 1977.

New, P.F.J. : Computed tomography; A major diagnostic advance. Hosp. Prac., *10* : 55-64, 1975.

New, P.F.J. : Computer assisted tomography. JAMA, *232* : 941-943, 1975.

New, P.F.J. : Computed tomography; Experience at the Massachusetts General Hospital. In : Cerebral vascular diseases (edited by Whisnant, J.P., Sandok, B.A.), Grune & Stratton Inc. New York, 1975, p.203-221.

New, P.F.J. and Aronow, S. : Attenuation measurement of whole blood and blood fractions in computed tomography. Radiology, *121* : 635-640, 1976.

New, P.F.J., Davis, K.R. and Ballantine, H.T., Jr. : Computed tomography in cerebral abscess. Radilogy, *121* : 641-646, 1976.

New, P.F.J., McKusick, K.A., Pendergrass, H.P., et al. : Impact of computerized axial tomography upon radionuclide brain scanning for neoplasms. J. Nucl. Med., *15* : 519, 1974.

New, P.F.J., Scott, W.R. and Schnur, J.A. : Computed tomography; Immobilization of the head by dental holder. Radiology, *114* : 474-476, 1975.

New, P.F.J., Soctt, W.R., Schnur, J.A., et al. : Computerized axial tomography with the EMI scanner. Radiology, *110* : 109-123, 1974.

New, P.F.J., Scott, W.R., Schnur, J.A., et al. : Computed tomography with the EMI scanner in the diagnosis of primary and metastatic intracranial neoplasms. Radiology, *114* : 75-87, 1975.

Norman, D., Enzman, D.R., Levin, V.A., et al. : Computed tomography in the evaluation of malignant glioma before and after therapy. Radiology, *121* : 85-86, 1976.

Obrador, S. and Martin-Rodriguez, J.G. : Biological factors involved in the clinical features and surgical management of cerebellar hemangioblastomas. Surg. Neurol., *7* : 79-85, 1977.

O'Conner, D.J., Chang, D.T. and Shey, M.I. : Computed tomography in a community hospital. Radiology, *119* : 601-602, 1976.

Oldendorf, W.H. : Isolated flying spot detection of radiodensity discontinuities displaying the lateral structural pattern of a complex object. IRE Transactions on Bio-Medical Electronics. vol. BME8, 68-72, 1961.

Oldendorf, W.H. : Spin-migration; an early attempt at radiographic transmission section scanning. Bull. Los Angeles Neurol. Soc., *39* : 138-143, 1974.

Ommaya, A.K. : Computerized axial tomography of the head. The EMI-scanner; a new device for direct examination of the brain "in vivo." Surg. Neurol., *1* : 217-222, 1973.

Ommaya, A.K. : X-ray densitography. Lancet, *1* : 464, 1974.

Ommaya, A.K., Murray, G., Ambrose, J., et al. : Computerized axial tomography; estimation of spatial and density resolution capabillity. Br. J.Radiol., *49* : 604-611, 1976.

Ostertag, C., Hemmer, R., and Mundinger, F. : Observation on the differentiation of hydrocephalus occlusus in infancy and childhood using computerized axial tomography. Neuropaediatrie, *7* : 322-326, 1976.

560

Palacios, E., Kia, B.A. and Love, L. : Computerized axial tomography with the EMI-scanner at Loyola University Medical Center. Ill. Med. J., *146* : 392-393, 1974.

Paxton, R. and Ambrose, J. : The EMI scanner. A brief review of the first 650 patients. Br. J. Radiol., *47* : 530-565, 1974.

Pay, N.T., Carella, R.J., Lin, J.P., et al. : The usefulness of computed tomography during after radiation therapy in patients with brain tumors. Radiology, *121* : 79-83, 1976.

Pendergrass, H.P., McKusick, K.A., New, P.F.J., et al. : Relative efficacy of radionuclide imaging and computed tomography of the brain. Radiology, *116* : 363-366, 1975.

Penn, R.D., Walser, R., Kurtz, D., et al. : Tumor volume, luxury perfusion and regional blood volume changes in man visualized by subtraction computerized tomography. J, Neurosurg., *44* : 449-457, 1976.

Perry, B.J. and Bridges, C. : Computerized transverse axial scanning (tomography), Part 3. Radiation dose consideration. Br. J. Radiol., *46* : 1048-1049, 1973.

Peters, T.M. : Enhanced display of three-dimensional data from computerized x-ray tomograms. Comput. Biol. Med., *5* : 49-52, 1975.

Peters, T.M. : Principles of computerized tomography. Australas. Radiol., *19* : 118-126, 1975.

Peters, T.M., Smith, P.R. and Gibson, R.D. : Computer aided transverse body-section radiography. Br. J.Radiol., *46* : 314-317, 1973.

Peterson, N.T., Duchesneau, P.M., Westbrook, E.L., et al. : Basilar artery ectasia demonstrated by computed tomography. Radiology, *122* : 713-715, 1977.

Pevsner, P.H., Garcia-Bunuel, R., Leeds, N., et al. : Subependymal and intraventricular hemorrhage in neonates; Early diagnosis by computed tomography. Radiology, *119* : 111-114, 1976.

Phelps, M.E., Gado, M.H. and Hoffman, E.J. : Correlation of effective atomic number and electron density with attenuation coefficients measured with polychromatic x-rays. Radiology, *117* : 585-588, 1975.

Phelps, M.E., Hoffman, E.J. and Ter-Pogossian, M.M. : Attenuation coefficients of various body tissues, fluids and lesions at photon energies of 18 to 136 keV. Radiology, *117* : 573-583, 1975.

Phelps, M.E. and Kuhl, D.E. : Pitfalls in the measurement of cerebral blood volume with computed tomography. Radiology, *121* : 375-377, 1976.

Philips, R.L. and Stephens, D.H. : Computed tomography of liver specimens. Radiology, *115* : 43-46, 1975.

Phillips, D.F. and Lillé, K. : Putting the leash on "CAT". Hospitals, *50* : 45-49, 1976.

Pickering, R.S., Hattery, R.R., Hartman, G.W., et al. : Computed tomography of the excised kidney. Radiology, *113* : 643-647, 1974.

Pohutsky, L.C. and Pohutsky, K.R. : Computerized axial tomography of the brain: a new diagnostic tool. Am. J.Nurs. *75* : 1341-1342, 1975.

Porot, A. : Radio-anatomie générale de la tête. 37 coupes anatomiques de la tête dans les trois plans. Masson et Cie, Paris, 1955.

Pressman, B.D., Gilbert, G.E. and Davis, D.O. : Computerized transverse tomography of vascular lesions of the brain. Part 2. Aneurysm. Am. J. Roentgenol. Radium Ther. Nucl. Med., *124* : 215-219, 1975.

Pressman, B.D., Kirkwood, J.R. and Davis, D.O. : Computerized transverse tomography of vascular lesions of the brain. Part 1. Arteriovenous malformations. Am. J. Roentgenol. Radium Ther. Nucl. Med., *124* : 208-214, 1975.

Pressman, B.D., Kirkwood, J.R. and Davis, D.O. : Posterior fossa hemorrhage. Localization by computerized tomography. JAMA, *232* : 932-933, 1975.

Prochaska, J.M. and Lowry, J.L. : Computed cranial tomography. J.Tenn. Med. Assoc., *68* : 800-801, 1975.

Rådberg, C. and Söderlundh, S. : Computer tomography in cerebral death. Acta Radiol., Suppl. (Stockh.), *346* : 119-129, 1975.

Reese, D.F., O'Brien, P.C., Beeler, G.W. Jr., et al. : An investigation for extracting more imformation from computerized tomography scans. Am. J. Roentgenol. Radium Ther. Nucl. Med., *124* : 177-185, 1975.

Reich, N.E., and Seidelmann, F.E. : Computed tomography using the EMI scanner; Part II. Intracranial pathology. J. Am. Osteopath. Assoc., *74* : 1133-1138, 1975.

Reich, N.E., Zelch, J.V., Alfidi, R.J., et al. : Computed tomography in the detection of juxtasellar lesion. Radiology, *118* : 333-335, 1976.

Riding, M., Bergström, M., Bergvall, U., et al. : Computer intravenous angiography. Acta Radiol., Suppl. (Stockh.), *346* : 82-90, 1975.

Robertson, G.H., Brismar, J., Weiss, A., et al. : CSF enhancement for computerized tomography. Surg. Neurol., *6* : 235-238, 1976.

Roberts, M.A. and Caird, F.I. : Computerized tomography and intellectual impairment in the elderly. J. Neurol. Neurosurg. Psychiatry, *39* : 986-989, 1976.

561

References

Roberts, M.A., Caird, F.I., Grossart, K.W., et al. : Computerized tomography in the diagnosis of cerebral atrophy. J.Neurol. Neurosurg. Psychiatry, *39* : 909-915, 1976.

Roberts, M. and Hanaway, J. : Atlas of the human brain in section. Lea & Febiger, Philadelphia, 1970.

Rosenberger, A. and Adler, A. : Computer assisted tomography of the head. Harefuah., *88* : 421-422, 1975.

Rothner, A.D., Duchesneau, P.M. and Weinstein, M. : Agenesis of the corpus callosum revealed by computerized tomography. Dev. Med. Child Neurol., *18* : 160-166, 1976.

Rottenberg, D.A., Talman, W. and Chernik, N.L. : Location of pyramidal tract questioned. Neurol., *26* : 291-292, 1976.

Roy-Camille, R : Coupes horizontales du tronc. Masson et Cie, Paris, 1959.

Rüegsegger, P., Elsasser, U., Anliker, M., et al. : Quantification of bone mineralization using computed tomography. Radiology, *121* : 93-97, 1976.

Rutherford, R.A., Pullan, B.R. and Isherwood, I. : Calibration and response of an EMI scanner. Neuroradiology, *11* : 7-13, 1976.

Rutherford, R.A., Pullan, B.R. and Isherwood, I. : Measurement of effective atomic number and electron density using an EMI scanner. Neuroradiology, *11* : 15-21, 1976.

Rutherford, R. A., Pullan, B.R. and Isherwood, I. : X-ray energies for effective atomic number determination. Neuroradiology, *11* : 23-28, 1976.

Rutherford, R.A., Pullan, B., Isherwood, I., et al. : Proceedings; Quantitative aspects of computer assisted tomography. Br. J.Radiol., *48* : 605, 1975.

Sabin, T.D. and Mark, V.H. : Computerized axial tomography and electroencephalography. JAMA, *236* : 138, 1976.

Sackett, J.F., Messina, A.V. and Petito, C.K. : Computed tomography and magnification vertebral angiotomography in the diagnosis of colloid cysts of the third ventricle. Radiology, *116* : 95-100, 1975.

Sagel, S.S., Stanley, R.J. and Evans, R.G. : Early clinical experience with motionless whole-body computed tomography. Radiology, *119* : 321-330, 1976.

Saleman, M. : CT-scan symbols. New Engl. J. Med., *295* : 1262, 1976.

Saleman, M., Hilal, S., Brisman, R., et al. : Computerized tomography correlated with CSF protein concentration Surg. Neurol., *5* : 57-58, 1976.

Salvolini, U., Menichelli, F. and Pasquini, U. : Computer assisted tomography in 90 cases of exophthalmos. Computed Tomography, *1* : 81-100, 1977.

Sanders, M.D. : Computer-assisted tomography (EMI scan) in orbital and neuro-ophthalmologic diagnosis. Trans. Pac. Coast Ophthalmol.Soc., *56* : 17-42, 1975.

Sanders, M.D. and Gawler, J. : Computerized tomographic scanning (EMI scan) in neuro-ophthalmology. Trans. Ophthalmol. Soc. UK., *95* : 237-245, 1975.

Schellinger, D., Di Chiro, G., Axelbaum, S.P., et al. : Early clinical experience with the ACTA scanner. Radiology, *114* : 257-261, 1975.

Schields, R.A., Isherwood, I. and Pullan, B.R. : The use of an off-line static display system with a computerized transverse axial tomographic unit. Br. J. Radiol., *47* : 893-895, 1974.

Schoenberg, B.S., Glista, G.G. and Reagan, T.J. : The familial occurrence of glioma. Surg. Neurol., *5* : 139-145, 1976.

Schoultz, T.W., Morrison, J.R. and Calhown, J.D. : Atlas of the human brain for use in diagnosis by computerassisted tomography. Surg. Neurol., *5* : 255-266, 1976.

Scott, W.R., New, P.F.J., Davis, K.R., et al. : .Computerized axial tomography of intracerebral and intraventricular hemorrhage. Radiology, *112* : 73-80, 1974.

Seidelmann, F.E. and Reich, N.E. : Computed tomography using the EMI scanner; Part 1. The apparatus, the normal scan, and its variants. J.Am. Osteopath, Assoc., *74* : 1125-1132, 1975.

Sheedy, P.F.II., Stephens, D.H., Hattery, R.R., et al. : Computed tomography of the body; initial clinical trial with the EMI prototype. Am. J. Roentgenol., *127* : 23-51, 1976.

Shepp, L.A. and Loan, B.F. : The Fourier reconstruction of a head section. IEEE, NS-*21* : 21-42, 1974.

Shipps, F.C., D'Agostino, A. and Raaf, J. : Brain-cutting device for correlation of brain scan and autopsy sections. J. Neurosurg., *44* : 759-760, 1976.

Sigel, R.M. and Messina, A.V. : Computed tomography; the anatomic basis of the zone of diminished density surrounding meningiomas. Am. J.Roentgenol., *127* : 139-141, 1976.

Small, J.G., Dian, D.A., Milstein, V., et al. : CAT scans in children with behavior disorders. Am. J. Psychiatry, *133* : 584, 1976.

Smith, D.R., Pressman, B.D., Lawrence, W.H., et al. Computerized tomography; a new clinical modality. Va. Med. Mon., *102* : 827-834, 1975.

Smith, P.R., Peters, T.M., Müller, H.R., et al. Towards the assessment of the limitations on computerized axial tomography. Neuroradiology, *9* : 1-8, 1975.

Söderström, C.E., Kjellin, K.G. and Cronqvist, S. : Computer tomography compared with spectrophotometry of cerebrospinal fluid in cerebrovascular diseases. Acta Radiol., Suppl. (Stockh.), *346* : 130-142, 1975.

562

Stanley, R.J., Sagel, S.S. and Levit, R.G. : Computed tomography of the body; early trends in application and accuracy of the method. Am. J. Roentgenol., *127* : 53-67, 1976.

Stefoski, D., Bergen, D., Fox, J., et al. : Correlation between diffuse EEG abnormalities and cerebral atrophy in senile dementia. J. Neurol. Neurosurg. Psychiatry, *39* : 751-755, 1976.

Steiner, L., Bergvall, U. and Zwetnow, N. : Quantitative estimation of intracerebral and intraventricular hematoma by computer tomography. Acta Radiol., Suppl. (Stockh.), *346* : 143-154, 1975.

Stephens, D.H., Hattery, R.R. and Sheedy, P.F. : Computed tomography of the abdomen; Early experience with the EMI body scanner. Radiology, *119* : 331-335, 1976.

Svendsen, P. : Computer tomograpy of traumatic extracerebral lesions. Br. J.Radiol., *49* : 1004-1012, 1976.

Synek, V. and Reuben, J.R. : The ventricular-brain ratio using planimetric measurement of EMI scans. Br. J. Radiol., *49* : 233-237, 1976.

Synek, V., Reuben, J.R. and Du Boulay, G.H. : Comparing Evans' index and computerized axial tomography in assessing relationship of ventricular size to brain size. Neurol., *26* : 231-233, 1976.

Tanaka, E. and Iinuma, T.A. : Correction function and statistical noises in transverse section picture reconstruction. Compt. Biol. Med., *6* : 295-306, 1976.

Terbrugge, K., Scotti, G., Ethier, R., et al. : Computed tomography in intracranial arteriovenous malformations. Radiology, *122* : 703-706, 1977.

Ter-Pogossiam, M.M. : The challenge of computed tomography. Am. J.Roentgenol., *127* : 1-2, 1976.

Ter-Pogossian, M.M., Phelps, M.E., Hoffman, E.J., et al. : A positron-emission transaxial tomograph for nuclear imaging (PETT). Radiology, *114* : 89–98, 1975.

Thomson, J.L.G. : The computed axial tomograph in acute herpes simplex encephalitis. Br. J.Radiol., *49* : 86-87, 1976.

Thomson, J.L.G. : Computerized axial tomography and the diagnosis of glioma; a study of 100 consecutive histologically proven cases. Clin. Radiol., *27* : 431-441, 1976.

Till, K. : Computerized axial tomography in paediatric neurology and neurosurgery. Proc. R. Soc. Med., *68* : 713-716, 1975.

Till, K. : Computerized axial tomography; Particular applications and advantages in paediatric neurosurgery. Childs Brain, *2* : 46-53, 1976.

Torack, R.M., Alcala, H., Gado, M., et al. : Correlative assay of cranial tomography CCT, water content and specific gravity in normal and pathological postmortem brain. J. Neuropathol. Exp. Neurol., *35* : 385-392, 1976.

Towfighi, J., Bilaniuk, L.T., Zimmerman, R.A., et al. : Hemorrhage in bilateral choroid plexus hemangiomas demonstrated by computed tomography; Case report. J.Neurosurg., *45* : 218-222, 1976.

Tsai, C.M. and Çho, Z.H. : Phisics of contrast mechanism and averaging effect of linear attenuation coefficients in a computerized transverse axial tomography (CTAT) transmission scanner. Phys. Med. Biol., *21* : 544-559, 1976.

Trokel, S.L., and Hilal, S.K. : Axial tomography. Am. J. Ophthalmol., *81* : 535-536, 1976.

Tutton, R.H. : Computerized axial tomography (EMI scanner). J. La. State Med. Soc., *126* : 327-328, 1974.

Twigg, H.L., Axelbaum, S.P. and Schellinger, D. : Computerized body tomography with the ACTA scanner. JAMA, *234* : 314-317, 1975.

Uttley, D. : The EMI scan in head injury. Acta Neurochir. (Wien), *31* : 258, 1975.

Vermess, M., Di Chiro, G., Newby, N.R., et al. : Positional shift of intraventricular blood clots demonstrated by computed tomography. Radiology, *118* : 341-342, 1976.

Vigouroux, B.P., Baurand, C., Gomez, A., et al. : Intérêt de la tomographie axiale commandée par ordinateur (tacographie) dans les traumatismes crânio-cérébraux. Neuro-Chirurgie, *22* : 281-291, 1976.

Walser, R.L. and Ackerman, L.V. : Determination of volume from computerized tomograms; Finding the volume of fluid-filled brain cavities. Computed Tomography, *1* : 117-130, 1977.

Walshe, T.M., Hire, D.B. Davis, K.R. : The diagnosis of hypertensive intracerebral hemorrhage; The contribution of computed tomography. Computerized Tomography, *1* : 63-69, 1977.

Warren, K.G., Ball, M.J., Paty, D.W., et al. : Computer tomography in disseminated sclerosis. Can. J. Neurol. Sci., *3* : 211-216, 1976.

Watson, R.C. : The whole body scan. Computed tomography (CT)—a major advance in the diagnosis of cancer. Clin. Bull., *6* : 47-51, 1976.

Weinstein, M.A., Berlin, A.J., Jr. and Duchesneau, P.M. : High resolution computed tomography of the orbit with the Ohio Nuclear Delta head scanner. Am. J.Roentgenol., *127* : 175-177, 1976.

Weinstein, M.A., Duchesneau, P.M. and MacIntyre, W.J. : White and gray matter of the brain differentiated by computed tomography. Radiology, *122* : 699-702, 1977.

Weinstein, M.A., Rothner, A.D., Duchesneau, P., et al. : Computed tomography in diastematomyelia. Radiology, *117* : 609-611, 1975.

Welborn, S.G. : Anesthesia for EMI scanning in infants and small children. South Med. J., *69* : 1294-1295, 1976.

References

Wever, D.A. : Computerized axial tomography. Am. J. Dis. Child, *130* : 16, 1976.

Wiggans, G., Schein, P.S., MacDonald, J.S., et al. : Computed axial tomography for diagnosis of pancreatic cancer. Lancet, *2* : 233-235, 1976.

Wiggli, U., Muller, H.R. and Elke, M. : Formes d'hydrocéphalie en tomographie axiale assistée par calculateur (TAC). Neuro-Chirurgie, *22* : 177-184, 1976.

Wiggli, U., Muller-Brand, J., Muller, H.R., et al. : L'apport de la tomographie axial computérisée (TAC) au diagnostic de l'hydrocéphalie arésorptive. Rev. Neurol. (Paris), *132* : 405-414, 1976.

Wilson, G.H. : Computed cerebral tomography : West. J.Med., *122* : 316-317, 1975.

Wing, S.D., Norman, D. and Pollock, J.A. : Contrast enhancement of cerebral infarcts in computed tomography. Radiology, *121* : 89-92, 1976.

Wittenberg, J., Maturi, R.A., Ferrucci, J.T., et al. : Computerized tomography of in Vitro abdominal organs—Effect of preservation methods on attenuation coefficient. Computerized Tomography, *1* : 95-101, 1977.

Wolf, B.S., Nakagawa, H. and Staulcup, M.S. : Feasibility of coronal views in computed scanning of the head. Radiology, *120* : 217-218, 1976.

Wortzman, G. : Computerized transaxial tomography; Its role in the post-operative tumor case. Can. J. Neurol. Sci., *3* : 51-58, 1976.

Wortzman, G., Holgate, R.C. and Morgan, P.P. : Cranial computed tomography. An evaluation of cost effectiveness. Radiology, *117* : 75-77, 1975.

Wright, J.E., Lloyd, G.A.S. and Ambrose, J. : Computerized axial tomography in the detection of orbital spaceoccupying lesions. Am. J. Ophthalmol., *80* : 78-84, 1975.

Wüllenweber, R., Winkel, K. zum, Grumme, Th., et al. : Differentialdiagnose des Schlagenfalles im Computer-Tomogramm. Neurochirurgia, *19* : 1-9, 1976.

Yamamoto, Y.L., Thompson, C.J., Meyer, E., et al. : Dynamic positron emission tomography for study of cerebral hemodynamics in a cross section of the head using positron-emiting ^{68}Ga-EDTA and ^{77}Kr. Computed Tomography, *1* : 43-56, 1977.

Yock, D.H. and Marshall, W.H., Jr. : Recent ischemic brain infarcts at computed tomography; Appearances pre-and postcontrast infusion. Radiology, *117* : 599-608, 1975.

Zatz, L.M. : The effect of the kVp level on EMI values. Radiology, *119* : 683-688, 1976.

Zelch, J.V., Duchesneau, P.M., Meaney, T.F., et al. : The EMI scanner and its application to clinical diagnosis. Cleve. Clin. Q. *41* : 79-91, 1974.

Zilkha, E., Ladurner, G., Iliff, L.D. et al. : Computer subtraction in regional cerebral blood-volume measurements using the EMI-scanner. Br. J. Radiol., *49* : 330-334, 1976.

Zimmerman, R.A., Bilaniuk, L.T., Shipkin, P.M., et al. : Evolution of cerebral abscess; Correlation of clinical features with computed tomography. Neurol., *27* : 14-19, 1977.

Zimmerman, R.D., Leeds, N.E. and Naidich, T.P. : Ring blush associated with intracerebral hematoma. Radiology, *122* : 707-711, 1977.

Zimmerman, R.A., Patel, S. and Bilaniuk, L.T. : Demonstration of purulent bacterial intracranial infections by computed tomography. Am. J.Roentgenol., *127* : 155-165, 1976.

Index

Pages are indicated in parentheses